ORAL AND MAXILLOFACIAL
DIAGNOSTIC IMAGING

ORAL AND MAXILLOFACIAL DIAGNOSTIC IMAGING

Allan G. Farman
B.D.S., Ph.D.(Odont.), Dip. A.B.O.M.R., Ed.S., M.B.A.

Professor and Director of Radiology
and Imaging Sciences, School of Dentistry
University of Louisville
Louisville, Kentucky

Christoffel J. Nortjé
B.Ch.D., Ph.D.(Odont.), Dip. A.B.O.M.R.

Professor and Head
Department of Maxillofacial Radiology
Faculty of Dentistry
University of Stellenbosch
Tygerberg, Cape, Republic of South Africa

Robert E. Wood
D.D.S., M.Sc., Dip. Oral Rad., M.R.C.D.(C).

Oral and Maxillofacial Radiologist
The Princess Margaret Hospital
Toronto, Ontario, Canada

With 972 illustrations

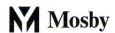 Mosby

St. Louis Baltimore Boston Chicago London Philadelphia Sydney Toronto

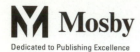
Mosby
Dedicated to Publishing Excellence

Editor-in-Chief: Don E. Ladig
Executive Editor: Linda L. Duncan
Assistant Editors: Melba Steube, Susan Baxter
Project Manager: Mark Spann
Production Editor: Julie Zipfel
Designer: John Rokusek
Cover Designer: Julie Taugner
Manufacturing Supervisor: Theresa Fuchs
Cover photographs: Marius Jooste

Printed in the United States of America

Mosby-Year Book, Inc.
11830 Westline Industrial Drive
St. Louis, Missouri 63146

Library of Congress Cataloging in Publication Data

Farman, Allan G.
    Oral and maxillofacial diagnostic imaging / Allan G. Farman,
Christoffel J. Nortjé, Robert E. Wood.— 1st ed.
      p.   cm.
    Includes bibliographical references and index.
    ISBN 0-8016-1549-6
    1. Jaws—Imaging.   2. Face—Imaging.   3. Jaws—Abnormalities-
-Diagnosis.   4. Jaws—Diseases—Diagnosis.   5. Mouth—Diseases-
-Diagnosis.   I. Nortjé. Christoffel J.   II. Wood, Robert E.
III. Title.
      [DNLM: 1. Diagnostic Imaging.   2. Stomatognathic Diseases-
-diagnosis.   WU 141 F233o]
    RD526.F37   1993
    617.5'220757—dc20
    DNLM/DLC   92-49868
    for Library of Congress   CIP

93 94 95 96 97 CL/MY 9 8 7 6 5 4 3 2 1

CONTRIBUTORS

Sharon L. Brooks, D.D.S., M.S.

Professor
Department of Oral Medicine/Pathology/Surgery
University of Michigan
School of Dentistry
Ann Arbor, Michigan

Isamu Kashima, D.D.S., Ph.D.

Professor and Chairman
Department of Oral Radiology
Kanagawa Dental College
Yokosuka, Kanagawa, Japan

Linda Lee, D.D.S., M.Sc.

Assistant Professor
Department of Oral Radiology
University of Toronto
Faculty of Dentistry
Toronto, Ontario, Canada

Walter G. Maxymiw, D.D.S.

Chief of Dentistry
Princess Margaret Hospital
Toronto, Ontario, Canada

Timothy E. Moore, M.D., Ch.B., F.R.A.C.R.

Associate Professor of Diagnostic Radiology
University of Iowa College of Medicine
Iowa City, Iowa

M.E. Parker, B.Ch.D., M.Sc.

Professor and Head
Department of Maxillofacial and Oral
    Radiology
University of the Western Cape
Faculty of Dentistry
Belville, Cape Town, South Africa

Michael J. Pharoah, B.Sc., D.D.S., M.Sc.

Associate Professor and Head
Department of Oral Radiology
University of Toronto
Faculty of Dentistry
Toronto, Ontario, Canada

Axel Ruprecht, D.D.S., M.Sc.D.

Professor and Director
Oral and Maxillofacial Radiology
Department of Oral Pathology and Medicine
University of Iowa
College of Dentistry
Iowa City, Iowa

Douglas W. Stoneman, D.D.S.

Professor Emeritus
Department of Oral Radiology
University of Toronto
Faculty of Dentistry
Toronto, Ontario, Canada

Steven J. Willing, M.D.

Assistant Professor of Radiology
Department of Radiology
University of Alabama at Birmingham
School of Medicine
Birmingham, Alabama

Dedicated to our families, mentors and students

PREFACE

Maxillofacial diagnostic imaging is an important subsection of head and neck radiology. It is of specific interest not only to medical and dental radiologists but also to oral surgeons, otorhinolaryngologists, plastic surgeons and persons in other health-related specialties. This book is designed to be both a rapid reference and a more comprehensive guide to the radiologic features of the common maxillofacial pathologic processes.

The book is divided into several main segments. The first chapter briefly outlines the philosophy to be followed in this publication concerning the role of imaging in the diagnosis of oral and maxillofacial pathologic processes. This is followed by a comprehensive grouping of signs with comprehendible line diagrams and lists of conditions to be considered when developing differential diagnoses. The remainder is an atlas that demonstrates the various diagnostic imaging features of oral and maxillofacial lesions primarily grouped by pathologic process. Variations in radiologic features are stressed. Three areas are treated specifically by site; the salivary glands, the paranasal sinuses, and the temporomandibular joint.

While lead authors have been assigned to each chapter, to ensure a commonality of style, lack of repetition and selection of the best available cases from the rich collections available to the authors, final responsibility for the contents lies with the primary authors. The primary authors accept full responsibility for the correct diagnosis in all cases presented and for the final editing of all contributions. The aim has been to present cases that have not been published elsewhere. Imaging modalities displayed have been selected according to their diagnostic utility for the described conditions.

ACKNOWLEDGMENTS

The authors are thankful for the close cooperation given by staff from Mosby-Year Book during the development of this publication; especially Sandy Reinhardt, Susan Baxter, Melba Steube, Mark Spann, Tim O'Brien, April Nauman, and Julie Zipfel.

The authors would also like to acknowledge the valued artistic contributions of Arend Louw, Dip. Comm. Art, Department of Graphic Arts, Faculty of Dentistry, University of Stellenbosch. He prepared the line illustrations in Chapter 2.

Allan G. Farman
Christoffel J. Nortjé
Robert E. Wood

CONTENTS

Contents

1

PRINCIPLES OF IMAGE INTERPRETATION

THE SYSTEMATIC APPROACH

Radiography is only one part of the diagnostic process in maxillofacial diagnosis. Though it is useful to train one's ability to perceive features in isolated radiographs, the interpretation of these features is rarely pathognomonic. Furthermore it would be ethically unsound to make radiographs without following appropriate selection criteria, because patients should not be exposed to unnecessary radiation. A thorough case history and clinical examination should precede selection of the radiographs and other diagnostic images needed for each patient. Laboratory tests may also be required for diagnosis.

Case History

The necessity of a thorough case history cannot be overemphasized. History taking, like radiographic interpretation, needs to be approached in a rational and systematic way. In addition to demographic details such as patient name, address, age, and gender, history taking should include the patient's chief complaint (if any), a history of the present condition, the patient's past medical and dental history, and a brief note on how the investigation will proceed. The precise technique for history taking is beyond the scope of this book, but it should be as thorough as possible. A thorough case history is an invaluable record that

can be referred to when clinical, radiologic, histologic, and other laboratory test evidence has been gathered.

Clinical Examination

Radiographs should not be taken before a thorough clinical examination has been performed and the findings recorded in detail in the patient's chart. A visual examination helps the clinician select the radiographic projections most likely to provide useful information to contribute to the evaluation (and eventual diagnosis) of the patient's condition. The examination should not be restricted to the area of chief complaint. It should include a thorough extraoral and intraoral inspection. A clinical evaluation is essential even in asymptomatic patients undergoing routine dental reviews. The decision as to which radiographs are needed will vary for different patients, depending on clinical findings such as oral health status, presence or absence of teeth, and dental alignment. Adjustments in radiographic technique may be necessary to compensate for anatomic variations such as tori, a shallow palate, and ankyloglossia (tongue-tie). It is the clinician's job to select and prescribe the appropriate radiographs necessary for assessing the oral and maxillofacial health status of the individual patient. This responsibility should not be delegated.

1

Existing Diagnostic Radiographs

An effective way to reduce the patient's unnecessary exposure to ionizing radiation is to avoid taking radiographs that are already available. If the patient is not certain which views have already been made, it is the clinician's responsibility to see that this information is obtained from earlier health care providers.

Even when previous radiographs are too old to reliably replace new exposures, they are still of value. By comparing old and new radiographs, the clinician can evaluate changes over a specific time. This information on the progression of a radiographic feature can be of great value in helping to differentiate among disease entities and between normal and disease states. It also provides a dynamic assessment of the rate of development of common chronic diseases such as dental caries and periodontal disease.

Image Selection

Professional judgment should be used to determine the type, frequency, and extent of each radiographic examination. As noted earlier, this requires history taking, a thorough clinical examination, and the acquisition of information from existing radiographs.

Symptomatic patients: For patients with signs or symptoms of disease, all radiographs professionally judged to be necessary to evaluate the patient's condition should be made. Failure to obtain the necessary radiographs is negligent and constitutes failure to provide the appropriate standard of care. If a patient refuses to have necessary radiographs made, the clinician should document the fact and not proceed with treatment.

The type of radiograph obtained depends on the site to be evaluated, the dimensions of the probable lesion, and clinical practicality. For the more common dental conditions, intraoral periapical and bitewing films provide the best resolution and also cover the area of interest. When a patient is unable to open his or her mouth because of trismus, extraoral alternatives to intraoral radiographs must be sought. Such alternatives include lateral oblique projections of the jaw and panoramic radiographic views. These alternatives are also often needed when the lesion extends beyond the dimensions of standard intraoral film. Special series of radiographs are often necessary to examine traumatic injuries, progressive dysfunction of the temporomandibular joint, dental malocclusion requiring orthodontic evaluation, syndromes of the head and neck, and multifocal or systemic pathoses.

Asymptomatic patients. For asymptomatic patients undergoing routine dental checkups, selection of radiographs again depends largely on professional judgment. In these patients the principal reasons for taking radiographs are to detect incipient interproximal dental caries and to evaluate clinically detected progressive periodontal disease. Guidelines for selecting radiographic examinations for such patients have been developed by the Center for Devices and Radiological Health of the Food and Drug Administration. Professional judgment is important in the selection of radiographs. No radiographs should be taken merely as a routine or for administrative purposes.

Initial Examination of Images

When radiographs have been obtained, they first need to be evaluated for proper exposure, positioning, and processing. They should be examined for adequate density to illustrate specific structures in specific circumstances. Different densities are acceptable in certain instances but unacceptable in others. Adequate contrast will also depend on the individual clinical situation. For example, a long scale of contrast is desirable for evaluating periodontal disease, but a shorter scale of contrast is generally preferred for evaluating dental caries. Exposure and processing techniques influence density and contrast and may be altered to improve these properties. Technically inferior radiographs should not be used.

The clinician must then determine if the radiographs obtained show the structures of interest. If not, the clinician decides what further radiographs are needed. Because radiographs are two-dimensional representations of three-dimensional structures, a single radiograph is often inadequate for optimal interpretation. For pathologic lesions, which are the main focus of this atlas, it is often necessary to obtain a minimum of two radiographs at right angles to one another. On occasion the patient may need to be referred for assessment by more advanced imaging modalities, such as computed tomography or magnetic resonance imaging.

Viewing Environment

The proper environment should be available for reading radiographs. The best environment has dim lighting and is free from distractions. The darker the room, the better, as fine details may go unnoticed in normal room lighting. Such viewing conditions are present in most medical facilities; however, some practitioners only view radiographs at the chairside, in normal lighting and with all the distractions of the clinic. You are strongly urged to get into the habit of evaluating radiographs under appropriate viewing conditions.

The viewing area should have a viewbox of sufficient size that is brightly and evenly illuminated and in a position comfortable for the operator. A bright light, or dense-spot viewer, is indispensable for sufficient viewing of dark portions of radiographs. Magnifying glasses should be available to allow the examiner to focus on important areas of the film. Opaque masks should be available to block out extraneous light from the viewbox, as it is difficult for the observer's eyes to accommodate the range of light intensities transmitted through the radiographs and directly from the viewbox.

Clinicians should view all patients' radiographs at one time when there are no distractions, such as at the beginning of the day before patients arrive or at the end of the day when the patients are gone. The improved interpretation and treatment planning are certainly worth the extra effort.

OBSERVATION AND INTERPRETATION

Identification

All radiographs should be identified with the patient's name, information to discriminate among patients having the same name (e.g., date of birth, social security number, hospital number, or address), and the date of exposure of the radiograph. This information should be carefully checked before writing a report. The legal and medical literatures are full of cases in which this simple precaution has not been taken. It is best not to rely on unlabeled radiographs when making a diagnosis.

Localization

Localizing radiographs should be a simple matter if the clinician performed the imaging procedure; however, this is not always the case. A clinician might need to orient radiographs taken by other clinicians. Orientation generally is achieved by a knowledge of normal anatomic landmarks and the use of special markers to distinguish between the right and left side of the patient. Metallic markers are generally used for extraoral radiographs. When obtaining intraoral radio-

graphs, however, there is no room for such markers. For these cases the manufacturers of x-ray film include an embossed dot on the film. The convexity of this dot points toward the source of the radiation. Care should be taken to assure correct orientation of films, as confusion between the right and left sides could lead to negligent patient treatment and would be impossible to defend in a court of law.

Evaluation Sequence

The evaluation sequence commences with history taking, clinical examination, and selection of appropriate tests, including radiographs. The radiographs are examined under suitable viewing conditions. Observations are listed before the clinician attaches significance to them and determines the likely nature of any disease process that may be present. A radiographic differential interpretation is formulated based on the radiographic features alone. These features are then correlated with the patient's clinical information, history, and the results of other tests, including histologic assessment, to make a working diagnosis. It cannot be overemphasized that radiographic interpretation is only one factor in the ultimate diagnosis: it is an *interpretation,* not the diagnosis. Further special tests, possibly including additional diagnostic imaging, may be needed before the clinician can make a definitive diagnosis, plan treatment, and begin treatment. The evaluation sequence is summarized in the box below.

THE EVALUATION SEQUENCE

Take history and perform clinical examination.
Select radiographs and assure quality.
Examine radiographs.
Make observations.
Attach significance, or hypothesize about likely disease nature.
Formulate differential interpretation.
Integrate patient history and clinical and other findings.
Formulate working diagnosis.
Consider additional tests.
Formulate definitive diagnosis and treatment plan.
Perform necessary treatment.

Normal Versus Abnormal

After the clinician assures the identity of the patient whose images are being evaluated and determines image quality and orientation, the clinician decides whether the radiographic features are normal. Such a determination is predicated on a thorough knowledge of normal anatomy and the factors involved in the production of radiographs, including image casting, radiodensity, the law of tangency, and the law of summation. It should also be remembered that normal is a range; it is relative rather than restrictive. In consequence, one needs to determine what should be recorded as being beyond the normal range and which observations require further investigation or treatment. In general, relative bilateral symmetry tends to suggest a normal structure, and lack of change in features between radiographs taken at long intervals tends to support a conservative approach.

Listing of Observations

Observations should be listed in a systematic manner. When examining a radiograph for the purposes of interpretation, the clinician must examine all parts of the radiograph. As radiographs are usually taken to evaluate clinical impressions, it is all too easy to examine a few parts of the image and neglect the rest of it. Often, when an abnormality is found, the observer will not complete the examination of the remainder of the radiograph and thereby neglect potentially important information. Hence, when an abnormality is found, it is wise to ignore it for a time and examine the rest of the radiograph for a second or even a third area of abnormality. A system of analysis is useful to ensure that all parts of a radiograph are examined. This takes self-discipline, and each practitioner needs to develop a personal method for assuring that the whole of the radiograph is assessed.

For a full mouth series of periapical and bitewing radiographs, a systematic approach includes the following:

1. The radiographs should be mounted in an opaque mount to mask out extraneous light from around the films. It is usual to view the films with the embossed dot convexities facing the observer, so that the patient's right side is mounted on the observer's left, as if he or she were looking at the patient. Before progressing the clinician checks the embossed dots and normal anatomic details to assure that the films are correctly mounted. Failure to do so could lead to misdiagnosis and inappropriate treatment. Also, the clinician checks the patient's name and the date of the radiographs to make sure they are the appropriate set.

2. The observer begins by viewing the posterior bitewing radiographs, starting with the right side in the maxilla and continuing across the maxilla, then, for the mandibular teeth, viewing from the left side to the right. The posterior teeth are assessed for primary or recurrent dental caries, with special attention given to the enamel surfaces just below the interproximal contact points. When in doubt, the clinician should refer to the adjacent periapical views for additional information. It is important to view the surfaces of every tooth.

3. The anterior periapical radiographs are evaluated for primary or recurrent dental caries.

4. The clinician then checks for the periodontal margin level of all interproximal alveolar crests in a systematic manner, starting with the right maxillary molar teeth and working around the arches, first to the left side of the maxilla, then from the left side of the mandible to the right. The presence of dental calculus is charted at this time.

5. The pulp chamber and periodontal ligament space of each tooth are assessed in turn, starting with the right side of the maxilla and progressing around the arches tooth by tooth.

6. The clinician then evaluates the normal anatomic bony landmarks, including but not limited to both maxillary sinuses, the outlines of the nasal passages, the anterior nasal spine, the incisal fossa, the mental foramen, and the mandibular canals.

For a lesion to be demonstrated radiographically, there needs to be a change in the tissues profound enough to be visualized. This change may be in the general architecture of the involved tissues or in radiodensity.

A comprehensive description of each significant lesion is needed. This description should be written in the patient's clinical notes and include the lesion site, size, shape, symmetry, borders, content, and associations. The following descriptors will be applied to lesions affecting bone; however, they can be extended to include the dental structures and soft tissues.

Site: The position of the lesion should be designated as accurately as possible, preferably in both standard diagrams and narrative description. The epicenter of the lesion may help in determining its origin. For instance, lesions arising in the body of the mandi-

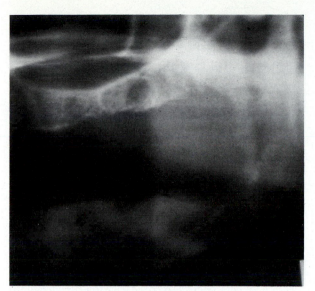

Fig. 1-1 Saucerized appearances tend to indicate that the lesion probably arose in soft tissue.

ble above the mandibular canal are more likely to be odontogenic in origin than are those arising below the canal. The clinician should also determine whether the lesion is solitary or multiple and whether it affects one bone or is multifocal. This will help in differentiating between a local or systemic etiology and pathogenesis for the disease.

Size: The size of the lesion as measured on the radiographs should be indicated in millimeters rather than by reference to objects such as peas or plums. Peas and plums vary in size, and even if they did not one cannot rely on one's eyes to perceive dimensions accurately. The size is an important factor for potential treatment planning and for judging dynamic change with time. A ruler should be kept at the side of the viewbox. Clinicians must remember that radiographic projections are subject to some dimensional distortion and that there is generally magnification in the image.

Shape: To describe the shape of the lesion, clinicians should refer to at least two radiographs taken at right angles when possible. The shape often provides clues to origin. For example, a "brandy glass" appearance tends to indicate a lesion that commenced in bone and secondarily extended to soft tissues. On the other hand, a saucer appearance tends to indicate a lesion originating in the soft tissues and secondarily involving bone (see Fig. 1-1). Usually lesions grow in the direction of least resistance, which will be reflected in their shape.

Symmetry: Bilateral symmetry usually indicates a condition that is either a variant of normal or an inherited condition (Fig. 1-2). In general, asymmetry is more worrisome than symmetry.

Borders: There are several factors to be considered when assessing the border, or outline, of a lesion in bone. First, before a lesion can be demonstrated, there must be sufficient change for it to be detected radiographically in architecture or resorption or deposition of bone. Early stages of disease processes may be too subtle to detect radiographically, as in the case of an initial carious lesion of enamel in which loss of mineral salts is insufficient to result in a perceptible radiodensity change. It should also be remembered that specific cell types need to be present before bone can be resorbed; thus an acute periapical abscess may not be seen on a radiograph, as cells that resorb bone are not present until chronic inflammation ensues. Second, it should be recognized that the border of a lesion is perhaps its most significant feature, as the active process in any lesion tends to be at the periphery. Just as the histopathologist gains the best information about a biopsy specimen from the growing edge of the lesion where abnormal meets normal, so the diagnostic radiologist can obtain a great deal of information from interpretation of the radiographic outline of a lesion.

The border may be well demarcated, moderately demarcated, poorly demarcated, or undemarcated. Benign conditions (with the exception of inflammatory lesions) tend to take the two extremes, cysts and tumors being well-demarcated (Fig. 1-3) and developmental conditions, such as late fibrous dysplasia, being undemarcated (Fig. 1-4). In the latter cases, structural architecture is changed. The degree of cortication of the border will vary depending on the type of lesion. Lesions that are poorly demarcated tend also to be poorly corticated. A radiolucent zone in a well-corticated, well-demarcated border suggests encapsulation of the lesion—a feature most consistent with a benign process (Fig. 1-5).

Detectable borders on lesions can be further subtyped. The sharp sclerotic margin of benign cysts and neoplasms (Figs. 1-3 and 1-5) and the diffuse border that melds with normal bone (Fig. 1-4) have already been illustrated. Some benign lesions—usually the more aggressive types, such as ameloblastoma and odontogenic keratocyst—tend to be crenated or multilocular rather than unilocular in outline (Fig. 1-6). Infiltrative (bays within bays) borders suggest malig-

(Text continued on page 8).

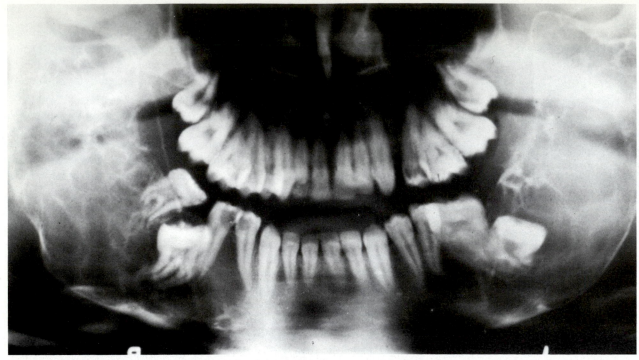

Fig. 1-2   Bilateral symmetry suggests either a variant of normal or an inherited condition. Symmetry in mandibular lesions is a common feature in cherubism, a dominantly inherited condition.

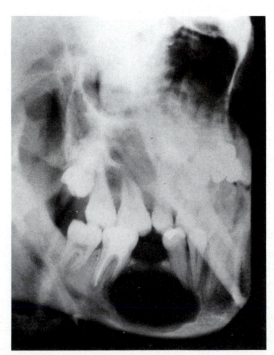

Fig. 1-3   Well-demarcated benign cystic process.

Opposite page:

Fig. 1-4 (top),   Undermarcated lesion of late fibrous dysplasia can be seen through effect on jawbone architecture.

Fig. 1-5 (bottom left),   Encapsulated benign lesion. Note the radiolucent halo separating the well-corticated outline from the lesion. The condition demonstrated here is a cementoblastoma.

Fig. 1-6 (bottom right),   Multilocular radiolucent outlines are often found in more locally aggressive benign cysts and neoplasms of the jaws. The condition demonstrated here is an ameloblastoma.

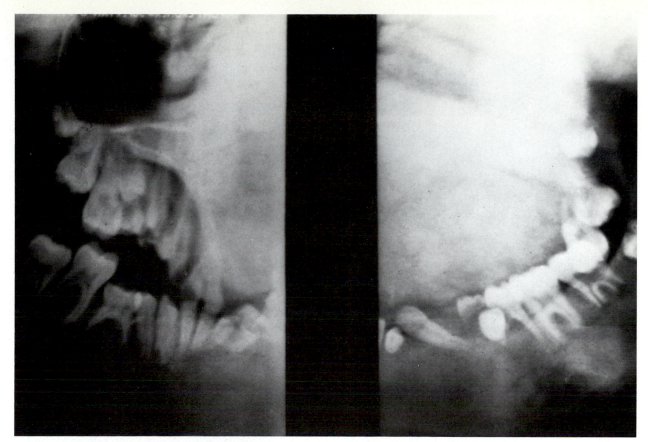

Fig. 1-4.

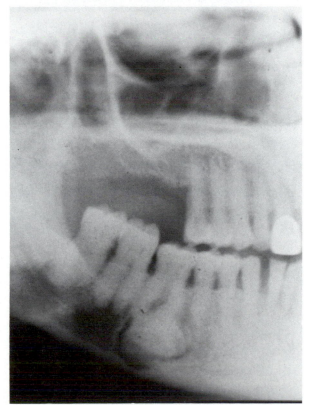

For legends see opposite page.

Fig. 1-5.

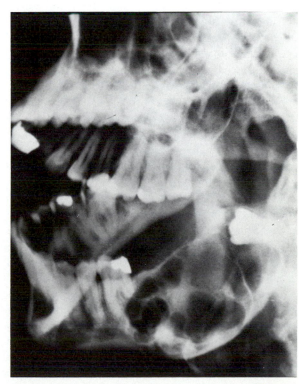

Fig. 1-6.

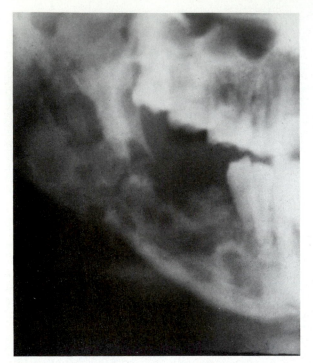

Fig. 1-7 Poorly defined lesion with "moth-eaten" appearance in primary leiomyosarcoma of the mandible.

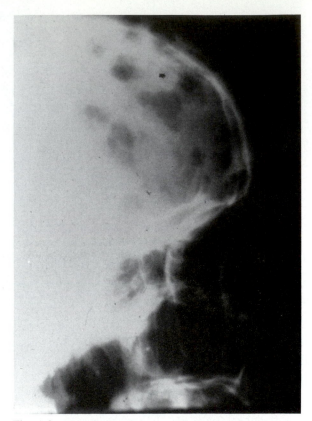

Fig. 1-8 "Punched-out" lesions of multiple myeloma.

nancy, whereas a ragged, "moth-eaten" (or "worm-eaten") border can be found both in severe inflammatory conditions and malignant neoplasia (Fig. 1-7). Well-demarcated, "punched-out" lesions with uncorticated margins are typically found in the idiopathic histiocytosis and in myeloma (Fig. 1-8).

Content: Lesions may be entirely radiolucent, homogeneously radiopaque, or mixed radiolucent and radiopaque. One should, however, be very careful when applying these terms. The terms *radiolucent* and *radiopaque* are relative, depending on the relative density and thickness of adjacent structures and the radiographic technique used (Fig. 1-9). Also, a lesion that appears as a radiolucency or a mixed radiolucency and radiopacity using one technique may appear as a homogeneous radiolucency on another view (Fig. 1-10). Comparisons of radiodensity are fraught with error if the bulk of the tissue being examined is not considered.

Another facet to consider is the pathogenesis of the radiologic features. Most lesions start with a radiolucent appearance, some progress to become mixed radiolucent and radiopaque, and some progress to become homogeneously radiopaque. The actual appearance of a lesion can vary with the stage of pathogenesis. For example, periapical cemental dys-

Text continued on page 10.

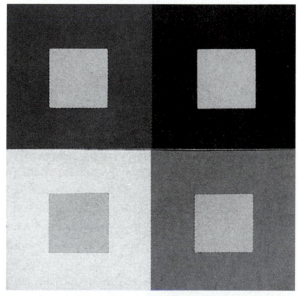

Fig. 1-9 *Radiolucent* and *radiopaque* are relative terms. The inner squares in this example all have equal density. Note their relative density changes depending on the density of their surroundings.

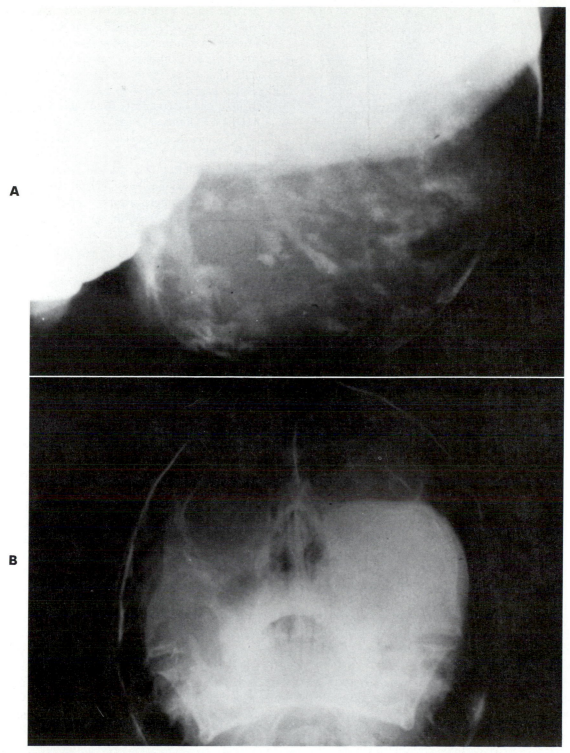

Fig. 1-10 On the occlusal film **(A)** a cementifying fibroma is seen as a mixed radiolucency and radiopacity. On the Waters' **(B)** view of the sinus the lesion appears as a homogeneous radiopacity. In the latter view the beam passed through a much greater bulk of the tumor tissue, resulting in increased attenuation.

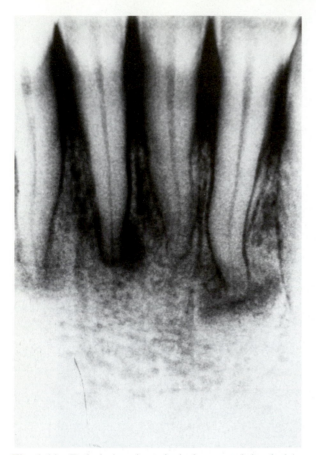

Fig. 1-11 Early lesions in periapical cemental dysplasia are radiolucent.

plasia starts with the appearance of multiple radiolucencies that progressively calcify to become radiopaque (Figs. 1-11 and 1-12).

Essentially, a radiolucent lesion suggests that lysis of normal bone has occurred. The development of a calcified product in a lesion results in varying degrees of radiopacity, depending on the nature of the calcified product (e.g., cementum, dentin, or enamel), the degree of calcification, the size of the lesion, and the distribution of the calcified product (Fig. 1-13). Foreign bodies can sometimes be much more opaque than calcified products manufactured by the body. They are usually easy to identify (Fig. 1-14).

Also important to consider are the size and distribution of trabeculation, or the trabecular pattern, in general or in the affected site. The normal trabecular pattern is usually coarser and more angular, with relatively larger marrow spaces in the mandible than in the maxilla. Black patients tend to have denser bone than whites. However, "normal" is a wide range.

Particularly thin trabeculation and rarefied bone patterns of the jaws in general can be associated with systemic conditions, such as hyperparathyroidism, early stages of Paget disease of bone (osteoporosis circumscripta), and osteoporosis. Unusually dense, generalized trabeculations are found in osteopetrosis and a number of other less frequently encountered conditions.

Trabecular patterns in a discrete lesion can be in the form of septa creating varying degrees of multilocularity. When such septa are few, and the loculi are relatively rounded and large, the term *soap bubble appearance* is sometimes applied. This is the type of trabeculation commonly seen in the ameloblastoma, the central giant cell granuloma, and the odontogenic keratocyst (see Fig. 1-6). Narrower, "honeycomb" separations with angular interstices are more typically found in the odontogenic myxoma and intraosseous hemangiomas (Fig. 1-15).

Some lesions show particular trabecular patterns that help in the diagnosis. The "hair-on-end" appearance of trabeculations in the skull are typical of the hemolytic anemias, β-thalassemia, and sickle cell anemia (Fig. 1-16). The coarse trabeculation leaves space for hemotopoietic marrow to persist. An irregular "sunburst" appearance of trabeculations in a destructive or productive lesion is one of the typical features of the osteogenic sarcoma (Fig. 1-17). Here the product is completely uncoordinated from the stress-bearing needs of the bone. Dense patches of sclerotic bone can form in response to local inflammatory stimulus, as in condensing osteitis (Fig. 1-18), and can be more widespread, as the "cotton ball" appearance in late stages of Paget disease of bone or in florid osseous dysplasia (Fig. 1-19). In late stages of fibrous dysplasia the bone trabeculations are fine but dense. This gives rise to an "orange peel" appearance on intraoral radiographs (Fig. 1-20). Because the resolution of extraoral radiographs is lower than that for intraoral radiographs, lesions with an orange peel appearance on the latter have a "ground glass" (or "frosted glass") appearance on the former (see Fig. 1-4).

Associations: The effects of a lesion on structures in the jaws (e.g., teeth, mandibular canal, maxillary sinuses) can be useful aids to interpretation. Lesions can be classified as tooth-associated or not tooth-associated. Conditions of odontogenic origin will tend to occur in the dental arches. Lesions surrounding, or en-

Text continued on page 14.

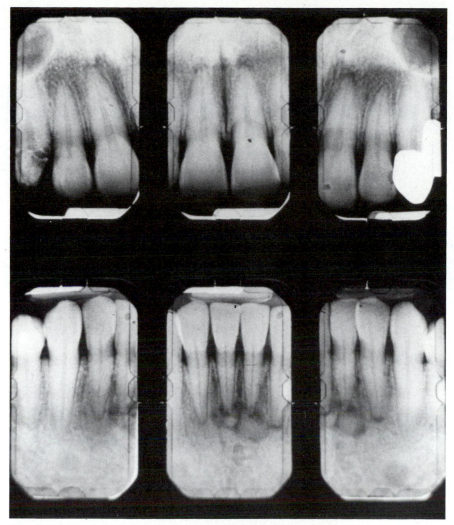

Fig. 1-12   Late lesions in periapical cemental dysplasia are radiopaque.

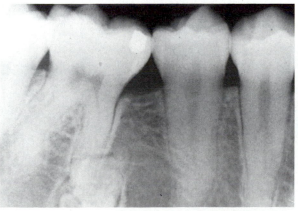

Fig. 1-13   Odontoma. Note that the calcified component
has the same opacity as the adjacent teeth.

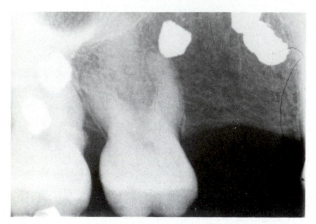

Fig. 1-14   Metallic foreign bodies.

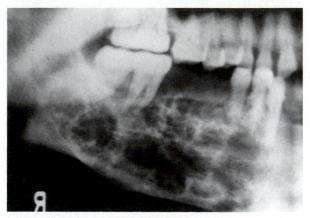

Fig. 1-15   "Honeycomb" appearance of multilocularity. This was an odontogenic myxoma.

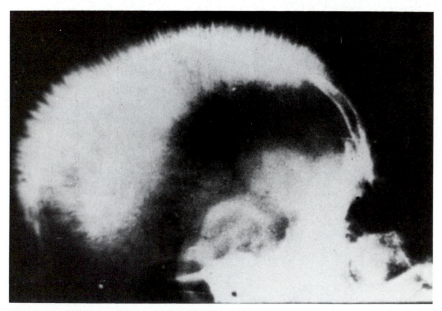

Fig. 1-16   "Hair-on-end" appearance typical of the hemolytic anemias.

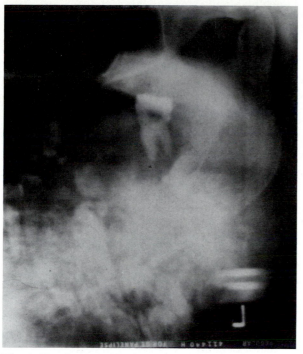

Fig. 1-17 "Sunburst" appearance typical of osteogenic sarcoma.

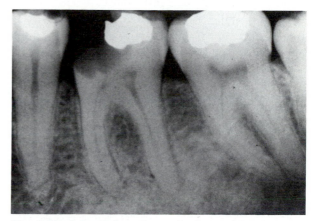

Fig. 1-18 Sclerotic bone in condensing osteitis.

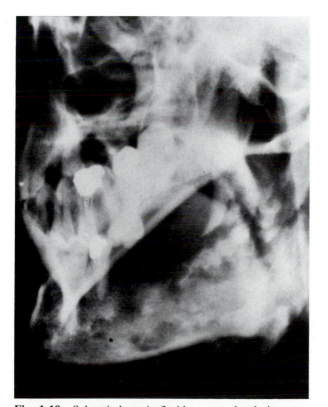

Fig. 1-19 Sclerotic bone in florid osseous dysplasia.

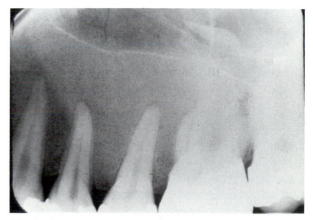

Fig. 1-20 "Orange peel" appearance in fibrous dysplasia.

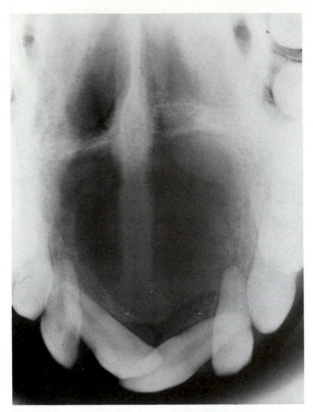

Fig. 1-21 Nasopalatine duct cyst displacing subjacent teeth.

veloping, the crown of the unerupted tooth may have developed from the reduced enamel epithelium (e.g., dentigerous cyst) or have invaded the dental follicle space (e.g., envelopmental odontogenic keratocyst). Lesions associated with a radiolucent widening of the apical periodontal ligament space are most frequently of dental origin following an insult to the pulp of the affected tooth.

Lesions may have one of three effects on the associated structures: no effect, displacement, or resorption.[3] The type of change can be used to aid in determining the nature of the disease process. As a rough generalization, the less aggressive benign cysts and tumors tend to displace adjacent structures (Fig. 1-21). Locally aggressive benign lesions *may* spread along the jaws without severe effects on the involved structures (Fig. 1-22). Malignancies and chronic infections *may* cause osseous erosion and even resorption of structures (Fig. 1-23).

Attaching Significance to Observations

Clearly, then, certain features are highly suggestive or even pathognomonic of a particular disease process; however, most radiographic features are pieces of contributory evidence rather than diagnostic. The combination of radiographic features provides a direction for further inquiry. These features can also be used with artificial intelligence computer programs (e.g., ORAD) to produce a list of possible diagnoses based on interpretation of the various radiographic features and other information. Whether or not computer-aided diagnosis is employed, the radiographic features need to be correlated with other diagnostic information before the clinician can make a working diagnosis and determine what further tests are needed. After these steps, the clinician can make a definitive diagnosis and decide whether biopsy of the lesion is indicated.

Radiographic Versus Surgical Sieve

The concept of the "surgical sieve" is a well-established schematic giving the broad classification of diseases (Table 1-1). Much of this sieve is based on the patient's history and clinical examination. Radiographic findings are correctly viewed as one piece of

TABLE 1-1 Broad Classification of Diseases (The " Surgical Sieve")

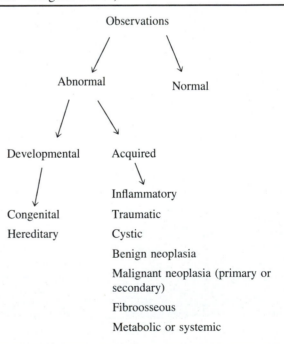

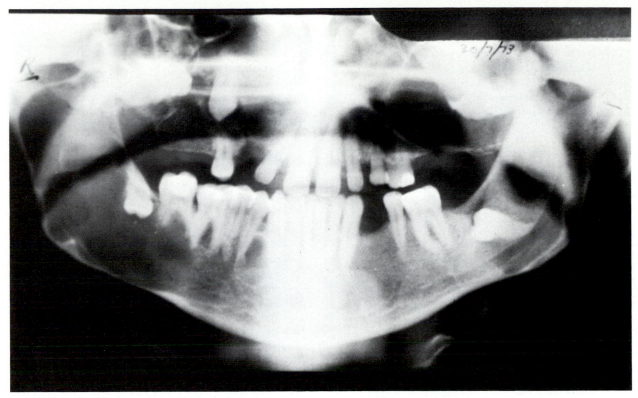

Fig. 1-22 Odontogenic keratocyst extending in the mandible with little effect on adjacent structures.

the puzzle. Rarely do radiographic findings contribute the only information in the diagnostic process. The broad classifications discussed in the section "Listing of Observations" can be used to produce a radiographic sieve with the described features applied to each section of the surgical sieve (Tables 1-2 and 1-3).

TABLE 1-2 The Radiographic Sieve

Normal vs Abnormal

Radiolucent vs Mixed opacity vs Radiopaque

Solitary vs Multiple

Well-defined vs Poorly defined

Unilocular vs Multilocular

Tooth-associated vs Tooth-independent

Adjacent structures unaffected vs Displaced vs Eroded

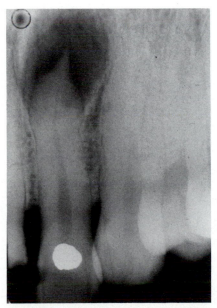

Fig. 1-23 Root resorption resulting from severe local inflammatory process.

TABLE 1-3   Method of Systematically Analysing Lesions That Exhibit Radiologic Signs.

Lesion analysis:
1. Overall degree of radiolucency/opacity
   — radiolucent?
   — radiopaque?
   — mixed lucent/opaque?
2. Position of the lesion
   — mandible?
   — maxilla?
   — both jaws?
   — dental tissue?
   — cortical bone?
   — cancellous bone?
   — soft tissue?
3. Origin of the lesion
   — where is the lesion centre?
   — is it from outside bone extending into it or from inside bone extending out of it?
   — is there a saucerized margin or a lipped margin?
   — is there an associated soft tissue mass?
4. What kind of lesion border or margin is there?
demarcation
   — well-demarcated?
   — moderately well-demarcated?
   — not well-demarcated?
   — undemarcated?
cortication
   — well-corticated?
          — thick cortex?
          — thin cortex?
   — moderately well-corticated?
   — poorly corticated?
   — uncorticated?
encapsulation
   — is there a partial or total capsule surrounding the lesion?
border sub-types
   — infiltrative (bays within bays) malignant border
   — smooth-edged
   — etched smooth hydraulic border
   — crenated undulating benign tumour border
   — ragged moth-eaten border
   — diffuse border that melds with normal bone
   — displaced border of normal girth
   — sharp sclerotic border
   — punched-out border
5. What is the nature of the internal structure?
radiolucency
   — solitary?
   — multiple separate?
   — rarefying osteitis?
   — blurring of trabeculae?
   — diminished density of trabeculae?
   — diminished number of trabeculae?

radiopacity
bone
   — sequestrum?
   — sclerosing osteitis?
   — granular bone?
   — increased trabecular size?
   — long spindly trabeculae?
   — septae or pseudo septae?
   — normal residual bone?
   — honeycombed bone pattern?
   — tubular bone pattern?
   — linear striations in bone?
dental tissues
   — globular cemental masses?
   — enamel?
   — dentin?
   — dental soft tissues?
   — mixtures of the above?
calcifications
   — metastatic or dystrophic?
   — vascular?
   — lymph node?
   — salivary?
   — in muscle planes?
foreign bodies
   — metallic
   — non-metallic
6. What is the effect of the lesion on adjacent structures?
bone
   — alterations in cortical definition or density?
   — alterations in trabecular bone?
   — density changes?
   — architecture changes?
   — thinning of cortices?
   — displaced cortices of normal size?
   — true hair on end periosteal reaction?
   — false hair on end ("T ended")?
   — Codman's triangle?
   — expansion with cortical breaching?
   — laminar periosteal new bone?
   — displaced and destroyed periosteal new bone?
teeth
   — hypercementosis?
   — resorption?
   — movement of teeth?
   — changes in eruption?
   — formation changes?
effects on other specific structures
   — mandibular canal

Radiographic Differential Interpretation

Ideally, one should read radiographs without knowing the other information that will eventually contribute to the diagnosis. In this way an unbiased list of possibilities based solely on radiographic features can be made. This is an interpretation rather than a diagnosis. The differential radiographic interpretation can then be integrated with the other available information to form a working diagnosis. There is less likelihood that salient features will be ignored if the radiographs are observed by a clinician who has not been biased by the history or clinical examination.

Synthesis of Diagnostic Information (Decision Making)

Synthesizing the diagnostic information requires integrating the radiographic interpretations with the other collected data, including the clinical observation, history, histopathologic evaluation, and other special tests. This synthesis allows for a narrowed group of differential diagnoses—the working diagnoses. Further special tests may be needed to develop the definitive diagnosis. These tests may include further radiographs or other diagnostic images. Effective, efficient treatment relies on establishing a definitive diagnosis.

Treatment

Radiographs are not only used for making the diagnosis; they are sometimes an integral component of the treatment process, too. For example, the various stages of endodontic therapy are evaluated radiographically. Furthermore, radiographs are used to check successful healing after endodontic treatment, dental implantology, and certain oral surgical procedures.

Expert Observation Versus Supervised Neglect

When a radiographic abnormality is detected, several pertinent questions must be asked: Should it be ignored? Should it be observed? Should it be tested further or treated? These are the "bottom line" questions facing all those responsible for interpreting radiographs. If one suspects a benign process that does not generally require treatment and the patient is reliable, one can occasionally place the patient under "expert observation" for a short period to assess whether the condition is progressive. If one suspects a benign process that will invariably require treatment, there is no sense in procrastinating. Because the patient is always entitled to be informed, it is much better to make a definitive diagnosis without unnecessary delay. It is unpleasant to feel uncertain about one's health, and most disease processes are easier to treat and have a better prognosis if treated early. When a condition is likely to be locally aggressive or malignant or to have other systemic consequences, there is no such thing as "expert observation." In such a situation, delay always constitutes "supervised neglect."

REFERENCES

American Dental Association Council on Dental Materials, Instruments, and Equipment: Recommendations in radiographic practices: an update, 1988, *J Am Dent Assoc* 118:115, 1989.

Center for Devices and Radiological Health: *The selection of patients for x-ray examinations,* HHS Pub No 88-8273, Rockville, Md, 1987.

Farman AG, Nortjé CJ, Grotepass FW: Pathological conditions of the mandible: their effect on the radiologic appearance of the inferior dental canal, *Br J Oral Surg* 15:64, 1977.

2

SIGNS IN MAXILLOFACIAL IMAGES

This chapter concentrates on radiologic signs rather than disease processes. It provides lists of the common, uncommon, and rare disease associations for each radiologic sign in the oral and maxillofacial region. Most of the listed conditions are covered in detail elsewhere in the text and can be studied once a working differential diagnosis has been developed.

DENTAL SIGNS

Large Teeth

Single

developmental abnormality, teeth most
   commonly involved:
     maxillary central incisor
     maxillary canine
     mandibular second premolar
     mandibular third molar
fusion
gemination
single central incisor–short stature
   syndrome

Multiple

normal variant (hereditary)
adjacent or contiguous benign vascular
   tumor
adjacent or contiguous benign neural
   tumor
adjacent lymphangioma
lipomatosis
pituitary gigantism
acquired unilateral hyperplasia
congenital unilateral hyperplasia

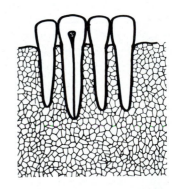

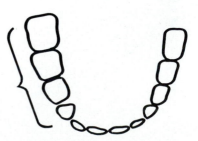

Small Teeth

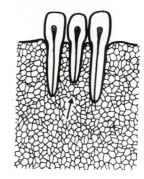

Single

developmental abnormality, teeth most
  commonly involved:
  maxillary lateral incisor
  maxillary third molar
  mandibular second premolar
supernumerary teeth

Multiple

normal variant
dentinogenesis imperfecta
trisomy 21
congenital facial hypoplasia
acquired facial hypoplasias
pituitary (Levi-Lorain) dwarfism
vascular tumors

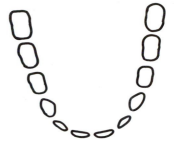

Single or a Few Teeth of Altered Form

Common:
infection from overlying primary tooth
  (Turner tooth)
dilaceration
taurodontism
enamel invaginations
peg-shaped lateral incisors
enlarged cingulum
enamel evaginations (tuberculated premolar)
shovel-shaped incisors

Uncommon:
fusion
concrescence
gemination
twinning
tuberculated maxillary lateral incisors
Hutchinson teeth—congenital syphilis
mulberry molars—congenital syphilis
premolarization of canines
molarization of premolars

Rare:
resulting from mutilative surgery
resulting from radiotherapy
resulting from chemotherapy

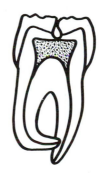
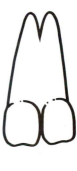

Hypercementosis

physiologic—secondary to passive
  eruption
idiopathic
periapical cemental dysplasia
periodontal disease
Paget disease
acromegaly
benign tumor
  cementoblastoma
  osteoblastoma

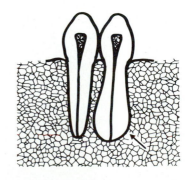

Hypodontia

Common:

previously extracted teeth
idiopathic
ectodermal dysplasias
previous radiotherapy
trisomy 21 (Down syndrome)

Uncommon:

chondroectodermal dysplasia
congenital unilateral facial hypoplasia
incontinentia pigmenti
orofaciodigital syndrome II (Mohr
   syndrome)
oculodentoosseous dysplasia

oculomandibulodyscephaly syndrome
   (Hallermann-Streiff syndrome)
oligodontia and primary mesodermal
   iris dysgenesis (Rieger syndrome)
PHC syndrome (Böök syndrome)
craniofacial dysostosis (Crouzon disease)
Ehlers-Danlos syndromes
focal dermal hypoplasia (Goltz syndrome)
pyknodysostosis
progeria (Hutchinson-Gilford syndrome)
hypoparathyroidism
Inverted Marfan syndrome

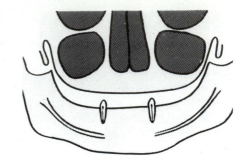

Hyperdontia

Common:

idiopathic
cleidocranial dysplasia
cleft palate
compound odontoma

Uncommon:

Gardner syndrome (intestinal polyposis type II)
oculomandibulodyscephaly syndrome
   (Hallermann-Streiff syndrome)
orofaciodigital syndrome
distomus
achondroplasia
Ehlers-Danlos syndromes

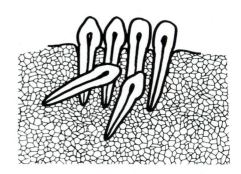

Failure of Eruption—Single

Common:

idiopathic
supernumerary tooth
nondevelopment of tooth

mechanical obstruction by other tooth
mechanical displacement by other
   teeth
retained primary tooth roots and teeth
dentigerous cyst or eruption cysts
odontogenic keratocyst
benign odontogenic tumor odontoma
ameloblastic fibroodontoma
ameloblastic fibroma
adenomatoid odontogenic tumor
cleft palate
ankylosis or submersion
inflammation coronal to erupting tooth
overlying tooth with pulpotomy

Uncommon:

odontogenic myxoma
cherubism
unicystic ameloblastoma
histiocytosis X
ossifying fibroma
malignancy
radiotherapy (usually delayed)
fibrous dysplasia
postextraction scar

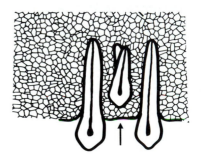

Failure of Eruption—Multiple

Common:

fibromatosis gingivae
drug-induced gingival hyperplasia
cleidocranial dysplasia
condylar hypoplasia and ankylosis
cherubism

Uncommon:

Gardner syndrome (intestinal polyposis type II)
Apert syndrome (acrocephalosyndactyly type I)
gingival hyperplasia syndromes
chondroectodermal dysplasia (Ellis-van Creveld syndrome)

trisomy 21
focal dermal hypoplasia (Goltz syndrome)
osteopetrosis
regional odontodysplasia
progeria (Hutchinson-Gilford syndrome)
pseudohypoparathyroidism
pyknodysostosis
juvenile hypothyroidism (cretinism)
ectodermal dysplasias
vitamin D deficiency syndromes

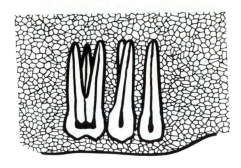

Premature Eruption

Common:

normal variant
early loss of primary teeth

Uncommon:

adjacent benign vascular tumors
adjacent benign neural tumors
underlying malignant tumor

underlying osteomyelitis
hyperthyroidism
pituitary gigantism
previous radiotherapy
hypergonadism
Cushing syndrome
adrenogenital syndrome

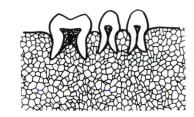

Early Loss of Teeth

Common:

rampant dental caries
dentofacial trauma
juvenile periodontitis

Uncommon:

histiocytosis X
factitial injury
cyclic neutropenia
malignancy
    leukemia
    lymphoma
    rhabdomyosarcoma
    neuroblastoma
hyperkeratosis palmoplantaris and periodontoclasia in childhood (Papillon-Lefèvre syndrome)
acrodynia (pink disease)
other heavy-metal poisoning
acatalasia
hyperparathyroidism

Rare:

acroosteolysis
severe rickets
pituitary cachexia syndrome (Simmond syndrome)
Chédiak-Higashi syndrome

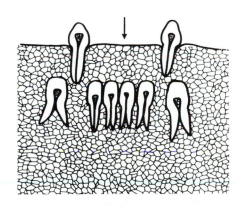

Moved Teeth and Tooth Buds

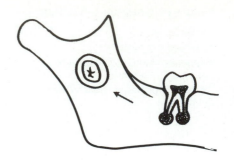

Common:

normal variant
malocclusion
dentigerous cysts
other cysts
traumatic displacement
submergence

Uncommon:

cherubism
lateral inflammatory odontogenic cyst
benign giant cell tumor
ameloblastoma

melanotic neuroectodermal tumor of
  infancy
other benign odontogenic and nonodontogenic tumors
osteomyelitis
histiocytosis X
malignancy adjacent to tooth bud
  Burkitt lymphoma
  lymphosarcoma
  neuroblastoma
rhabdomyosarcoma
osteomyelitis of maxilla in newborn

Enlarged Pulps

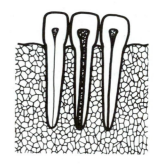

Common:

projection effects—maxillary incisors
normal variant—large cornua
taurodontism
dentinogenesis imperfecta
internal resorption
marcrodontia
fusion
gemination
enamel evagination

Uncommon:

vitamin D–resistant rickets
shell teeth
hypophosphatasia
renal osteodystrophy
enamel pearl with pulpal extension

Small Pulps

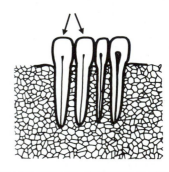

Common:

traumatically induced
normal variant

Uncommon:

branching canals
dentinogenesis imperfecta
dentinal dysplasias
arborization of root end
calcification of pulp

Enamel Aberrations

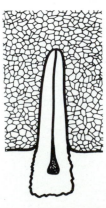

Common:

Turner tooth (single tooth)
amelogenesis imperfecta—
  hypocalcific type
amelogenesis imperfecta—hypoplastic
  type
environmental enamel hypoplasias
  neonatal disease
  exanthematous fevers
  nutritional deficits
  metabolic disease

drug induced
  tetracycline
  heavy metal toxicity
  fluorosis

Uncommon:

mucopolysaccharidosis IV (Morquio
  syndrome)
Ehlers-Danlos syndrome
hypophosphatasia
hypoparathyroidism
radiation therapy during development

Dentin Aberrations

Common:
dentinogenesis imperfecta
regional odontodysplasia

Uncommon:
osteogenesis/dentinogenesis imperfecta
dentin dysplasia
shell teeth
Ehlers-Danlos syndrome
radiotherapy during development

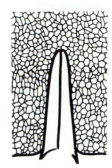

Persistent Open Apex of Tooth

variation of normal
nonvital tooth
periapical infectious pathology (e.g.,
    cyst, granuloma, abscess)
dens evaginatus
delayed development
internal resorption

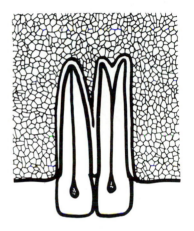

Prematurely Closed Apex

previous trauma to tooth
previous radiotherapy of jaws
dentinogenesis imperfecta

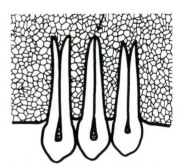

Calcified Pulp Tissue

Common:
normal variant for age
projection effect—root overlap on
    molar teeth
calcareous degeneration
previously restored tooth

Uncommon:
traumatically induced pulp calcifica-
    tion
enamel pearl superimposed over pulp
    chamber
dentinogenesis imperfecta

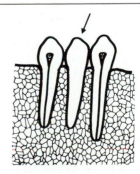

External Resorption

Normal:
physiologic resorption—primary teeth
normal variant mesial root of lower
  first molar
pulpotomy of primary tooth
projection effect
normally short roots

Common pathologic:
previous root amputation
periapical infection
unerupted tooth
excessive orthodontic forces
idiopathic
early pulpal death
root canal therapy
benign odontogenic tumors
cysts
intentional reimplantation
traumatic occlusion

Uncommon:
factitial injury
inostosis
malignant tumors (lymphoma)
oxalosis
idiopathic hypoparathyroidism
periodontal disease
foreign body reaction
internal resorption

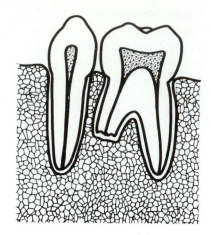

Internal Resorption

idiopathic
traumatically induced
caries induced
enlarged pulps
pulpal diverticuli
external resorption
odontomalacia

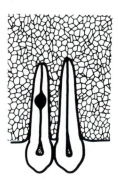

Loss of Lamina Dura—Localized

Common normal variations:
apex of maxillary canine
rotated tooth
maxillary premolars—before maturation
projection over maxillary sinus
projection over mandibular canal
projection over mental foramen

Pathologic:
inflammatory periapical disease
periapical granuloma
radicular cyst
simple bone cyst
periapical cemental dysplasia
osteomyelitis

Uncommon:
malignant tumor
fibrous histiocytoma
histiocytosis X

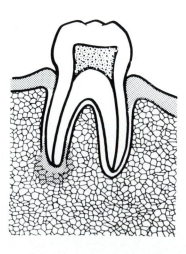

Loss of Lamina Dura—Generalized

Common:

idiopathic
Paget disease of bone
leukemia

Uncommon:

metastatic malignancy (especially breast)
hyperparathyroidism
multiple myeloma
osteomalacia
Rickets (including vitamin D–resistant rickets)
Cushing syndrome
hypoparathyroidism
hypothyroidism
postmenopausal osteoporosis

renal acidosis
acromegaly
oxalosis
hypervitaminoses D
hypovitaminoses C
systemic sclerosis (scleroderma)
hyperphosphatasia

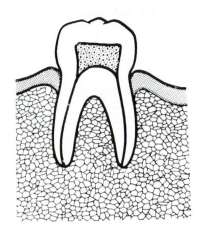

Accentuation of Lamina Dura

normal variant
systemic sclerosis (scleroderma)

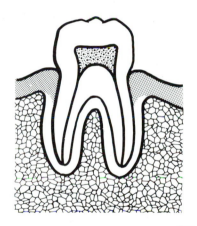

Increased Width of Periodontal Ligament Space

Common:

projection effect
normal finding around necks of teeth
root shadow cast over sinus
periapical inflammation
periodontal inflammation (including furcation disease)
systemic sclerosis (scleroderma)
traumatic loosening of teeth
traumatic occlusion
fractured root
fracture through socket

Uncommon:

intentional reimplantation (early changes)
osteomyelitis
actinomycotic infection
periodontosis
malignant tumors (especially osteosarcoma)
fibrous histiocytoma
diabetes
cystinosis

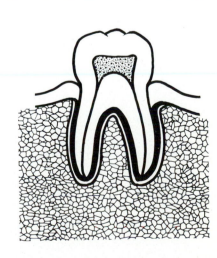

Suspected Ankylosis of Tooth

Common:
late sequela to reimplantation of
    avulsed tooth
trauma
overlying obscuring sclerosing osteitis

Uncommon:
infection
inostosis
false ankylosis (socket sclerosis)
idiopathic osteosclerosis

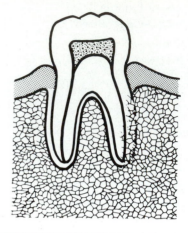

Crestal Radiolucency Leading to Decreased Alveolar Bone

Common:
hyperemic decalcification
periodontitis
juvenile periodontitis
factitial injury
acute necrotizing ulcerative gingivitis

Uncommon:
histiocytosis X
hyperkeratosis palmoplantaris and pe-
    riodontoclasia in children (Papillon-
    Lefèvre syndrome)
leukemia
local malignancy
    peripheral
    central

previous radiotherapy
hypothyroidism (cretinism/myxedema)
hyperthyroidism
hyperparathyroidism
peripheral giant cell tumor
giant cell epulides
other epulides
cyclic neutropenia
hypophosphatasia
acrodynia
acroosteolysis
self-mutilative syndromes
acatalasia
pituitary cachexia syndrome (Sim-
    mond disease)
Chédiak-Higashi syndrome

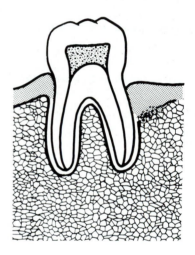

RADIOLUCENCIES OF THE JAWS

Periapical Radiolucency

False (variations of normal):
marrow spaces
dental papillae of developing teeth
maxillary sinus
incisive foramen
nasolacrimal canals
submandibular fossa
sublingual fossa
mandibular canal and mental foramen
thin bone in anterior mandible
tomographic plane artifacts (including panoramic artifacts)
processing errors (e.g. developer splash)

True (pathologic):
Common:
periapical granuloma
radicular cyst
fibrous healing defect
chronic or acute alveolar abscess
early stages of periapical cemental dysplasia
periodontal abscess

Uncommon:
osteomyelitis
dentigerous cyst of underlying tooth
simple bone cyst
other cysts
primary malignant tumors (e.g., leukemia)
underlying benign odontogenic tumors
early cementifying or ossifying fibroma
central giant cell granuloma
histiocytosis X
lingual salivary gland depression (Stafne defect)
multiple myeloma
metastatic malignancy (especially breast metastases)
early cementoblastoma or osteoblastoma
dentin dysplasia
odontogenic myxoma
early odontomas

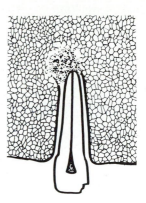

Pericoronal Radiolucency

Common:
normal follicular space
dentigerous cyst
odontogenic keratocyst
adenomatoid odontogenic tumor
early odontoma or ameloblastic fibro-odontoma

Uncommon:
ameloblastic fibroma
ameloblastoma
Hurler syndrome (mucopolysaccharidosis IH)
early calcifying odontogenic cyst

Multiple:
occasional normal finding
odontogenic keratocyst – basal cell nevus syndrome (Gorlin-Goltz syndrome)
Gardner syndrome (intestinal polyposis type II)
other mucopolysaccharidoses

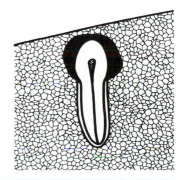

Lucency at the Side of a Tooth Root

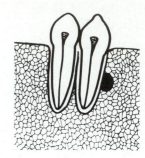

Common:
periodontal abscess
extension of disease from adjacent tooth
perforation of root during endodontic therapy
lateral periodontal cyst
periodontal cyst of inflammatory origin

Uncommon:
lateral canal periapical cyst
odontogenic keratocyst
neurofibroma
giant cell granuloma
unilocular ameloblastoma
neurilemmoma
histiocytosis X
hyperparathyroidism

Single Lucency, Well-Defined, Not Necessarily Contacting Teeth

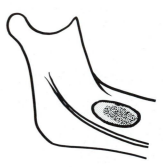

Common:
normal anatomic variation (marrow space, follicle nutrient canals, foramina)
residual cyst
postextraction healing defect
simple bone cyst
postsurgical defect

fibrous dysplasia
eosinophilic granuloma
neurofibroma
odontogenic myxoma
central hemangioma

Uncommon:
odontogenic keratocyst
ameloblastoma
giant cell granuloma
nasopalatine cyst
early cementifying fibroma

Rare:
aneurysmal bone cyst
chondrosarcoma
central true fibroma
tuberculous infection (geographic or socioeconomic variations)
hydatid cyst
calcifying epithelial odontogenic tumor

Single Lucency with Ragged Borders

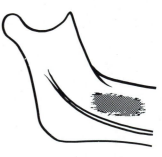

Common:
chronic osteitis
osteomyelitis
squamous cell carcinoma of oral cavity
infected radicular, residual, or other cyst

chondrosarcoma
fibrosarcoma
lymphosarcoma
rhabdomyosarcoma
leiomyosarcoma
melanotic neuroectodermal tumor of infancy
leukemia
benign giant cell tumor
aneurysmal bone cyst
neurofibroma
odontogenic myxoma
Ewing sarcoma

Uncommon:
fibrous dysplasia
metastatic carcinoma
malignant salivary gland tumours involving bone
osteolytic osteosarcoma
multiple myeloma

Lucency in Region of Maxillary Lateral Incisor

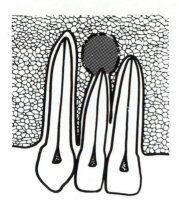

Common:
incisive fossa
canine fossae
periapical cyst or granuloma
periapical rarefying osteitis from adjacent central incisor

Uncommon:
clefts
aberrant foramen in anterior maxilla
nasopalatine duct cysts
odontogenic keratocyst
depression from nasolabial cyst
postsurgical defects

Noncystlike Lucency of Bone

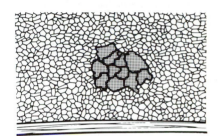

focal osteoporotic defect
large marrow space
lucent but normal maxillary tuberosity
normal sparse trabeculation in jaws of child
maxillary sinus
foramina
submandibular fossa
sublingual fossa
postcoronoid depression
sigmoid notch shadow
acute osteomyelitis
healing surgical defect
decalcification caused by overlying inflammation

Rarefying Osteitis (Focal Osteomyelitis)

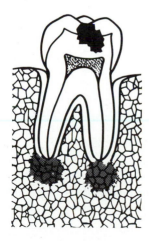

Common:
foramina
dental papilla
inferior canal and mental foramen
large marrow space
periodontal abscess
dental cyst or granuloma
early forms of periapical cemental dysplasia
antrum or nasal fossa
healing surgical defect

Uncommon:
actinomycotic infection
postradiotherapy change
leukemia
metastatic malignancy, especially breast
histiocytosis X

Generalized Rarefaction

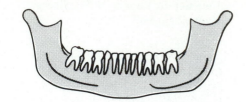

Common:
osteoporosis
cortisone therapy–induced rarefaction
rheumatoid arthritis
prolonged immobilization
malignant and other cachectic diseases

Uncommon:
Cushing syndrome
hyperparathyroidism
vitamin D deficiency syndromes
acromegaly
pancreatitis
malnutrition
pregnancy-related changes
diabetes
scurvy
inherited anemias
leukemia
histiocytosis X
multiple myeloma
Paget disease of bone
osteogenesis imperfecta
renal acidosis

Rare:
hypophosphatasia
hyperphosphatasia
hypoparathyroidism
thyrotoxicosis
hypogonadism
agranulocytosis
oxalosis
postradiation changes

Blurring of Trabecular Pattern

osteomyelitis
decalcification caused by inflamed
    adjacent tissues
poor-quality radiography (e.g., motion
    unsharpness, bend distortion)

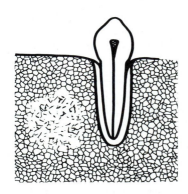

Diminished Number of Trabeculae

Common:
normal variant in children
inflammation
osteopenic metabolic diseases

Uncommon:
anaplastic anemias
postradiation changes
vitamin D deficiency syndromes
thalassemia
sickle cell anemia
neurofibroma

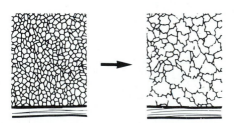

Decreased Size of Individual Trabeculae

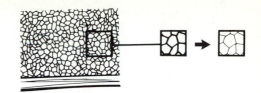

Common:
infection and inflammation
disuse atrophy of alveolus
normal variation

Uncommon:
postradiation change
vitamin D deficiency syndrome
thalassemia

Multilocular Radiolucency

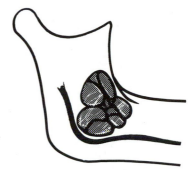

Common:
aberrant normal anatomic appearance
ameloblastoma
odontogenic keratocyst
central giant cell granuloma
cherubism
odontogenic myxoma
multilocular radicular or residual cyst

Uncommon:
mucoepidermoid tumor
aneurysmal bone cyst
central hemangioma
ameloblastic fibroma
arteriovenous malformation
calcifying odontogenic cyst
fibrous dysplasia
developing odontoma
histiocytosis X

Rare:
calcifying epithelial odontogenic tumor
central fibroma
central chondroma
sporotrichosis
cerebroside lipidosis (Gaucher disease)

Bilateral:
cherubism
cerebroside lipidosis (Gaucher disease)
odontogenic keratocyst–basal cell nevus syndrome (Gorlin-Goltz syndrome)

Ameloblastoma-like Radiolucency

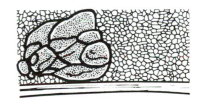

Common:
ameloblastoma
odontogenic keratocyst
giant cell granuloma
dentigerous cyst
multilocular large radicular or residual cyst

Uncommon:
ameloblastic fibroma
simple bone cyst
histiocytosis X
ossifying fibroma
fibrous dysplasia
calcifying odontogenic cyst
sporotrichosis
oxalosis

Lucency below Mandibular Canal

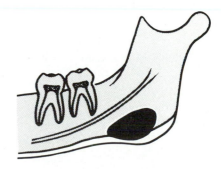

Common:
submandibular fossa
lingual salivary gland depression (Stafne defect)
variation of normal

Uncommon:
eosinophilic granuloma
benign tumor of salivary gland origin
subperiosteal neurofibroma
benign vascular tumor

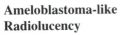

Expansile Jaw Lesions

Common:

laminar periosteal new bone

ameloblastoma
radicular or residual cyst
benign giant cell tumor
dentigerous cyst
fibrous dysplasia

Uncommon:
hemangioma
neurofibroma

osteosarcoma
lymphosarcoma
ossifying fibroma
aneurysmal bone cyst

Rare:
simple bone cyst
Burkitt lymphoma

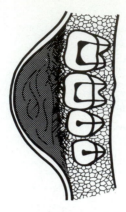

Lesions with Undulating or Crenated Margins

ameloblastoma
central giant cell granuloma
odontogenic myxoma
other benign odontogenic and nonod-
    ontogenic tumors
odontogenic keratocyst
botyroid lateral periodontal cyst

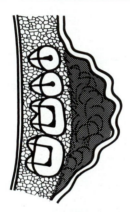

Lytic Lesions with Wide Bandlike Borders

Common:
infected cyst
lateral inflammatory odontogenic cyst
    of mandible

Rare:
osteoblastoma
osteoid osteoma

Uncommon:
fibrous dysplasia
benign giant cell tumor
aneurysmal bone cyst
ossifying fibroma

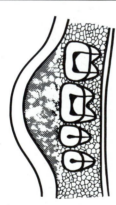

Widened Mandibular Canal

Common:
normal variant
neurilemmoma
neurofibroma
vascular tumor, hamartoma, or mal-
    formation

Uncommon:
malignant neoplasm entry into man-
    dibular canal
lymphoma

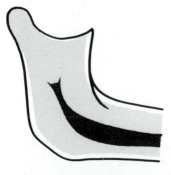

Scattered Bone Destruction Separated by Normal or Near-normal Bone

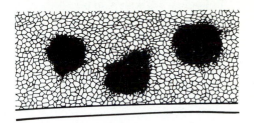

Common:
acute osteomyelitis
multiple myeloma
squamous cell carcinoma involving
  bone

Uncommon:
actinomycotic infections
osteoradionecrosis
metastatic carcinoma
oxalosis
tuberculous osteomyelitis

Short Linear Area of Radiolucency in Inferior Cortex

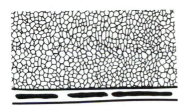

acute osteomyelitis
squamous cell carcinoma involving
  bone
other local malignant destruction
  (e.g., osteogenic sarcoma)

Cystlike Lucency with Windowlike Cortical Breaching

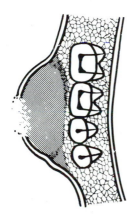

ameloblastoma
large radicular or residual cysts
odontogenic myxoma
central giant cell granuloma
neurofibroma

Thinned Inferior Mandibular Cortex

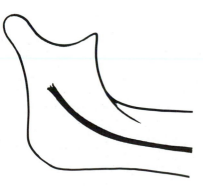

Common:
multiple myeloma
rheumatoid arthritis
diseases associated with generalized
  rarefaction

Uncommon:
histiocytosis X
hyperparathyroidism
thalassemia
sickle cell anemia

Rare:
hemifacial atrophy (Romberg disease)
osteogenesis imperfecta

Ballooned Inferior Cortex

Common:
osteomyelitis
ameloblastoma
dentigerous cyst
odontogenic myxoma
large radicular or residual cysts
fibrous dysplasia

Uncommon:
benign giant cell tumour
neurofibroma—blister lesion
hyperparathyroidism—blister lesion
hemangioma
calcifying odontogenic cyst
ameloblastic fibroma

Rare:
central true fibroma
Burkitt lymphoma
calcifying epithelial odontogenic tumor
osteogenic sarcoma
aneurysmal bone cyst

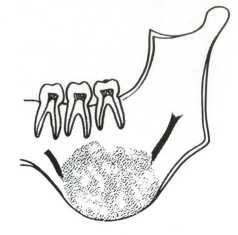

Attenuation of Shadow of Follicle Wall

Common:
localized infection of primary tooth
eruption cyst
acute osteomyelitis

hyperparathyroidism
Burkitt lymphoma

Uncommon:
vitamin D deficiency syndromes
histiocytosis X
leukemia
lymphosarcoma other than Burkitt
  lymphoma

Rare:
melanotic neuroectodermal tumor of
  infancy
rhabdomyosarcoma
neuroblastoma

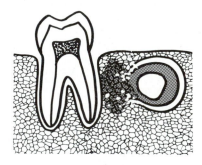

Discontinuity of Antral or Nasal Wall

Common:
localized periapical infection
fortuitous arrangement of shadows

invasive salivary gland malignancy
gross long-standing antritis
previous antral surgery

Uncommon:
osteomyelitis of the maxilla
odontogenic myxoma
ameloblastoma
invasive oral or antral squamous cell
  carcinoma

Rare:
osteogenic sarcoma
histiocytosis X
lymphosarcoma
true mucocele of antrum

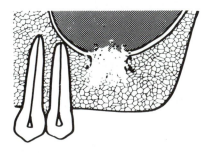

Suspected Daughter Cysts

Common:
odontogenic keratocyst
ameloblastoma

Uncommon:
central mucoepidermoid tumor
central hemangioma
botyroid lateral periodontal cyst

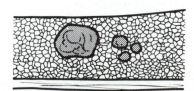

External Erosion of Bone

adjacent squamous cell carcinoma
systemic sclerosis (scleroderma)
result of polyvinylchloride poisoning
idiopathic
result of pulsatile vessel
Hodgkin disease
eosinophilic granuloma
malignant adjacent lymph node
carcinoma metastatic to mandible
local malignant tumor (e.g., osteosar-
    coma)
cystic hygroma

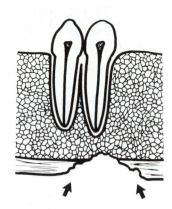

Lesion with No Internal Structure

Common:
odontogenic and nonodontogenic cysts
simple bone cyst

Uncommon:
ameloblastoma
odontogenic myxoma

hemangioma
neurofibroma
osteolytic osteogenic sarcoma
ameloblastic fibroma
early calcifying pathologic conditions
    (e.g., periapical cemental dysplasia,
    ossifying fibroma)

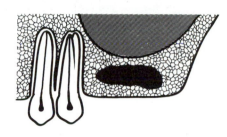

Multiple Separate Well-defined Lucencies

Common:
variations of normal
multiple periapical pathology of infec-
    tive origin
odontogenic keratocyst–basal cell ne-
    vus syndrome (Gorlin-Goltz syn-
    drome) early stages of periapical
    cemental dysplasia

Uncommon:
cherubism
multiple myeloma
metastatic carcinoma

histiocytosis X
lymphosarcoma
leukemia

Rare:
syndrome associated: Niemann-Pick
    disease or cerebroside lipidosis
    (Gaucher disease)
mucopolysaccharidoses
hyperparathyroidism

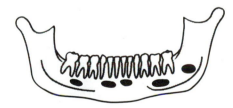

Multiple Osteolytic Lesions with Punched-out Margins

multiple myeloma
histiocytosis X
metastatic carcinoma
lymphosarcoma
hemangioma
Burkitt lymphoma

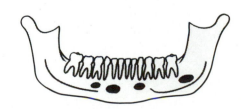

PRIMARY OPAQUE OR MIXED LUCENT/OPAQUE CONDITIONS

Periapical Mixed Lucent/Opaque

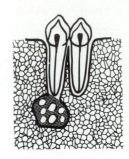

Common:
calcifying crown of developing tooth
tooth root with rarefying osteitis
rarefying and sclerosing osteitis
periapical cemental dysplasia
foreign body (e.g., cement)

Uncommon:
cementifying or ossifying fibroma
cementoblastoma
Paget disease
complex and compound odontoma
calcifying odontogenic cyst

Pericoronal Mixed Lucent/Opaque

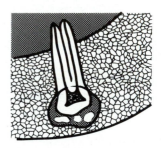

Common:
complex or compound odontomas
adenomatoid odontogenic tumor

Uncommon:
ameloblastic fibroodontoma
calcifying odontogenic cyst
odontogenic fibroma
cystic odontoma
calcifying epithelial odontogenic tumor

Periapical Opacities

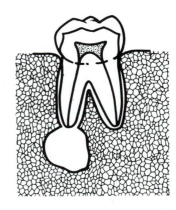

Common:
anatomic superimpositions
tori and/or exostoses
retained roots
film artifact
sclerosing osteitis
mature periapical cemental dysplasia
unerupted tooth
foreign bodies
hypercementosis

Uncommon:
superimposed soft tissue calcifications
cementoblastoma
osteoblastoma
cementifying fibroma
mature complex odontoma
osteoblastic metastases
Paget disease

Single, Mixed Lucent/Opaque, Not Necessarily Contacting Teeth

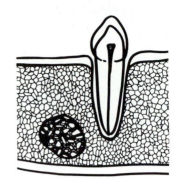

Common:

dense bone island
osseous excrescence
fibrous dysplasia and its variants
periapical cemental dysplasia
healing surgical defect
sclerosing osteitis
developing odontomas
cementifying and ossifying fibroma

ameloblastic fibroodontoma
complex and compound odontoma
calcifying odontogenic cyst
superimposed soft tissue calcification

Rare:

osteoblastoma and osteoid osteoma
carcinoma with superimposed infection
osteogenic sarcoma
chondrosarcoma
osteoblastic metastases

Uncommon:

chronic osteomyelitis
Paget disease

Increased Girth of Individual Trabeculae

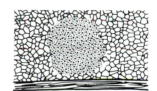

Common:

sclerosing osteitis (focal sclerosing osteomyelitis)
hemangioma
neurofibroma

Uncommon:

fluorosis
myelosclerosis
osteoblastic metastases

Granular Bone

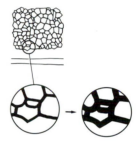

Common:

bone replacing former sequestrum
postsurgical defect
fibrous dysplasia
osteomyelitis
Paget disease

ossifying fibroma
osteogenic sarcoma
chondrosarcoma
Hodgkin disease
recovery phase of renal osteodystrophy

Uncommon:

thalassemia

Solitary Opacity Not Contacting Teeth

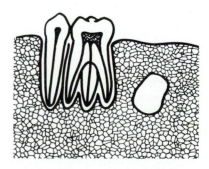

Common:

anatomic superimposition
artifact—fixer stain
dense bone island
tori and exostoses
unerupted teeth
retained roots
sclerosing osteitis
benign cemental masses
residual periapical cemental dysplasia

complex or compound odontoma
foreign body

Uncommon:

cementifying and ossifying fibroma
so-called osteoma
chondrosarcoma
osteoblastoma
overlying soft tissue calcification
osteogenic sarcoma

Compound Odontoma

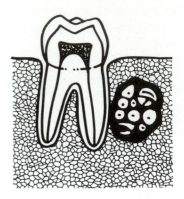

Common:
odontoma
supernumerary tooth
complex odontoma
ameloblastic fibroodontoma

Uncommon:
ameloblastic odontoma
distomus
teratoma
epignathus

Mixed Lucent/Opaque Lesion of Condylar Head

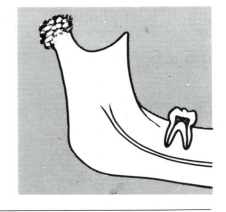

osteochondroma
osteomyelitis from middle ear
traumatic or other ankylosis of the
   temporomandibular joint
fibrous dysplasia
ossifying fibroma
osteoblastoma
osteogenic sarcoma
chondrosarcoma

Rare:
eosinophilic granuloma
Charcot joint

Sclerosing Osteitis (Focal Sclerosing Osteomyelitis)

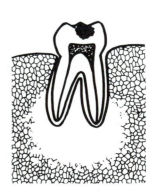

Common:
normal variation of trabecular pattern
superimposed normal structure
sclerosing osteomyelitis of inflammatory origin
periodontal disease
fibrous dysplasia
late stages of periapical cemental dysplasia
superimposed tori
Paget disease

Uncommon:
superimposed osteoma
idiopathic hypercalcemia
secondary hyperparathyroidism
superimposed submaxillary gland calculus

Rare:
osteopetrosis
melorheostosis
healing syphilitic gumma
metaphyseal dysplasia
infantile cortical hyperostosis
osteoid osteoma and osteoblastoma
osteogenic sarcoma
osteoblastic metastases
myelosclerosis
leukemia (rarely)
Hodgkin disease
sequela to radiation therapy

Complex Odontoma

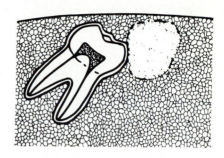

Common:
complex odontoma
periapical cemental dysplasia
ameloblastic fibroodontoma

Uncommon:
cementifying and ossifying fibroma
osteochondroma
osteogenic sarcoma
sclerosing osteitis
fibrous dysplasia
ameloblastic odontoma

Opacity Denser than Normal Bone

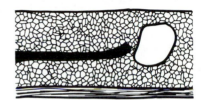

Common:
odontomas
periapical cemental dysplasia (late
    stages)
foreign body

osteogenic sarcoma
focal sclerosing osteomyelitis
oculodentoosseous dysplasia
Gardner syndrome (intestinal polypo-
    sis type II)

Uncommon:
osteopetrosis
fibrous dysplasia
cementifying and ossifying fibroma
osteoma

Multiple Separate Opacities

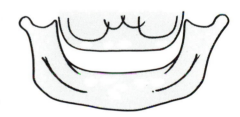

Common:
tori and exostoses
multiple retained roots
multiple socket sclerosis
periapical cemental dysplasia
multiple impacted teeth

osteosclerosis
calcinosis cutis
Gardner syndrome (intestinal polypo-
    sis type II)
enchondromatosis and hemangiomato-
    sis (Maffucci syndrome)
overlying soft tissue calcification

Uncommon:
gigantiform cementoma

Rootlike Density in Bone

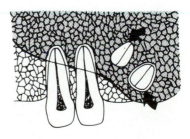

Common:
retained root
dense bone island
coronoid superimpositions
root in soft tissue
socket sclerosis
focal osteosclerosis

Uncommon:
antrolith superimposition
hamulus superimposition
antral bony spicule
submandibular duct calculus superim-
    posed
other soft tissue calcification
root or tooth pushed into fascial plane
superimposed osteochondroma

Suspected Foreign Body—Metallic

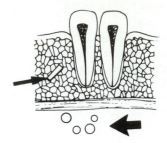

Common:
amalgam
other instruments and materials
artifactual—scratched cassette, fixer
   artifact

Uncommon:
needles
shotgun pellets
auto glass fragments
fragments of lead lining in x-ray cone
   (closed end cones only)

Suspected Foreign Body—Nonmetallic

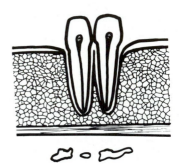

Common:
calcified acne
tooth root or crown fragment
sialolith
sclerosing osteitis
subclinical fibrous dysplasia
superimposed calcified lymph node

Uncommon:
cysticercosis
phleboliths
calcified lymph node
myositis ossificans
other soft tissue calcifications

Sequestra-like Density

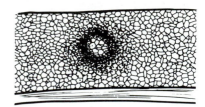

Common:
acute osteomyelitis
chronic osteomyelitis
osteoradionecrosis
other single large opacities
osteogenic sarcoma

Uncommon:
tuberculosis
actinomycosis
syphilis—large
mercury poisoning
phosphorus poisoning

Radiopacity with Peripheral Shadow—Target Lesion

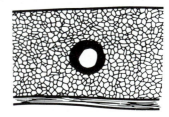

Common:
retained deciduous tooth root
infected residual permanent root tip
sequestra
periapical cemental dysplasia
odontomas

Uncommon:
cemeloblastoma
cementifying or ossifying fibroma
fibrous dysplasia

Rare:
Brodie abscess
osteoblastoma
osteoid osteoma

Excrescence with the Density of Bone

Common:
idiopathic bony excrescence(s)
osteochondroma
tori
ossifying fibrous epulis
soft tissue calcifications

Uncommon:
hyperostosis
fibrous dysplasia
Gardner syndrome (intestinal polyposis type II)
peripheral chondroma
chondrosarcoma

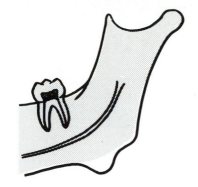

Thickened Inferior Cortex

secondary to preexisting osteomyelitis
phosphorus poisoning
fluorosis
sickle cell anemia
myelosclerosis
sclerosteosis
rare normal variant

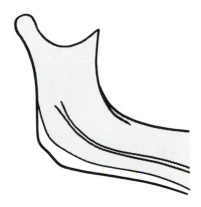

Laminar Periosteal New Bone

Common:
osteomyelitis
periostitis of the mandible of inflammatory origin

Uncommon:
infantile cortical hyperostosis
actinomycotic infection
tuberculosis of jaws
syphilitic lesions of jaws

eosinophilic granuloma
hypervitaminosis A
scurvy
leukemia—single layer
osteogenic sarcoma
Ewing sarcoma (rarely)
neostosis resulting from hemodialysis
idiopathic periostitis with dysproteinemia

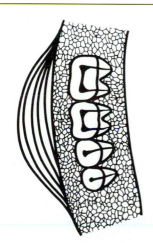

New Periosteal Bone with Internal Destruction

chronic osteomyelitis
tuberculous osteomyelitis
osteogenic sarcoma

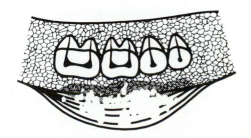

New Bone Perpendicular to Original Cortex

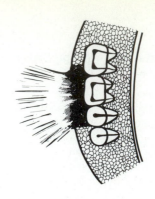

Common:

osteogenic sarcoma
osteoblastic metastases
chondrosarcoma
reticulum cell sarcoma
neuroblastoma

hemangioma
ossifying fibrous epulis
osteoma
sickle cell anemia
thalassemia
spherocytosis
Ewing sarcoma
Burkitt lymphoma

Uncommon:

syphilitic periostitis
meningioma

Lesions with Internal Spindly Trabeculae

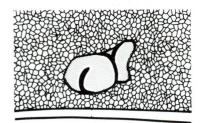

odontogenic myxoma
central giant cell granuloma
ameloblastoma
hemangioma
calcifying odontogenic cyst

Lesions with Septae or Pseudoseptae

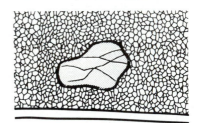

Common:

ameloblastoma
central giant cell granuloma
odontogenic myxoma
odontogenic keratocyst
simple bone cyst
cherubism

Uncommon:

central hemangioma
fibrous dysplasia
chondroma

Lesions with Honeycomb-like Internal Structure

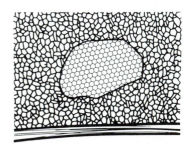

Common:

ameloblastoma
hemangioma
central giant cell granuloma
aneurysmal bone cyst
odontogenic myxoma
Ewing sarcoma

Uncommon:

neurofibroma
fibrous dysplasia
osteogenic sarcoma

Lesions with Wispy Internal Structure

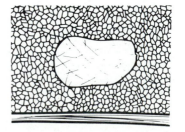

central giant cell granuloma
odontogenic myxoma
fibrous dysplasia
neurofibroma

Lesions with Internal Residual Bone

Common:
odontogenic myxoma
invasive squamous cell carcinoma
ameloblastoma
hemangioma

Uncommon:
fibrous dysplasia
ossifying fibroma
osteochondroma
Hodgkin disease
lymphoma

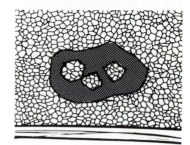

Lesions with Tubular Internal Structure

Common:
normal vascular channels
hemangioma or arteriovenous malformations

Uncommon:
central giant cell granuloma
ameloblastoma
neurofibroma

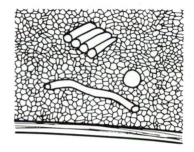

Lesions with Internal Rounded Dense Opacities

Common:
odontomas and their variants
periapical cemental dysplasia
fibrous dysplasia
cemental masses
Paget disease

Uncommon:
osteogenic sarcoma
chondrosarcoma

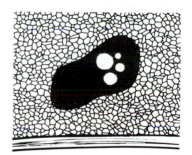

Linear Striations within Jaw Bone

Paget disease
normal variant in young mandible
bone replacing sequestrum
craniometaphyseal dysplasia (Pyle disease)

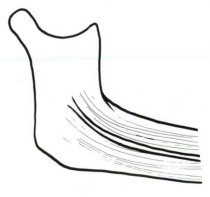

CRANIOFACIAL SIGNS

Small Skull

anencephaly
Cockayne syndrome
craniostenosis syndromes
cri du chat syndrome
de Lange syndrome
dysautonomia (Riley-Day syndrome)
focal dermal hypoplasia (Goltz syndrome)
hypospadias-dysphagia (G syndrome)
homocystinuria
idiopathic small brain
incontinentia pigmenti (Block-Sulzberger syndrome)
myotonic dystrophy
nanocephalic dwarfism (Seckel syndrome)
normal variant
pancytopenia-dysmelia (Fanconi syndrome)
phenylketonuria
prenatal irradiation or infection
Smith-Lemli-Opitz syndrome
trisomy 13 syndrome
trisomy 18 syndrome
trisomy 21
tuberous sclerosis (Bourneville-Pringle syndrome)

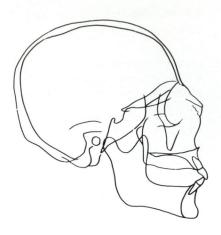

Large Skull

achondrogenesis
achondroplasia
cerebral gigantism (Soto syndrome)
cleidocranial dysplasia
congenital anemias
congenital hydrocephalus (Dandy-Walker syndrome)
craniometaphyseal dysplasia (Pyle disease)
craniostenosis
diaphyseal dysplasia (Engelmann disease)
familial macroencephaly
hydrocephalus
intracranial tumor
Beckwith-Wiedemann syndrome
mucopolysaccharidoses
pituitary dwarfism
osteogenesis imperfecta
Russell-Silver syndrome
subdural hematoma

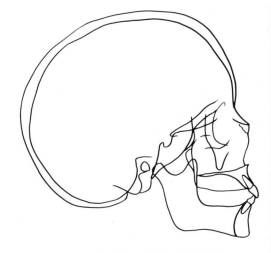

Frontal Bossing

achondroplasia
anemia
cleidocranial dysplasia
healed rickets
odontogenic keratocyst—basal cell nevus syndrome (Gorlin-Goltz syndrome)
mucopolysaccharidoses
oculomandibulodyscephaly (Hallermann-Streiff syndrome)
congenital syphilis
orofaciodigital syndrome
osteopetrosis
otopalatodigital syndrome
Rubinstein-Taybi syndrome

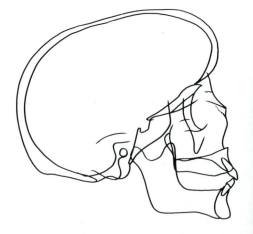

Craniostenosis

abnormal postsurgical sequelae
acrocephalopolysyndactyly (Carpenter syndrome)
acrocephalosyndactyly type I
craniofacial dysostosis (Crouzon disease)
craniometaphyseal dysplasia (Pyle disease)
diaphyseal dysplasia (Engelmann disease)
hyperthyroidism

hypervitaminoses D
hypophosphatasia
idiopathic
idiopathic hypercalcemia
idiopathic microcephaly
mandibulofacial dysostosis (Treacher Collins syndrome)
mucopolysaccharidoses
Rubinstein-Taybi syndrome
van Buchem syndrome
trisomy 21

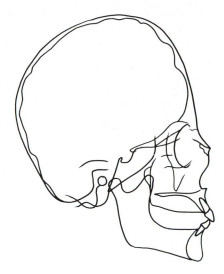

Basilar Invagination

achondroplasia
ankylosing spondylitis
cleidocranial dysplasia
Klippel-Feil syndrome
osteogenesis imperfecta
osteomalacia
Paget disease of bone
rickets
histiocytosis X

mucopolysaccharidoses
osteopetrosis
osteoporosis
pyknodysostosis
rheumatoid arthritis
syphilis
trauma
tuberculosis

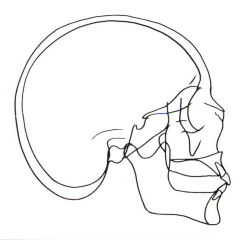

Hypoplasia of Skull Base

achondroplasia
chondroectodermal dysplasia

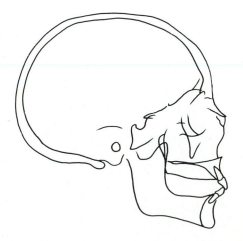

Generalized Increased Calvarial Density

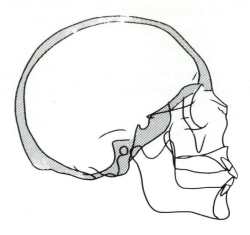

acromegaly
anemias
    sickle cell anemia
    thalassemia
    congenital spherocytosis or ellipto-
    cytosis
childhood cerebral atrophy
congenital cyanotic heart disease
chronic increased intracranial pressure
cranial hemiatrophy
craniometaphyseal dysplasia (Pyle disease)
craniostenosis
diaphyseal dysplasia (Engelmann disease)
dilantin medication
myotonic dystrophy
fibrous dysplasia
hyperostosis frontalis interna
hyperparathyroidism
hyperphosphatasia
hypervitaminoses D
hypoparathyroidism or pseudo-hypoparathyroidism
idiopathic
idiopathic hypercalcemia
melorrheostosis
meningioma
microcephaly
mucopolysaccharidoses
myelosclerosis
osteoblastic metastases
osteogenesis imperfecta
osteopetrosis
otopalatodigital syndrome
Paget disease of bone
sclerosteosis
secondary polycythemia
syphilitic osteitis
treated hydrocephalus
treated rickets
tuberous sclerosis (Bourneville-Pringle syndrome)
van Buchem syndrome

Localized Increase in Calvarial Density

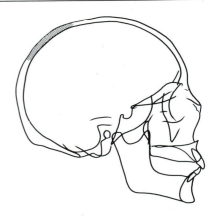

calcifying epithelioma of Malherbe
fibrous dysplasia
hyperostosis frontalis interna
late sequela to electrical burn
normal variant—dense bone island
osteoblastic metastases
superimposed soft tissue calcification
overlying carcinoma of scalp

Generalized Increased Opacification of Skull Base

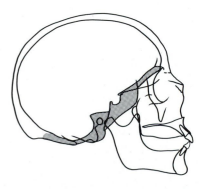

craniometaphyseal dysplasia (Pyle disease)
diaphyseal dysplasia (Engelmann disease)
fibrous dysplasia
fluorosis
healed vitamin D–resistant rickets
treated hyperparathyroidism
hypervitaminoses D
idiopathic hypercalcemia
juvenile hyperthyroidism (cretinism)
melorrheostosis
meningioma
neurofibromatosis
osteodysplasia
osteopetrosis
Paget disease
severe anemia

Localized Increased Opacification of Skull Base

acromegaly

chondrosarcoma

chordoma with calcification

chronic periostitis

fibrous dysplasia

lymphoma

mastoiditis

meningioma

nasopharyngeal carcinoma

osteoblastic metastases

osteochondroma

osteogenic sarcoma

sclerosteosis

sphenoid sinusitis

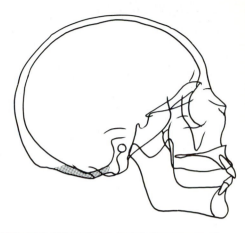

Generalized Thinning of Calvaria

chronic subdural hematoma

congenital arachnoid cyst

leptomeningeal cyst

localized temporal lobe hydrocephalus

neurofibromatosis

normal variant—parietal thinning

porencephalic cyst

slow-growing intracranial tumor

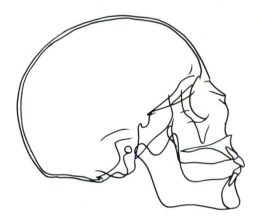

Localized Thinning of Calvaria

cleidocranial dysplasia

craniolacunia

hydrocephalus

hypophosphatasia

osteogenesis imperfecta

progeria (Hutchinson-Gilford syndrome)

vitamin D deficiency syndromes

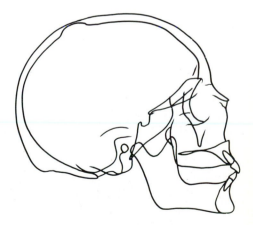

Granular Bone in Skull

congenital anemias (sickle cell, thalassemia, etc)
electrical burn
hyperparathyroidism—primary or secondary
leukemia
long-term steroid therapy
metastatic carcinoma
metastatic neuroblastoma

multiple myeloma
osteomalacia
osteomyelitis
osteoporosis
Paget disease
primary neoplasm of skull or meninges
radiation necrosis
syphilis

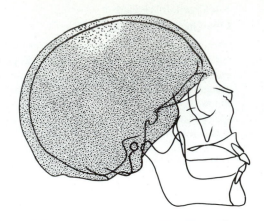

Erosion of Inner Diploë

arteriovenous malformation
chronic subdural hematoma
cisterna magna anomaly
eosinophilic granuloma
epidermoid cyst
glioma
hemangioma of skull

meningioma
metastasis
neoplasm of dura
pacchionian granulation
porencephaly
sinus pericranii

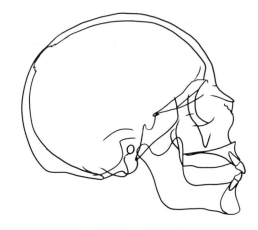

Radiolucent Defect in Skull of Child

arteriovenous malformation
central hemangioma
epidermoid cyst
fibrous dysplasia
hemophilic pseudotumor
soft tissue hemangioma
histiocytosis X

neurofibromatosis (blister lesion)
normal fontanelle
normal variant—venous lake
osteomyelitis
metastatic neuroblastoma
osteogenic sarcoma
surgical burr hole

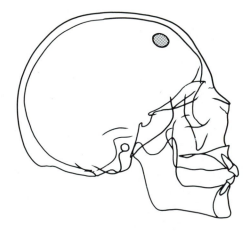

Multiple Calvarial Radiolucent Defects

cerebroside lipidosis (Gaucher disease)
craniolacunia
histiocytosis X
hyperparathyroidism
leukemia
lipid histiocytosis (Niemann-Pick disease)
lymphoma
metastatic malignancy
multiple myeloma
pacchionian granulations
postradiotherapy necrosis
osteomyelitis
normal variant—parietal foramina
sarcoidosis
surgical burr hole
syphilis
tuberculosis

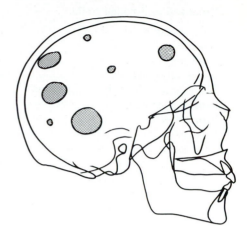

So-called Button Sequestra

eosinophilic granuloma
hemangioma
metastatic carcinoma
osteomyelitis
radiation necrosis
surgical burr hole
syphilis
tuberculosis

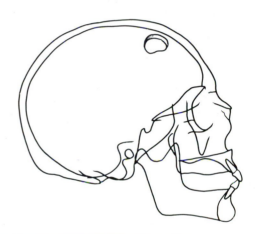

Solitary Radiolucent Calvarial Lesion

arachnoid cyst
arteriovenous malformation
benign tumor of scalp
carcinoma of scalp
cholesteatoma
dermal sinus
fibrous dysplasia
fracture
hemangioma
histiocytosis X
hyperparathyroidism
idiopathic
lymphoma
meningocele
metastasis
multiple myeloma
neurofibromatosis
normal variant—venous lake
osteogenic sarcoma
osteomyelitis
postsurgical defect
sarcoidosis
syphilis
tuberculosis

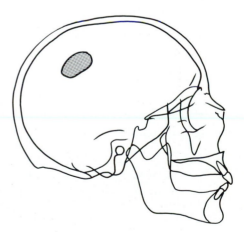

Enlarged or Eroded Sella

benign tumor of base of skull
chordoma
craniopharyngioma
empty sella syndrome
enlargement of internal carotid artery
hyperparathyroidism
hypogonadism
increased intracranial pressure
juvenile intracranial pressure
juvenile hypothyroidism (cretinism)
juxtasellar or suprasellar tumors
Hurler syndrome (mucopolysacchari-
    dosis IH)
metastatic malignancy
nasopharyngeal or sphenoid sinus
    neoplasm
optic sheath tumor
osteomyelitis
pituitary tumor
postsurgical sequelae
Rathke pouch cyst
tumor of frontal lobe of brain

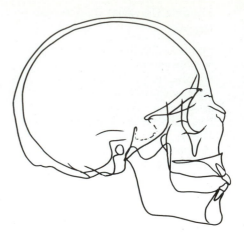

Small Sella

Cushing syndrome
genetic dwarfism
hypopituitarism juvenile hypothyroid-
    ism (cretinism)
myotonic dystrophy
normal variant
postpartum pituitary necrosis (Sheehan
    syndrome)
Prader-Willi syndrome
previous radiotherapy (during child-
    hood)
trisomy 21

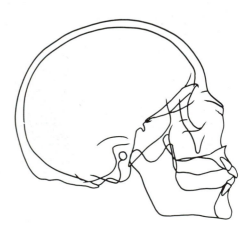

J-shaped Sella

Hurler syndrome (mucopolysacchari-
    dosis IH)
hydrocephalus
juvenile hypothyroidism (cretinism)
neurofibroma
normal variant
pituitary tumor
suprasellar tumor

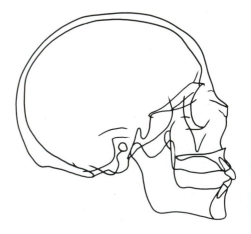

Multiple Calvarial Wormian Bones

cleidocranial dysplasia
hypophosphatasia
juvenile hyperthyroidism (cretinism)
normal variant
oculomandibulodyscephaly
    (Hallermann-Streiff syndrome)
osteogenesis imperfecta
otopalatodigital syndrome

pachydermoperiostitis
Prader-Willi syndrome
progeria (Hutchinson-Gilford syndrome)
pyknodysostosis
trisomy 21
vitamin D deficiency syndromes

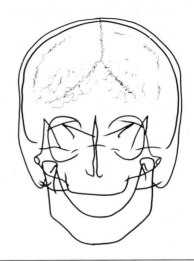

Presence of Fontanelle Shadows

cerebrohepatorenal syndrome
cleidocranial dysplasia
cutis laxa
dysplasia epiphysealis punctata (Conradi disease)
hypophosphatasia
intracranial tumors
juvenile hyperthyroidism (cretinism)
oculomandibulodyscephaly
    (Hallermann-Streiff syndrome)
osteodysplasia
osteogenesis imperfecta

otopalatodigital syndrome
pachydermoperiostosis
pediatric rubella infection
progeria (Hutchinson-Gilford syndrome)
pyknodysostosis
Rubinstein-Taybi syndrome
Russell-Silver syndrome
trisomy 13 syndrome
trisomy 18 syndrome
trisomy 21

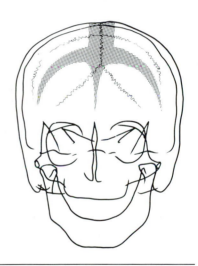

Defective Cranial Ossification

cleidocranial dysplasia
histiocytosis X (Letterer-Siwe variant)
hydrocephalus
hypophosphatasia
juvenile hyperthyroidism (cretinism)
neurofibromatosis
osteogenesis imperfecta

pachydermoperiostosis
prematurity
progeria (Hutchinson-Gilford syndrome)
pyknodysostosis
renal osteodystrophy
vitamin D deficiency syndromes

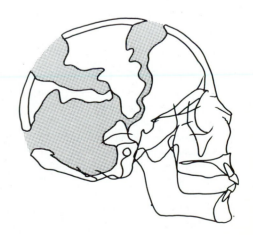

Hair on End Calvarial Density

congenital anemias
    hereditary spherocytosis or ellipto-
    cytosis
    thalassemia
    sickle cell anemia
congenital heart disease
Ewing sarcoma
hemangioma

iron deficiency anemia
meningioma
metastatic neuroblastoma
metastatic thyroid carcinoma
multiple myeloma
osteogenic sarcoma
polycythemia vera

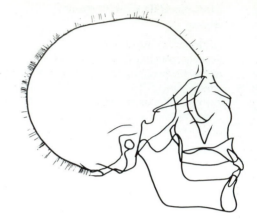

Solitary Intracranial Opacity

arachnoid granulation
arteriosclerosis
arteriovenous malformation
calcified cerebral infarct
calcified choroid plexus
calcified diaphragma sellae
calcified dura — falx, tentorium, sagit-
    tal sinus
calcified hematoma
calcified petroclinoid or interclinoid
    ligaments
chondrosarcoma of base of skull
chordoma
craniopharyngioma
cysticercosis
Sturge-Weber syndrome (encephalot-
    rigeminal angiomatosis)

ependyoma
epidermoid or dermoid cyst
foreign body
granuloma
healed brain abscess
hemangioma
idiopathic
meningioma
metastatic neoplasm
osteochondroma
pineal gland
pituitary adenoma
postradiotherapy necrosis
rubella
syphilitic gumma
tuberous sclerosis (Bourneville-Pringle
    syndrome)

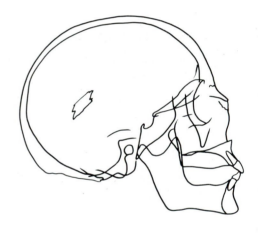

Multiple Intracranial Opacities

aneurysm
arteriosclerosis
basal ganglia calcifications
idiopathic
Sturge-Weber syndrome (encephalot-
    rigeminal angiomatosis)
healed brain abscess
carbon monoxide intoxication
Cockayne syndrome
cytomegalovirus inclusion disease
encephalitis
hematomas
hepatolenticular degeneration (Wilson
    disease)

hyperparathyroidism
hypervitaminoses D
lipoid proteinosis
metastatic malignancy
multiple tumors (e.g., meningioma)
neurofibromatosis
odontogenic keratocyst – vasal cell
    nevus syndrome (Gorlin-Goltz syn-
    drome)
parasitic disease
toxoplasmosis
tuberous sclerosis

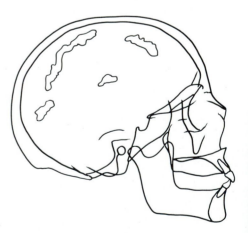

Basal Ganglia Calcification

birth anoxia
carbon monoxide poisoning
Cockayne syndrome
encephalitis
hemorrhage
hypoparathyroidism
idiopathic

lead intoxication
Parkinsonism
previous radiation therapy
pseudohypoparathyroidism
pseudopseudohypoparathyroidism
toxoplasmosis
tuberous sclerosis

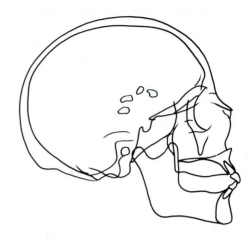

Hypertelorism

Apert syndrome (acrocephalosyndactyly type I)
anterior meningocele
central facial hypoplasia
cerebral gigantism (Soto syndrome)
cleidocranial dysplasia
craniofacial dysostosis (Crouzon disease)
craniostenosis
cri du chat syndrome
de Lange syndrome
dysplasia epiphysealis punctata (Conradi disease)
facial duplication
fibrous dysplasia
hypertelorism-hypospadias syndrome
idiopathic
Larsen syndrome

metaphyseal chondrodysplasia
metaphyseal dysplasia
midline dermoid or teratoma
Hurler syndrome (mucopolysaccharidosis IH)
odontogenic keratocyst—basal cell nevus syndrome (Gorlin-Goltz syndrome)
multiple pterygium (Bonnevie-Ulrich
syndrome)
Noonan syndrome
orofaciodigital syndrome
osteogenesis imperfecta
otopalatodigital syndrome
thalassemia
mandibulofacial dysostosis (Treacher
Collins syndrome)
Turner syndrome

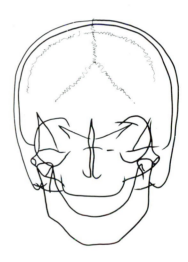

Destructive Orbital Lesion with Exophthalmos

chloroma
histiocytosis
lymphoma
metastatic neuroblastoma
metastatic carcinoma
primary carcinoma
Burkitt lymphoma

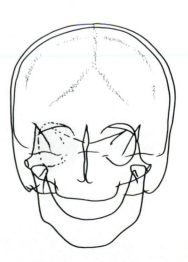

Enlargement of Superior Orbital Fissure

aneurysm of internal carotid artery
chordoma
craniopharyngioma
extension of orbital malignancy
histiocytosis X
meningioma
metastatic carcinoma to sphenoid bone

middle cranial fossa mass
neurofibroma
neurofibromatosis
normal variant
pituitary tumor
posterior orbital encephalocele

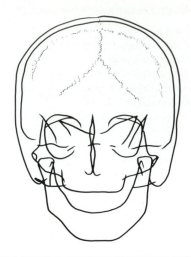

Hypotelorism

arhinencephalia
glycogen storage diseases
oculodentoosseous dysplasia
phenylketonuria
trigonocephaly
trisomy 13 syndrome
trisomy 21

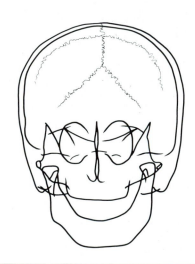

Unilateral Exophthalmos

craniostenosis
dermoid cyst
epidermoid cyst
fibrous dysplasia
fracture with retroorbital blood or air
hemangioma
hyperthyroidism
lacrimal gland tumor
meningioma
metastatic disease
mucocele

mucormycosis
neurofibromatosis
orbital meningocele
ossifying fibroma
osteoma of paranasal sinus
osteomyelitis
Paget disease
primary orbital soft tissue disease
pseudotumor of orbit
retroorbital abscess or cellulitis
sinusitis

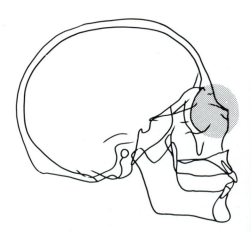

Prognathism

Common:
normal variation
edentulous mandible
relative prognathism (e.g., retrog-
    nathic midface secondary to cleft)
acromegaly

Uncommon:
Paget disease
pituitary gigantism
congenital or acquired hemifacial hy-
    perplasia

lymphangioma of tongue (cystic hy-
    groma)

Rare:
odontogenic keratocyst–basal cell ne-
    vus syndrome (Gorlin-Goltz syn-
    drome)
craniometaphyseal dysplasia (Pyle dis-
    ease)
Beckwith-Wiedemann syndrome
XXXXY syndrome
Waardenburg syndrome

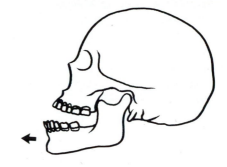

Retrognathism

Common:
normal variant
relative retrognathism (protrusion of
    midface)
ankylosis of temporomandibular
    joint(s)
juvenile rheumatoid arthritis

Uncommon:
micrognathia
hemifacial hypoplasia
subluxation of infant jaw
hypopituitarism
progressive hemiatrophy
agenesis or dysgenesis of mandible
agnathia

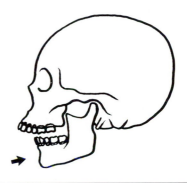

Micrognathia

Common:
mandibulofacial dysostosis (Treacher
    Collins syndrome)
gonadal dysgenesis (Turner syndrome)
juvenile rheumatoid arthritis (Still dis-
    ease)
cleft lip, micrognathia, and glossopto-
    sis (Pierre Robin syndrome)

Uncommon:
oculoauricularvertebral dysplasia
    (Goldenhar syndrome)
XX and XY phenotypes of Turner
    syndrome (Noonan syndrome)
oculomandibulodyscephaly
    (Hallermann-Streiff syndrome)
pyknodysostosis

Rare:
bird-headed dwarfism
congenital telangiectatic erythema with
    growth retardation (Bloom syn-
    drome)
cri du chat syndrome

chondrodysplasia punctata (Conradi-
    Hünermann syndrome)
de Lange syndrome
diastrophic dwarfism
G syndrome
cleft palate, flattened facies and multi-
    ple congenital dislocations (Larsen
    syndrome)
long arm 21 deletion syndrome
mesomelic dwarfism
orofaciodigital syndrome
osteodysplasia
progeria (Hutchinson-Gilford syn-
    drome)
Rubinstein-Taybi syndrome
Russell-Silver syndrome
short arm deletion 18 syndrome
Smith-Lemli-Opitz syndrome
thrombocytopenia
trisomy 13 syndrome
trisomy 18 syndrome

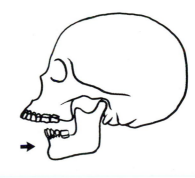

Prominent Areas of Muscle Attachment—Any Bone

acromegaly
normal variant
ankylosis
pseudoankylosis
masseteric hypertrophy

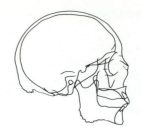

TEMPOROMANDIBULAR JOINT SIGNS

Unilateral Small Jaw

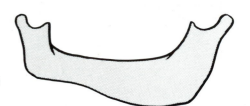

Common:

lateral facial dysplasia
unilateral temporomandibular joint
  ankylosis
forceps delivery trauma
early radiotherapy

Uncommon:
hemifacial hypoplasia

hemifacial atrophy (Romberg disease)
partial mandibular agenesis
linear scleroderma

Rare:
neurofibroma
hemangioma

Enlargement of Part of Jaw (Anatomically Correct)

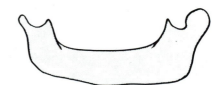

adjacent hemangioma
adjacent neurofibroma
fibrous dysplasia

hemifacial hyperplasia
Paget disease

Obtuse Gonial Angle

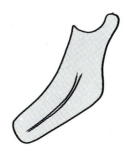

Common:
normal age change
edentulous mandible
condylar hyperplasia (contralateral
  condyle)
trisomy 21
systemic sclerosis (scleroderma)

Uncommon:
Hurler syndrome (mucopolysaccharidosis IH)
craniometaphyseal dysplasia (Pyle disease)
osteopetrosis
hemifacial hypoplasia

Aberrant Gonial Angle

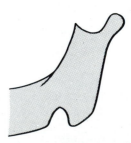

Common:
variation of normal
ankylosis of temporomandibular joint
juvenile rheumatoid arthritis
mandibulofacial dysostosis (Treacher
  Collins syndrome)
systemic sclerosis (scleroderma)
neurofibroma
trisomy 21

Uncommon:
Marfan syndrome
odontogenic keratocyst–basal cell
  nevus syndrome (Gorlin-Goltz
  syndrome)
isolated anomaly

Persistent Mandibular Midline Suture

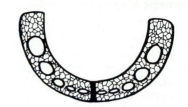

Common:
normal at less than 6 months of age
cleidocranial dysplasia
midline fracture

Uncommon:
normal variant
mandibular midline cleft

Absent or Diminished Coronoids

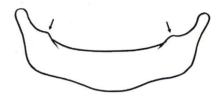

Common:
poor-quality panoramic radiograph
lateral facial dysplasia
previous surgery
systemic sclerosis (scleroderma)
radiotherapy in childhood

Uncommon:
hemifacial atrophy
erosion caused by local or metastatic
  malignancy
agnathia or agenesis

Unilateral Failure of Condyle to Develop

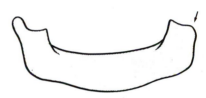

Common:
early trauma, including forceps delivery
childhood infection in temporomandibular joint region (mastoiditis, otitis media and externa, dental, or skin infection)
lateral facial dysplasia
childhood radiotherapy

Uncommon:
hemifacial hypoplasia
linear scleroderma
benign tumor
local malignant tumor destruction of
  growth center
metastatic malignancy

Bilateral Failure of Condyle to Develop

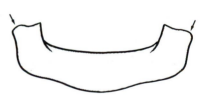

Common:
trauma
juvenile rheumatoid arthritis (Still disease)
mandibulofacial dysostosis (Treacher Collins syndrome)
cleft palate, micrognathia, and glossoptosis (Pierre Robin syndrome)

Uncommon:
oculomandibulodyscephaly
  (Hallermann-Streiff syndrome)
congenital dwarfisms
mucopolysaccharidoses
childhood radiotherapy
progeria (Hutchinson-Gilford syndrome)
agnathia or micrognathia
Cockayne syndrome

Condylar Hyperplasia

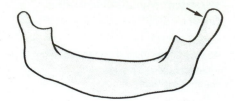

Common:
true condylar hyperplasia
benign tumor (e.g., osteochondroma)
influence of adjacent benign vascular
   or neural tumors
acromegaly
prognathism

Uncommon:
hypertrophic arthritis
malignant tumor (e.g., chondrosarcoma)
fibrous dysplasia
Paget disease

Pathologic Fractures

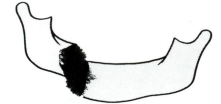

Common:
oral squamous cell carcinoma
central bone malignancy (e.g., multiple myeloma)
metastatic carcinoma
osteoradionecrosis

Uncommon:
severe osteomyelitis
marked alveolar atrophy
systemic sclerosis (scleroderma)
histiocytosis X

Multiple Fractures

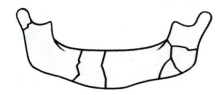

Common:
severe trauma
child abuse
osteogenesis imperfecta

Uncommon:
juvenile idiopathic osteoporosis
achondrogenesis

osteopetrosis
pyknodysostosis
mucolipidoses
metaphyseal dysplasia
homocystinuria
multiple idiopathic fractures

Increased Temporomandibular Joint Space

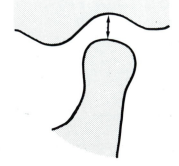

Common:
nonuniform patient positioning
projection effect from beam angulation
preferential positioning of jaw by patient
normal variant
displaced articular disk

Uncommon:
effusion into joint
hemorrhage into joint
loose body in joint
acute suppurative arthritis
displaced condyle or fossa from fracture
mandibular partial agenesis
mucopolysaccharidoses

Increased Anterior Temporomandibular Joint Space

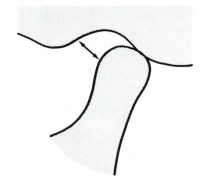

normal variant
artifact (beam angulation, patient position)
internal derangement in temporomandibular joint

backward placement of joint resulting from occlusion
deep overbite
overclosure of mandible
absent middle ear
rheumatoid arthritis

Decreased Temporomandibular Joint Space

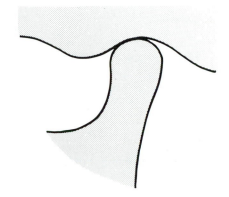

Common:
excess vertical angulation of beam in transcranial view
arthritis of any kind
gross disk displacement

Uncommon:
previous surgical removal of disk
bony or other true ankylosis

Limited Temporomandibular Joint Movement

Common:
normal variant
pain reaction
internal derangements of joint
true and false ankylosis

Uncommon:
scar tissue on face or in mouth
systemic sclerosis (scleroderma)

fractured zygomatic arch
coronoid hyperplasia
malignancy in region of joint
facial paralysis
torticollis
myositis ossificans progressiva
submucous fibrosis
caused by high-dose radiation therapy

Unusually Great Anterior Temporomandibular Movement

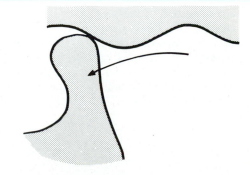

Common:
variation of normal
lax temporomandibular joint capsule

Uncommon:
recurrent dislocation
Ehlers-Danlos syndromes

True Temporomandibular Joint Ankylosis

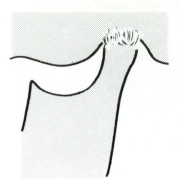

Common:

infection
    osteomyelitis
    tonsillitis
    otitis media or externa
    mastoiditis
    adjacent soft tissue infections
    dental infections
    tuberculosis

traumatic
    mandibular fracture
    forceps delivers

other
    Still disease (juvenile rheumatoid
      arthritis)
    rheumatoid arthritis
    ankylosing spondylitis

Uncommon:

infection
    typhoid
    masseter cellulitis
    rheumatic fever
    measles
    cancrum oris

traumatic
iatrogenic
    temporal muscle fibrosis
    chronic dislocation of mandible
neoplasia
    invasive malignancy
    osteochondroma

other
    result of thermal burn
    congenital fusion of gums
    congenital

False Temporomandibular Ankylosis

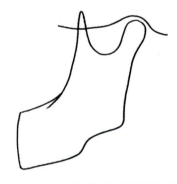

Common:

splinting from pain in temporomandib-
    ular joint
fibrous or bony union following malar
    fracture
coronoid hyperplasia
coronoid hyperplasia with
    pseudocampylodactyly
osteochondroma of coronoid process

Uncommon:

systemic sclerosis (scleroderma)
hysterical trismus
temporal muscle fibrosis
myositis ossificans progressiva
torticollis
congenital elevation of the scapula

Radiolucent Lesion of Condylar Head

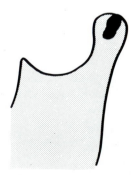

"Cyst" of degenerative joint disease
rheumatoid arthritis and its variants
projection effect of pterygoid pit
other normal variants of projection
superimposition of bifid condyle
superimposed air cell in zygomatic
    arch
old trauma to condylar head
villonodular synovitis

primary malignancies
osteosarcoma
lymphoma
synovial sarcoma
adjacent glandular carcinomas
rhabdomyosarcoma
secondary malignancies
    hypernephroma
    carcinoma of bowel or rectum
    multiple myeloma
central giant cell granuloma

MAXILLARY AND MAXILLARY SINUS SIGNS

Small Antrum (Normal in Shape)

Common:

normal variant
warm climate
related to fibrous dysplasia
following Caldwell-Luc procedure
nondevelopment

craniofacial dysostosis (Crouzon disease)
other congenital craniostenosis
thalassemia and other congenital anemias
hemifacial atrophy (Romberg disease)
oculomandibulodyscephaly (Hallermann-Streiff syndrome)
odontogenic keratocyst–basal cell nevus syndrome (Gorlin-Goltz syndrome)

Uncommon:

congenital hemifacial hypoplasia
craniometaphyseal dysplasia (Pyle disease)
cleidocranial dysplasia

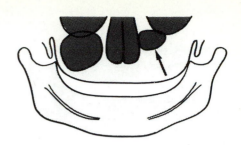

Suspected Antral Foreign Bodies

Common:

tooth roots in antrum
superimposed tooth roots
radiopaque dressings
antral stalagmite–like bony excrescence
overlying soft tissue calcification

Uncommon:

whole teeth
broken instruments
cements
drainage tubes
pellets, bullets, shrapnel, automobile glass
impression material
heavy cosmetics
aspergillosis

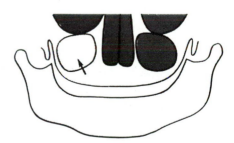

Antral Opacification with Normal Bony Walls

Common:

infectious antritis
allergic antritis
mucus retention phenomenon
gross mucositis caused by adjacent periapical disease
gross mucositis caused by adjacent periodontitis
traumatic hemorrhage into antrum

Uncommon:

polyp in antrum
blocked ostia
polyposis of antral lining
cystic fibrosis
dental cyst (rare appearance)
true mucocele (blocked ostia with antral enlargement)
aspergillosis

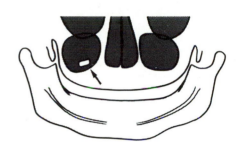

Antral Opacification with Abnormal Bony Walls

Common:

radicular cysts
other odontogenic cysts
fibrous dysplasia (thicker)
hypoplasia of antrum (thicker)
malignancy of antrum (carcinoma or lymphoma)

odontogenic myxoma
inverted papilloma

Uncommon:

osteomyelitis
thalassemia
agenesis of antrum
mucormycosis

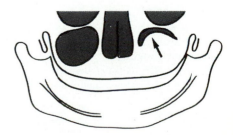

Antral Opacification with Breached Cortical Walls

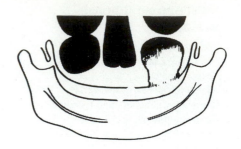

Common:

oral-antral fistula
malignancy
carcinoma of antrum
lymphoma
salivary gland carcinoma
oral squamous cell carcinoma
sarcoma
infected dental cyst
   radicular

residual
   other
odontogenic myxoma

Uncommon:

infectious antritis
infected antrolith
ameloblastoma of maxilla
true mucocele

Enlarged Maxilla

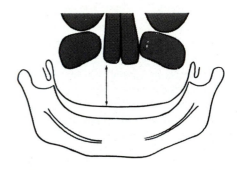

Common:

normal variant
relative to mandible—see retrognathism
influence of adjacent or contiguous
   vascular tumour
Paget disease
osteopetrosis
fibrous dysplasia

Uncommon:

juvenile hypothyroidism (cretinism)
thalassemia
influence of adjacent or contiguous
   neural tumor
craniopharyngioma

SOFT TISSUE SIGNS

Calcifications in Soft Tissues of Face

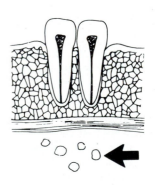

Common:

calcified acne
calcified lymph node (usually after
   tuberculosis)
phleboliths
calcified hematoma
calcified fat
noncalcification (e.g., tooth root in
   soft tissue)

Uncommon:

myositis ossificans (traumatic)
myositis ossificans progressiva
Ehlers-Danlos syndromes
systemic sclerosis (scleroderma)
calcinosis universalis
cysticercosis
hypervitaminoses D

Widespread Calcifications in Soft Tissue

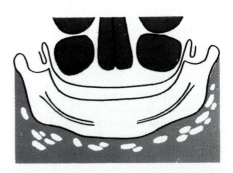

Common:

calcinosis universalis
hypoparathyroidism
systemic sclerosis (scleroderma)
vascular calcifications (multiple)

hyperparathyroidism
immobilization
lupus erythematosus
cysticercosis
tumoral calcinosis
idiopathic hypercalcemia
gross metabolic bone breakdown

Uncommon:

gout

Calcifications in Muscles and Subcutaneous Tissues

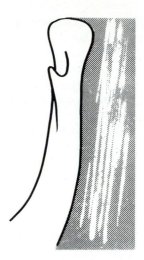

Common:

dermatomyositis and calcinosis
gout
systemic sclerosis (scleroderma)
vascular calcifications
rheumatoid arthritis
healing abscess

Ehlers-Danlos syndromes
idiopathic hypercalciuria
myositis ossificans (progressiva and
    traumatic)
paraplegia

Uncommon:

hyperparathyroidism
hypoparathyroidism
odontogenic keratocyst–basal cell ne-
    vus syndrome (Gorlin-Goltz syn-
    drome)

calcified parasites
carbon monoxide poisoning
fracture segment
tumoral calcinosis
caused by thermal burn or frostbite
benign or malignant soft tissue neo-
    plasm
lupus erythematosus

Vascular Calcification

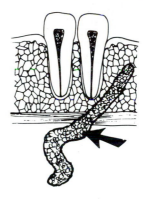

Common:

soft tissue hemangioma
phleboliths of arteriovenous malforma-
    tions
arteriosclerosis of familial type

Rare:

Mönckeberg sclerosis
enchondromatosis-hemangiomata syn-
    drome (Maffucci syndrome)
aneurysm
progeria (Hutchinson-Gilford syn-
    drome)
lipodystrophy

Uncommon:

secondary arteriosclerosis:
    diabetes
    Cushing syndrome
    nephrotic syndrome

renal homotransplantation
Werner syndrome
generalized calcification of infancy

Solitary Large Calcified Mass Adjacent to Bone

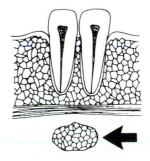

Common:

calcified fat
calcified hematoma

gout
hyperparathyroidism
soft tissue osteosarcoma or chondro-
    sarcoma

Uncommon:

systemic sclerosis (scleroderma)
osteochondroma

tumoral calcinosis
myositis ossificans
foreign body

Calcification in Lymph Nodes of Face

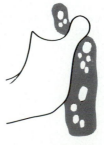

Common:

previous tuberculosis (asymptomatic
    or symptomatic)
idiopathic

previous bacille Calmette-Guérin vac-
    cination
coccidioidomycosis
filariasis
lymphoma
osteoblastic metastases

Uncommon:

histoplasmosis

Calcification in Region of Submandibular Gland

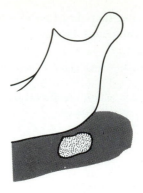

Common:
calcification in duct of gland
calcification in gland
root of a tooth superimposed in soft tissue
calcified lymph node
foreign body

phlebolith
calcinosis universalis
systemic sclerosis (scleroderma)

Rare:
chondrodystrophia calcificans congenita
myositis ossificans

Uncommon:
film artifact

Calcification in Region of Parotid Gland

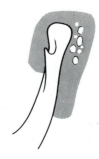

Common:
artifact
sialolith
phlebolith
foreign body

Uncommon:
calcinosis universalis
other soft tissue calcifications

Sialolith

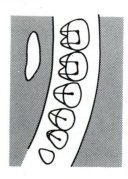

Common:
true sialolith
film artifact
superimposed root in soft tissue
superimposed root in bone
superimposed bone sclerosis
superimposed dense bone island
superimposed torus mandibularis

Uncommon:
calcified lymph node
calcifications in lymph follicles of tongue
foreign body

Soft Tissue Mass with Underlying Bone Erosion

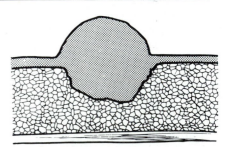

Common:
oral squamous cell carcinoma
nasolabial cyst
pregnancy tumor or pyogenic granuloma
inflammatory gingival epulides
neurofibromatosis (blister lesion)
salivary gland malignancy
metastatic malignancy growing from extraction site

denture-induced soft tissue hyperplasias
Kaposi sarcoma

Uncommon:
lymphoma in soft tissue
malignant lymph node
amyloidosis
angioma
fungal diseases
hemophilia
sarcoma of soft tissue

3

DEVELOPMENTAL DENTAL ABNORMALITIES

_____

HYPODONTIA

Overview

Definition: Hypodontia is defined as the presence of less than the normal complement of teeth. Although missing teeth can be either congenitally missing or lost through disease or extraction, hypodontia traditionally means the former. The term *anodontia* means congenital absence of all teeth. Sometimes the term *partial anodontia* is used as a synonym for hypodontia. *Pseudohypodontia* may be used to describe loss of teeth to disease or extraction.

Pathogenesis: A reduction in the normal number of teeth may result from hereditary failure of tooth development, destruction of tooth follicles, or early loss of mature teeth. Failure of teeth to develop usually affects only small portions of the dentition in a sporadic way that is not related to a more general syndrome. Less commonly, hereditary lack of tooth development is also seen in trisomy 21, the ectodermal dysplasias, chondroectodermal dysplasia, incontinentia pigmenti, congenital unilateral facial hypoplasia, orofaciodigital syndrome type II, oculodentoosseous dysplasia, oculomandibulodyscephaly, oligodontia and primary mesodermal iris dysgenesis, Böök syndrome, craniofacial dysostosis, Ehlers-Danlos syndrome, focal dermal hypoplasia, pyknodysostosis, progeria, hypoparathyroidism, Russell-Silver syndrome, inverted Marfan syndrome, monosuperocentroincisivodontic dwarfism, or as an isolated occurrence.

Destruction of developing tooth follicles occurs by one of four main processes: infection, adjacent malignancy, antitumor chemotherapy, or radiation therapy in which the jaws are within the radiation field.

Clinical Features

Demographics: Isolated missing permanent teeth are a common occurrence, with third molars being most frequently involved. The incidence of missing third molars ranges from 9% to 37%, whereas the frequency of other missing teeth ranges from 3.5% to 6.5%. The pattern of tooth absence depends on the patient's race but the most commonly missing teeth other than third molars are the maxillary lateral incisors, mandibular second bicuspids, and mandibular lateral incisors. The primary dentition may be normal with abnormal permanent dentition, or both dentitions may be defective. An abnormal deciduous dentition is rarely followed by a normal permanent one.

Signs and symptoms: Patients with less than the normal number of teeth often exhibit spacing of the remaining teeth and diminished size of the alveolar processes of the jaws. Clinical examination fails to reveal the normal gingival bulges of the underlying tooth buds. In patients with isolated missing teeth, the alveolar process may appear thinned where the missing tooth would have been. Furthermore, patients with missing teeth may exhibit deep bite and are more likely to have an Angle class I molar relationship. If the condition is long-standing, as in congenital absence of teeth, the changes will be more remarkable. In patients with multiple missing teeth, such as is common in the ectodermal dysplasias, the existing teeth are often misshapen and reduced in size.

RADIOLOGIC FEATURES

Cardinal Signs

Missing teeth, not accounted for by extraction
Retention of primary teeth, which may or may not exhibit external resorption

Ancillary Signs

Reduction in the size of the remaining alveolar bone in both vertical and horizontal dimensions
Drifting of adjacent teeth within the alveolar processes

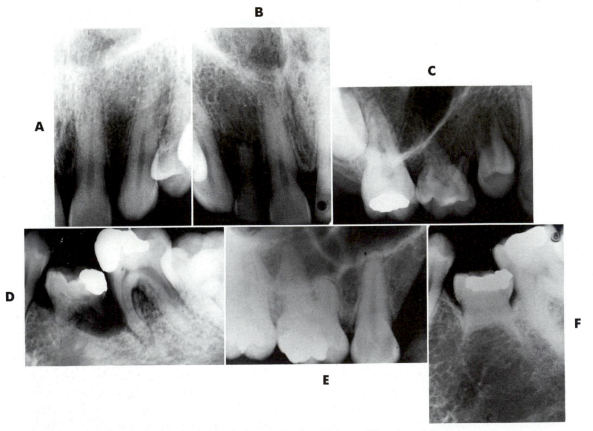

Fig. 3-1 A, Periapical radiograph illustrating hypodontia of left maxillary lateral incisor.
B, Hypodontia of right maxilary permanent lateral incisor. Retention of primary lateral incisor.
C, Hypodontia of right maxillary second premolar. Retention of primary second molar.
D, Hypodontia of left mandibular second premolar. Exfoliation of retained primary second molar in process. Note periodontal complications for first permanent molar. **E,** Missing maxillary first and second premolars allowing space for eruption of permanent canine and retention of primary canine. **F,** Missing mandibular second premolar with retained/ankylosed primary second molar.

Diminished density and number of trabeculae at the site of missing teeth

Misshapen crowns of remaining teeth

Diminished size of remaining teeth

General reduction in the size of the jaw

Differential Diagnosis

Pseudohypodontia through extraction

Ectodermal dysplasias

Childhood radiation therapy to jaws

SUPERNUMERARY TEETH (HYPERDONTIA)

Overview

Definition: All extra teeth may be termed *supernumerary,* although many authors taxonomically describe those resembling regular teeth in morphology as "supplemental." However, most supernumerary teeth are not of such shape as to be classed as supplemental.

Pathogenesis: The reason for the occurrence of excess teeth is obscure—it may be an atavistic phenomenon, although this has been questioned. Most supernumerary teeth are sporadic and idopathic. Occasionally, extra teeth are associated with syndromes such as cleidocranial dysostosis, osteomatosis-intestinal polyposis syndrome, oculomandibulodyscephaly, orofaciodigital syndrome, achondroplasia, distomus, or Ehlers-Danlos syndrome. Localized hyperdontia may also be seen with adjacent isolated cleft palate.

Clinical Features

Demographics: Hyperdontia is somewhat less common than hypodontia, being present in 0.1% to 3.6% of persons. Extra teeth may occur in any region of the jaws, although the anterior maxilla, maxillary molar, and mandibular premolar regions are the most common sites. Additional teeth are comparatively rare in the deciduous dentition; they are most common in the maxillary incisor (mesiodens) and the maxillary third molar regions (distamolars).

Signs and symptoms: If supernumerary teeth have erupted, their detection is uncomplicated: simple enumeration of erupted teeth reveals a greater than normal complement of teeth. A supernumerary tooth may hinder eruption of teeth, so that the presence of an extra tooth may be heralded by the clinical absence of teeth. Furthermore, examination may reveal deflections in the normal eruptive path of teeth or in the position of fully erupted teeth. Supernumerary teeth may also be recognized by the presence of an unexplained firm bulging of the oral mucosa or occasionally by mobility of adjacent normal teeth resulting from root resorption induced by the supernumerary tooth. However, the presence of supernumerary teeth is usually detectable only on radiographs.

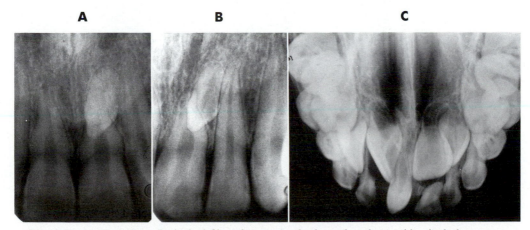

A   **B**   **C**

Fig. 3-2 A, Mesiodens. Periapical film taken at zero horizontal angle to midsagittal plane.
B, Mesiodens (same patient as in **A**). Periapical film taken at 20 degrees to midsagittal plane indicates lingual position of the supernumerary tooth using the buccal object rule.
C, Topographic occlusal radiograph of maxilla demonstrating mesiodens.

Continued.

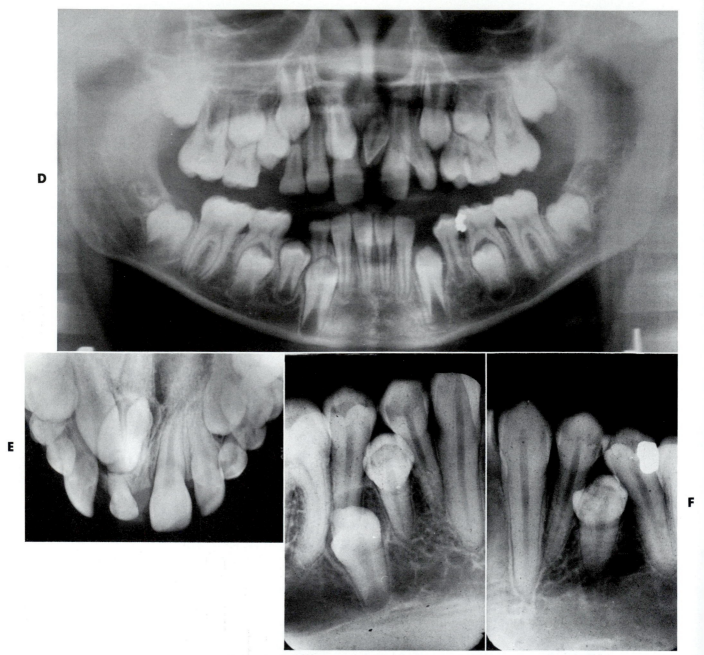

Fig. 3-2, cont'd. **D,** Panoramic radiograph showing mesiodens. **E,** Delayed eruption of central incisor resulting from inverted mediodens. **F,** Supplemental mandibular premolars.

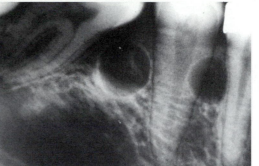

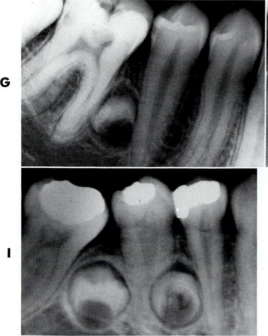

Fig. 3-2, cont'd. **G,** Postdentition supplemental supernumerary tooth. **H,** Postdentition supplemental supernumerary premolars. **I,** Patient in **H** after further development.

RADIOLOGIC FEATURES

Cardinal Signs

Greater than normal complement of teeth

Greater than normal complement of tooth follicles

Conical or tubercle-shaped radiopacity with surrounding radiolucent periodontal ligament shadow in the anterior maxillary, maxillary molar, or mandibular premolar region (The tooth may be inverted in position, erupted, and located either lingually or, less commonly, buccally.)

Prevention of eruption or altered eruptive pattern of a normal tooth associated with an adjacent radiopaque mass

Extra premolar-form tooth in the mandibular premolar-molar region

Ancillary Signs

Small radiopaque mass with surrounding thin zone of radiolucency in the maxillary or mandibular third molar region or buccal to the maxillary molar teeth

Resorption of adjacent normal teeth

Expansion of the follicular space about the crown of an unerupted extra tooth

Differential Diagnosis

Compound odontoma

MACRODONTIA (MEGADONTIA)

Overview

Definition: *Macrodontia* is the term applied to a single tooth (localized macrodontia) or many teeth (generalized macrodontia) that are of greater than normal size. In true macrodontia, the teeth are larger than normal-sized teeth of the same type; in relative macrodontia, a diminutive jaw gives the appearance of enlarged teeth.

Pathogenesis: Generalized true macrodontia can indicate pituitary gigantism, although in this condition enlargement of the jaw tends to mask the increased tooth size. Segmental or unilateral macrodontia results from the local hyperplastic influence of adjacent le-

Text continued on page 71.

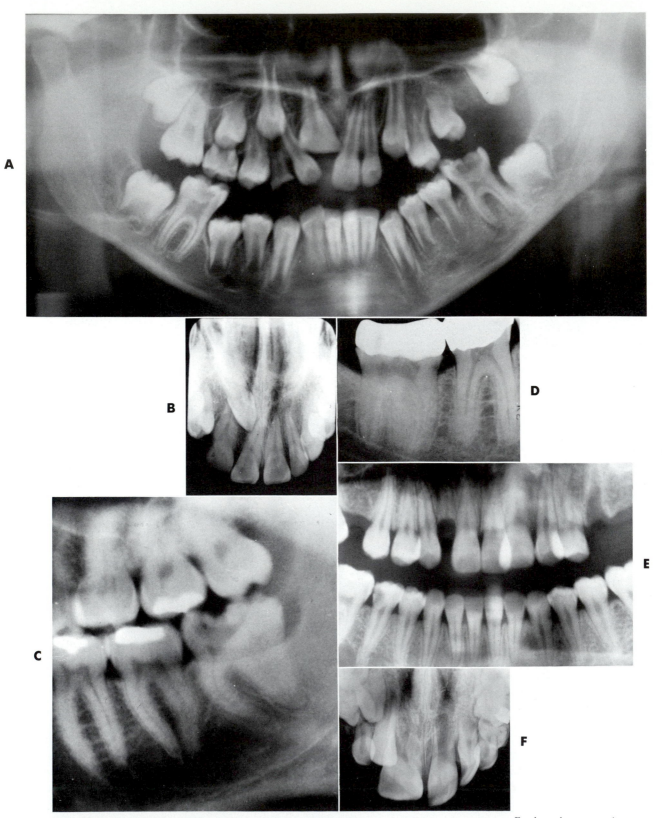

Fig. 3-3.

For legends see opposite page.

sions such as hemangioma, lymphangioma, neurofibroma, or lipomatosis. It may also occur in cases of congenital or acquired unilateral hyperplasia. Finally, isolated macrodontia may occur as an anomalous variant affecting the maxillary central incisor or canine, the mandibular second premolar, or the mandibular third molar. Single central incisor–short stature syndrome (monosuperocentroincisivodontic dwarfism) may be associated with an enlarged central incisor. Fusion and gemination of tooth buds may also give the clinical appearance of macrodontia.

Clinical Features

Signs and symptoms: Isolated macrodontia is easily revealed if the involved tooth is erupted, as clinical examination reveals a tooth that is incongruous with the patient's remaining teeth. In enlarged jaws, generalized true macrodontia may appear normal unless absolute tooth sizes are compared to normal values; in normal-sized jaws, generalized true macrodontia (relative macrodontia) will be manifested by severe overcrowding of the teeth.

RADIOLOGIC FEATURES

Isolated Macrodontia

Cardinal Signs

> Localized enlargement of a tooth with proportional enlargement of the pulp chamber, nerve canal, crown, and root
> Normal-sized adjacent teeth
> Normal complement of adjacent teeth (unless previously extracted)

Fig. 3-3 (opposite page), **A,** Panoramic radiograph illustrating isolated macrodontia of the partially erupted right maxillary permanent central incisor. **B,** Topographic occlusal view of maxilla. Macrodontia of right lateral incisor with impaction of right maxillary canine. **C,** Detail of panoramic radiograph showing macrodontia of mandibular third permanent molar. The tooth also demonstrates occlusal caries. **D,** Macrodontia of right mandibular second molar. This tooth also demonstrates a supernumerary third root. **E,** Macrodontia of left maxillary lateral incisor demonstrated on detail of panoramic radiograph. The maxillary right lateral incisor is missing, presumed extracted. **F,** Macrodontia of right maxillary central incisor.

Ancillary Signs

> Occasional deflection of adjacent teeth or crowding of teeth
> Altered tooth eruption pattern or impedance of eruption
> Development of dentigerous cysts about unerupted teeth

Multiple or Generalized Macrodontia

Cardinal Signs

> Multiple teeth or segments of teeth that are larger than their contralateral counterparts
> Enlargement of the jaw in the affected region

Ancillary Signs

> Coarseness of the trabecular bone pattern of the alveolar processes on the affected side as compared with the unaffected side
> Increased vertical depth of the jaw on the affected side

Differential Diagnosis

> Gemination
> Fusion

MICRODONTIA

Overview

Microdontia, like macrodontia, may be localized or generalized.

Definition: Microdontia is defined as an abnormal smallness of a single tooth or many teeth. Relative microdontia occurs when normal-sized teeth occupy a relatively large jaw; true microdontia is a genuine reduction in the size of the teeth compared to normal teeth.

Clinical Features

Signs and symptoms: Microdontia usually occurs as an isolated anomaly, as in peg-shaped lateral incisors or diminutive maxillary third molars. Generalized relative macrodontia is not rare and occurs when normal-sized or slightly small teeth appear in an enlarged jaw. True generalized microdontia may occur in patients with trisomy 21 or pituitary dwarfism and is also a feature of dentinogenesis imperfecta. Rarely, vascular tumors may contribute to the development of microdontia.

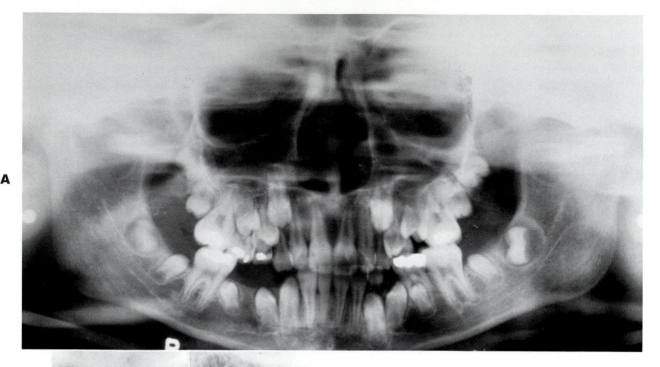

A

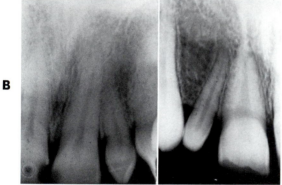

B   **C**

Fig. 3-4   **A,** Microdontia is most evident in the second molar regions and mandibular second premolar regions in this case. **B,** Microdontia of left lateral incisor, the so-called peg lateral. **C,** Peg-shaped lateral incisor.

Because microdontia is a developmental defect, it is clinically apparent from the time of tooth eruption. The teeth themselves may be small, normally shaped versions of normal teeth or misshapen. In the case of peg-shaped lateral incisors, the root is shorter than normal and the mesial and distal surfaces of the crown converge incisally. Alternatively, the entire incisor may be tapered in a cylindric fashion from gingival margin to incisal edge. Microdontia of premolar and molar teeth is evidenced by a marked reduction in tooth size, particularly in the roots of the teeth (rhizomicry).

RADIOLOGIC FEATURES

Isolated Microdontia

Cardinal Signs

Abnormally small-sized tooth compared to adjacent teeth

Abnormal shape of tooth, tending toward a more conical shape

Ancillary Signs

Greatly reduced root length and girth

Generalized Microdontia

Cardinal Signs

Abnormally small-sized teeth

Multiple spacing of teeth within the jaw

Ancillary Signs

Relative diminution of root width (slender roots)

Bulbous crowns with marked cervical constriction

Differential Diagnosis

Supernumerary tooth

Radiation therapy in childhood

CONCRESCENCE

Overview

Definition: Pindborg defined *true concrescence* as a cemental union of teeth formed by separate tooth buds during tooth formation and *acquired concrescence* as cemental union occurring after the complete development of the teeth. However, both Shafer et al. and Worth contend that concrescence is an acquired anomaly.

Pathogenesis: True concrescence may occur in regions with limited alveolar space or areas in which dislocation of tooth buds has occurred. Acquired concrescence results from hypercementosis, whether idiopathic or caused by chronic inflammation, or from trauma. Whatever the initiating process, the ultimate result is obliteration of intervening bone and periodontal ligament tissue and connection of the roots by a layer of cementum.

Clinical Features

Demographics: Concrescence may occur at any age, in either sex, and in any race. The most common site is the posterior maxilla involving the second and third molar teeth. More than two teeth are rarely involved.

Signs and symptoms: Clinically, teeth with concrescence are rigidly bound by a zone of cementum so that orthodontic or exodontic manipulation of one is accompanied by an associated reaction in both.

RADIOLOGIC FEATURES

Cardinal Signs

Close proximity of the roots of adjacent teeth with no detectable intervening periodontal ligament space shadow

A **B**

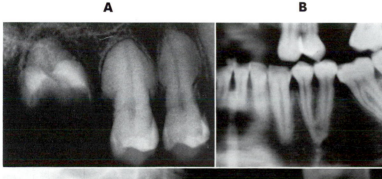

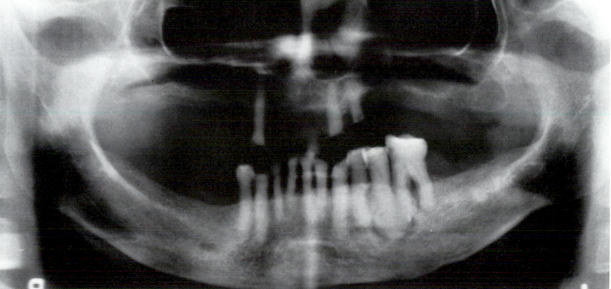

Fig. 3-5 **A,** Hypercementosis without concrescence. **B,** Concrescence of adjacent premolars shown on detail from panoramic radiograph. **C,** Panoramic radiograph. Concrescence of left mandibular second premolar and first molar.

C

Continued.

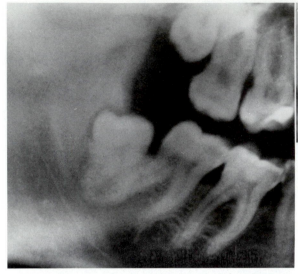

D

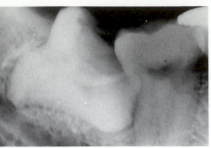

E

Fig. 3-5, cont'd. **D,** Detail from panoramic radiograph demonstrating concrescence of right mandibular second and third molars. **E,** Concrescence of mandibular third molar and supernumerary tooth (paramolar).

Radiopaque mass with the density of cemental tissue and lack of delineation of the periodontal ligament shadows in the roots of adjacent teeth

Continuity of the periodontal ligament space and lamina dura shadow around the contacting roots of two closely approximated teeth, with no extension between them

Gross hypercementosis of adjacent teeth with closely positioned roots.

Ancillary Signs

Occasional lack of eruption of one or all of the involved teeth

Differential Diagnosis

Fusion
Gemination
Hypercementosis
Bony ankylosis
Inostosis

FUSION

Overview

Definition: Pindborg defined fusion as a union between the dentin or enamel of two or more separate developing teeth, whereas Mader suggested that true fusion must involve the dentin of both teeth. Fusion may be partial, that is, involving a small section of the tooth, or total, the amount of tooth surface involved depending on the developmental stage at which the tooth buds unite. Because the net result of this process is the joining of two developing tooth buds to form a single dental unit, the number of teeth in the arch is reduced by one unless a supernumerary tooth is involved.

Pathogenesis: The cause of fusion is unknown, although compression of tooth buds, pressure necrosis of the tissue between tooth buds, or mere chance may be involved.

Clinical Features

Demographics: Fusion occurs more frequently in the primary dentition and in the anterior teeth. It may occur between two normal constituents of the dental arch or between normal and supernumerary teeth.

Signs and symptoms: When fusion occurs, the resultant combined dental unit often exhibits a groove on the labial surface or even an incisal notch. If posterior teeth are involved, the resultant cusp pattern is reminiscent of the forced combination of two adjacent teeth. Mader suggested that fused teeth cause clinical problems in that they are unattractive, may cause spacing problems, and may be subject to periodontal disease.

RADIOLOGIC FEATURES

Cardinal Signs

Radiographic evidence of joined dentin between two teeth

No evidence of an intervening periodontal ligament space shadow between two teeth with overlapping dentin shadows

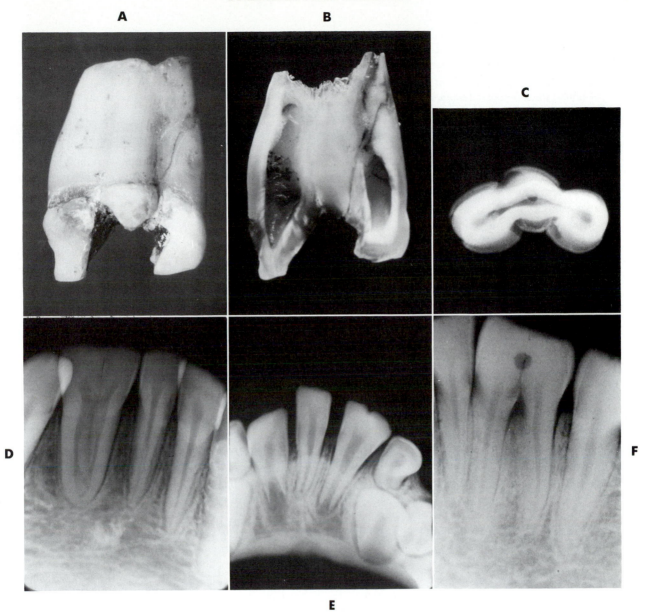

Fig. 3-6 **A,** Fused carious primary central incisors and mesiodens. **B,** Same patient as in **A.** Sectioned specimen showing fusion of supernumerary tooth to the two primary maxillary central incisors. **C,** Same patient as in **A.** Note the single pulpal complex linking the three fused teeth. **D,** Fusion of right mandibular permanent central and lateral incisors. **E,** Fusion of left mandibular permanent and lateral incisors. **F,** Fused mandibular central incisors.

Joined pulp chambers or shared pulp chamber complex

Diminished number of teeth (if the fused tooth complex is counted as one dental unit) in the dental arch

Evidence of incisal/occlusal notching of the fused crowns

Presence of supernumerary tooth as part of the fused tooth complex

Ancillary Signs

Occasionally, presence of separate pulp chamber complexes

Differential Diagnosis

Macrodontia

Gemination

Concrescence

Gemination may be difficult to separate from fusion unless the patient's extraction history is known and all the teeth are present. If this is the case, gemination will result in a normal number of dental units whereas fusion will result in a decreased number. The distinction is further complicated if the fusion is with a supernumerary tooth; hence, the term *connation* is sometimes used to include both fusion and gemination. Macrodontia may be differentiated from fusion in that macrodontia results in enlargement of the whole tooth, whereas fusion results in disproportionate enlargement of the tooth in a mesiodistal direction, without any great increase in root length. Concrescence may also be difficult to differentiate from fusion, although a normal number of dental units and the presence of excess cementum may help to confirm the diagnosis of concrescence.

GEMINATION

Overview

Definition: Although gemination may superficially resemble fusion, the process that leads to gemination is different. Levitas defined gemination as the development of two joined teeth in a single follicular sac. Gemination is an incomplete attempt by a single tooth bud to form two teeth. For some reason the process does not reach completion; if it does, a supplemental supernumerary twin tooth is the outcome. Unlike fusion, gemination will result in a normal number of dental units in the arch (if the geminated tooth is counted as a single dental unit).

Clinical Features

Demographics: Gemination is most prevalent in the permanent dentition and is most common in the maxillary anterior region. The condition is exceedingly rare, being present in from 0.08% to 0.5% of patients.

Signs and symptoms: Clinically, gemination occurs with the normal complement of teeth. Because the geminated tooth is of greater mesiodistal width than a normal tooth, a dental space problem will almost always be present. If the tooth becomes carious, it may present a restoration design problem. The tooth itself may exhibit a partial division with a confluent pulp chamber or separate crowns with a single root structure. The pulp chambers will almost always be confluent, and an incisal notch may be present between the coronal division.

RADIOLOGIC FEATURES

Cardinal Signs

Abnormally wide crown with normal or widened root

Radiographically visible incisal notch or labial groove

Radiographic evidence of a single radiolucent periodontal ligament shadow around the root system

Confluent or partially joined root canal system

Differential Diagnosis

Fusion

Concrescence

Macrodontia

DENS IN DENTE (DENS INVAGINATUS, ENAMEL INVAGINATION)

Overview

Definition: Dens in dente refers to invagination of tooth structure, generally on the cingular surface of maxillary anterior teeth.

Pathogenesis: The anomaly, also known as dens invaginatus, results from invagination of the enamel organ in coronal cases or of the Hertwig epithelial root sheath in radicular cases.

Clinical Features

Demographics: Amos demonstrated a 5% incidence of dens in dente in an examination of 1,000 patients. The maxillary lateral incisor is most commonly involved, and the condition is said to be rare in blacks. The precise cause is unknown, although lack of space in the jaws may be a contributing factor. Omnell[3] postulated that fusion of two tooth germs, dislocation of the enamel organ relative to the dental papilla, abnormal pressure from surrounding tissues during development, or defective enamel organ constituents may be responsible. More recently, De Smit, Jansen, and Dermaut stated that the condition was genetically predetermined.

Signs and symptoms: Unless the incisal region is carious, the lesions of dens in dente are asymptomatic. However, because of the angular, blind, enamel-lined sac that characterizes this disorder, caries is frequent. Careful probing of the lingual aspect

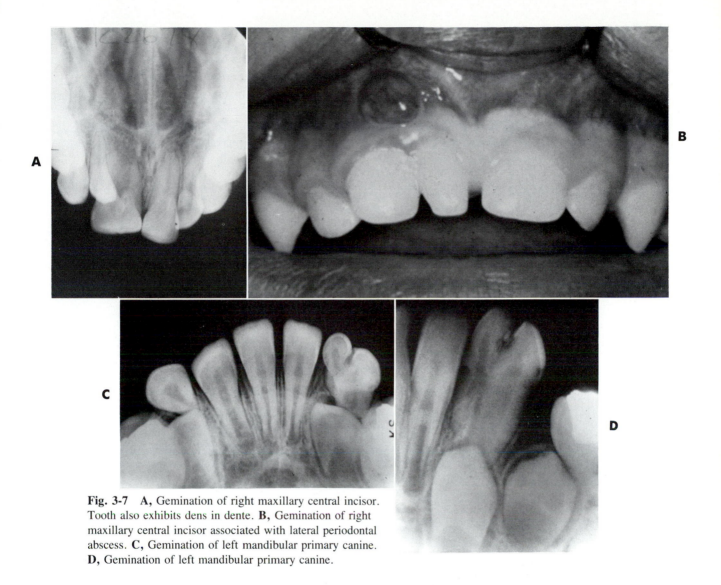

Fig. 3-7 **A,** Gemination of right maxillary central incisor. Tooth also exhibits dens in dente. **B,** Gemination of right maxillary central incisor associated with lateral periodontal abscess. **C,** Gemination of left mandibular primary canine. **D,** Gemination of left mandibular primary canine.

of maxillary incisors often discloses the sac, which varies from an accentuated cingulum to a deep invagination extending to the apex of the tooth. Hallett defined four gradations of invagination, but there is probably a continuum of severity. Dens in dente often remains undiagnosed until a radiographic survey is performed. Histologically the internal cleft is lined by enamel, which is often defective in quality so that the sac is confluent with the pulp of the involved tooth. It is therefore no mystery that these teeth often manifest apical inflammatory disease.

RADIOLOGIC FEATURES

Cardinal Signs

Angular cleft located at the junction of the cingulum and the lingual surface of a crown of a maxillary incisor tooth

Enamel lining of this cleft or sac, in whole or in part, so that the pulp of the tooth is overlayed with the thin enamel shadow of the sac lining

Ancillary Signs

Disturbances of the general shape of the tooth, ranging from clefting of the lingual surface to so-called dilated odontoma, in which the crown of the tooth is ballooned by the centrally located invagination

Invagination of the root surface into the apex of the tooth, in which case the invagination is not lined by enamel

Presence of a tooth-shaped, enamel-covered body within the pulpal tissue of an involved tooth

Apical rarefaction associated with the root of a maxillary incisor tooth

Carious destruction affecting the lingual region of a maxillary incisor

Occasionally, widening of the apical foramen of the involved tooth

Differential Diagnosis

Caries of the lingual surface of a maxillary incisor tooth

Pulpal diverticula

Pulp stones or pulpal calcifications

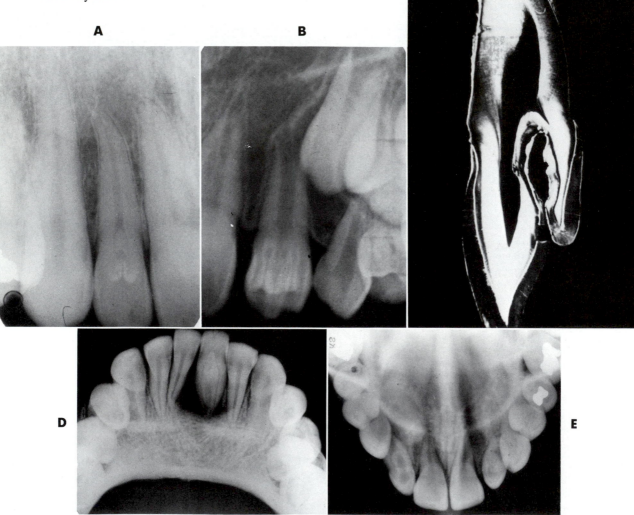

Fig. 3-8 **A,** Classic dens in dente in maxillary lateral incisor. **B,** Double dens in dente in maxillary lateral incisor. **C,** Ground section of tooth with dens in dente. **D,** Dens in dente in mandibular central incisor. **E,** Dens in dente in right maxillary lateral incisor.

DENS EVAGINATUS (OCCLUSAL TUBERCULATED PREMOLAR, LEUNG PREMOLAR, ENAMEL EVAGINATION, EVAGINATED ODONTOMA)

Overview

Definition: Dens evaginatus applies to the outfolding of the enamel-forming tissue on the occlusal surface of premolar and occasionally molar and cuspid teeth. The tuberculated tooth possesses a teatlike cusp projection. The condition is most common in mongoloid races, although it has been reported in caucasians.

Pathogenesis: The precise cause of dens evaginatus is not well known although it is probably hereditary in nature. It results from outfolding of the enamel organ during the process of tooth formation.

Clinical Features

Signs and symptoms: Clinically the projection usually lies in the center of the occlusal surface of a mandibular premolar. It is covered by enamel and has a pulpal extension of the main pulp chamber. Because of its occlusal position it is prone to fracture with subsequent pulp exposure and necrosis.

RADIOLOGIC FEATURES

Cardinal Signs

Occlusal table projection with the density of enamel
Small pulpal extension into this teatlike projection

Ancillary Signs

In many cases, apical rarefying osteitis as a result of fracture of the projection and secondary pulpal inflammation.

Differential Diagnosis

Normal cusp overlap (radiographic projection)
Normal pulpal extensions

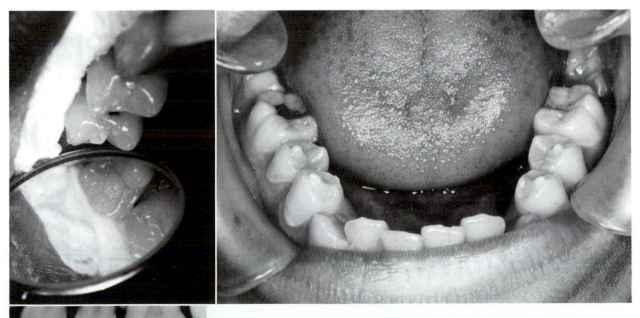

Fig. 3-9 **A,** Clinical picture of dens evaginatus. **B,** Clinical picture of dens evaginatus. **C,** Radiograph of dens evaginatus in mandibular second promolar.

TAURODONTISM

Overview

Definition: Taurodontism is an inherited morphologic anomaly of multirooted teeth caused by the failure of invagination of the Hertwig epithelial root sheath.

Pathogenesis: Taurodontism may be a specialized retrograde condition; a primitive pattern; a Mendelian recessive trait; an atavistic feature, or, according to Mangion, a mutation.

Clinical Features

Demographics: Taurodontism is more common in the permanent dentition, although it may occur in the deciduous teeth. The condition is usually bilateral and symmetric in distribution, although involvement of an isolated tooth is not rare. Taurodontism is common in American Indians and in the Cape Coloured population of South Africa.

Signs and symptoms: Clinical examination of crowns of involved teeth fails to reveal any abnormality.

RADIOLOGIC FEATURES

Cardinal Signs

Square- or rectangular-shaped teeth with the long axis of the rectangle oriented in an occlusal-apical direction.

Absence of normal cervical constriction of the root.

Lack of cervical constriction of the pulp chamber.

Increased occlusal-apical distance of the pulp chamber with extension of pulp horns far into occlusal dentin; pulp chamber may appear rectangular or square in shape

Diminished or absent bifurcation or trifurcation with reduced apical root length; furcation may not occur or may occur only a short distance from the apex.

Differential Diagnosis

No other conditions result in the characteristic radiographic pattern of taurodontism.

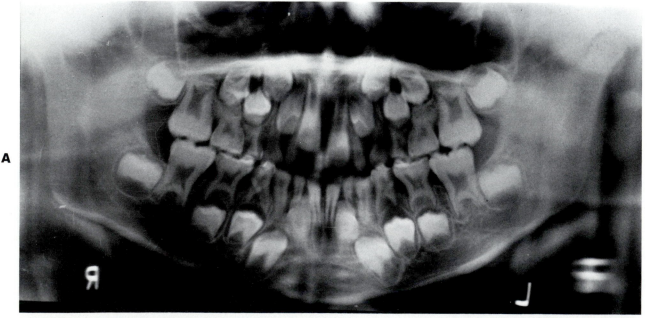

Fig. 3-10.   *For legend see opposite page.*

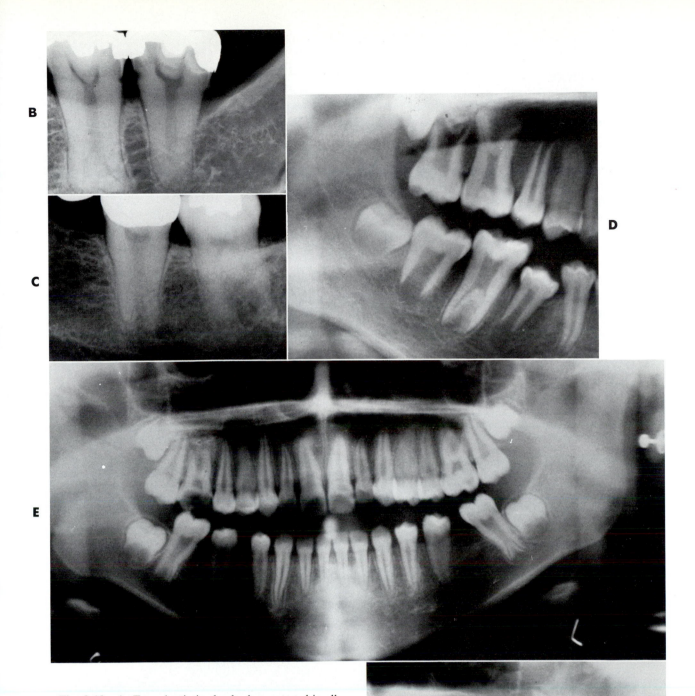

Fig. 3-10 **A,** Taurodontia is clearly demonstrated in all four first permanent and second primary molar teeth. Note the abnormally long pulp chambers. **B,** Taurodontia of mandibular first molar with pyramidal second molar. Both molars evidence cemental caries of the proximal surfaces. **C,** Taurodontia of mandibular first molar. The second molar has normal root morphology. **D,** Detail of panoramic radiograph demonstrating taurodontia of molars. **E,** Panoramic radiograph showing taurodontia of mandibular second molars (mandibular first molars are missing, presumed extracted). **F,** Taurodontia of primary and permanent molars.

DILACERATION

Overview

Definition: All tooth roots are curved to some degree, but the term *dilaceration* is reserved for instances of excess or abnormal root curvature. To make such a definition practical, the term should be restricted to cases in which the root curvature impedes conventional endodontic or exodontic therapy.

Pathogenesis: Any impediment to eruption may cause dilaceration, and the condition is frequently seen as a secondary feature of benign space-occupying lesions in positions coronal to unerupted teeth. It may also occur where a tooth root encounters the sinus floor, as an accompaniment to impaction, or as an unexplained anomalous variant.

Clinical Features

Demographics: Dilaceration is more common in the permanent dentition. It is thought to result from previous infection, trauma, or pressure, although this has yet to be proved. Maxillary incisor teeth are most commonly involved, although maxillary premolars and mandibular third molars are also frequently affected.

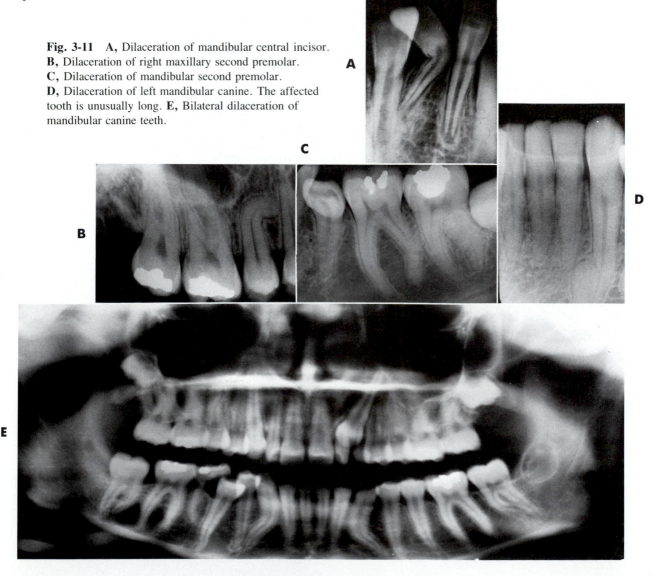

Fig. 3-11   A, Dilaceration of mandibular central incisor. **B,** Dilaceration of right maxillary second premolar. **C,** Dilaceration of mandibular second premolar. **D,** Dilaceration of left mandibular canine. The affected tooth is unusually long. **E,** Bilateral dilaceration of mandibular canine teeth.

Signs and symptoms: Clinically, the tooth often appears structurally and positionally normal; the abnormality is only visible on radiographic examination. Also, because conventional dental radiographs are two-dimensional images of three-dimensional objects, the direction of the dilaceration relative to the film plane will determine its radiographic representation.

RADIOLOGIC FEATURES

Cardinal Signs

Abnormal curvature of the root such that an endodontic file would be difficult to extend to the apex of the tooth or nonsurgical extraction would be onerous.

Position of dilaceration at any point along the root length or even double dilaceration.

Ancillary Signs

Presence of overlying space-occupying lesion or other impediment to normal eruption or uninterrupted root growth.

Presence of so-called "bull's-eye" root, in which the direction of the dilaceration is either from buccal to lingual or vice versa; bull's-eye root end is caused by a view down the root axis and shows the innermost pulp canal surrounded by root tissue, which in turn is encircled by the radiolucent periodontal ligament shadow and ultimately by the delimiting radiopaque lamina dura silhouette

Radiographic depiction of a crown with a view that is reminiscent of the perspective of the incisal edge of an anterior tooth and with a root projection extending from the edge of this image

Apparent increased opacity of the root ends of the teeth not caused by hypercementosis

Extra cusp or an incisal notch, if the dilaceration results from trauma during the development of the tooth

Visible, reconstituted fracture line, if the dilaceration resulted from trauma during the development of the tooth

Differential Diagnosis

Dilaceration in a mesial or distal direction will rarely be mistaken for anything else if the radiographic projections are of adequate quality.

Hypercementosis may be mistaken for labial/lingual dilaceration when the former occurs at the root ends of the teeth.

AMELOGENESIS IMPERFECTA

Overview

Although there are many documented subclassifications of amelogenesis imperfecta, from a radiographic standpoint there are two major divisions. The first includes disorders in which the basic mechanism of disease is defective calcification of the enamel matrix—hypocalcific amelogenesis imperfecta. The other major inheritable enamel disorder results from poor production of the enamel matrix itself—so-called hypoplastic amelogenesis imperfecta.

HYPOCALCIFIC AMELOGENESIS IMPERFECTA

Definition: Hypocalcific amelogenesis imperfecta results from defective calcification of a relatively normal enamel matrix. It may involve both dentitions.

Signs and symptoms: Clinically, the crowns of the teeth appear severely pitted, with portions either worn away or fractured off. The teeth are soft to probing and may have root surfaces in close proximity to one another as the result of mesial and distal coronal wear.

RADIOLOGIC FEATURES

Cardinal Signs

Moderate to severe pitting of all teeth, evidenced by mottled radiolucent flecks on the crowns

Radiographically normal dentin, cementum, pulp chambers and canals, and root shape (unless secondarily involved).

Severely worn teeth in a young individual without a valid reason for this wear.

Lack of radiographic contrast between dentin and enamel, so that the crowns appear radiographically homogeneous in density.

Differential Diagnosis

Hypoplastic amelogenesis imperfecta
Environmental enamel hypoplasia

HYPOPLASTIC AMELOGENESIS IMPERFECTA

Definition: Unlike hypocalcific amelogenesis imperfecta, in which the basic defect is poor mineralization of a normal matrix, in the hypoplastic type the matrix itself is abnormal. The degree of abnormality ranges from virtual absence of the enamel matrix, so-called enamel agenesis, to partial absence of the enamel matrix.

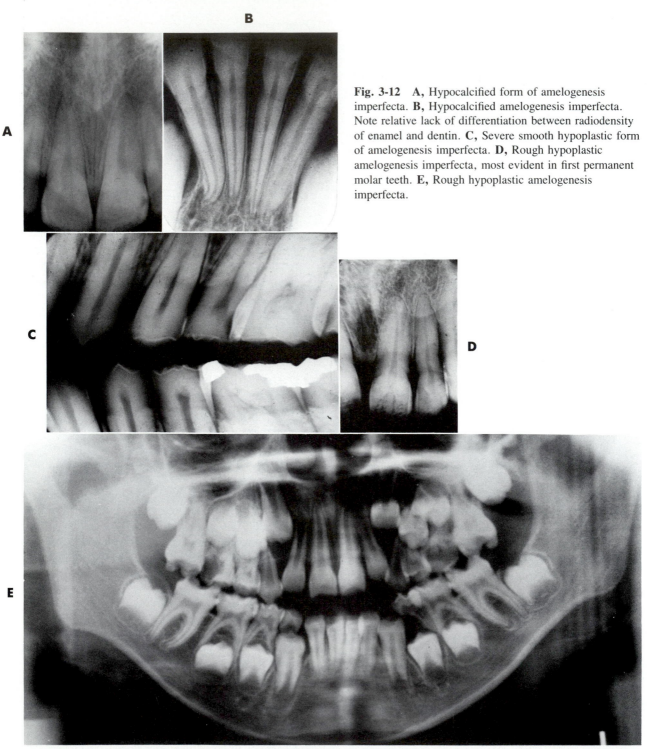

Fig. 3-12   **A,** Hypocalcified form of amelogenesis imperfecta. **B,** Hypocalcified amelogenesis imperfecta. Note relative lack of differentiation between radiodensity of enamel and dentin. **C,** Severe smooth hypoplastic form of amelogenesis imperfecta. **D,** Rough hypoplastic amelogenesis imperfecta, most evident in first permanent molar teeth. **E,** Rough hypoplastic amelogenesis imperfecta.

Continued.

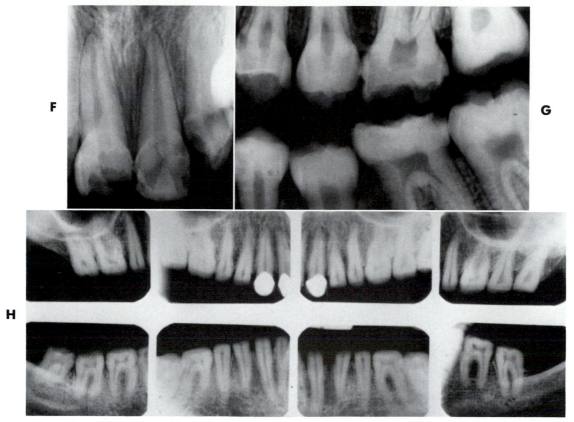

Fig. 3-12, cont'd. F, Rough hypoplastic amelogenesis imperfecta. **G,** Rough hypoplastic amelogenesis imperfecta. **H,** Smooth hypoplastic amelogenesis imperfecta.

Signs and symptoms: The disorder affects both dentitions; the different subtypes of enamel hypoplasia are delineated by Witkop and Sauk. The degree of severity of the hypoplasia determines the associated clinical signs. In severe cases in which the enamel matrix has completely failed to form, the teeth appear as if they had been prepared for full-coverage restorations. The teeth appear smaller than normal because of the absence of enamel and are square in shape. They are very soft to probing and prone to attrition because of the absence of a protective enamel cover. If the matrix has been partially formed, the teeth may appear small and shrivelled but with small zones of normal enamel calcification.

RADIOLOGIC FEATURES

Cardinal Signs

Apparent complete absence of enamel covering with square-shaped teeth, which may exhibit varying degrees of attrition.

Thin zone of enamel overlying the occlusal surfaces or at the mesial and distal margins; this enamel is normally mineralized and demonstrates a definite radiodensity difference between it and the underlying dentin.

Severe attrition with secondary pulp calcification to a degree dependent on the severity of the hypoplasia.

Differential Diagnosis

Pulpal calcification and severe attrition, which are present in some cases of hypoplastic amelogenesis imperfecta, may be mistaken for the changes seen in dentinogenesis imperfecta. However, dentinogenesis imperfecta usually results in shortened roots and more complete pulp calcification, whereas hereditary enamel hypoplasia exhibits more severe attrition.

ENVIRONMENTAL ENAMEL HYPOPLASIA

Overview

Definition: Whereas hereditary enamel defects often affect both dentitions, environmental effects depend on both the instance and duration of an environmental influence on the teeth. The final result may be seen in a single tooth or all teeth. In addition, environmental enamel defects are frequently accompanied by similar deleterious changes in the dentin.

Pathogenesis: Infection or trauma to the primary precursor tooth may cause localized enamel defects if the destructive stimuli act at the time of enamel formation. There are a multitude of systemic conditions that can lead to enamel hypoplasia. Nutritional deficits of vitamins A, C, and D; exanthematous fevers; congenital syphilis; hypocalcemic diseases; birth trauma, prematurity, and Rh incompatibility hemolytic disease; toxic chemical ingestion; cancer chemotherapy; and idiopathic causes may all lead to visible defects of enamel.

Clinical Features

Signs and symptoms: Clinically, the changes of environmental enamel hypoplasia vary from minor pitting and linear zones of defective enamel to gross malformation of all enamel with a concomitant reduction in crown size. In addition to the structural changes, the tooth may appear discolored.

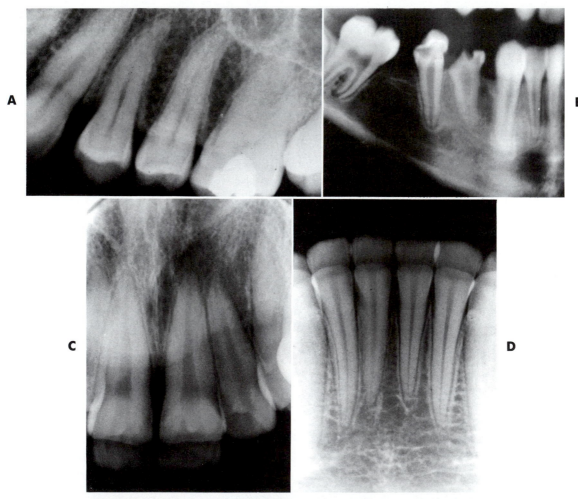

Fig. 3-13   **A,** Hypoplasia of maxillary second premolar (Turner tooth). **B,** Detail from panoramic radiograph showing environmental hypoplasia of right mandibular premolars. **C,** Neonatal line of maxillary incisors. **D,** Same patient as in **C,** Neonatal line of mandibular anterior teeth.

RADIOLOGIC FEATURES

Cardinal Signs

Apparent linear defect(s) in the crown(s) of affected teeth

Cleft or angular pit located on the mesial and distal surface of the involved tooth

Shriveled appearance of the crown of an affected tooth

In perinatal cases, the effect is usually restricted to the incisor and first molar teeth

In severe cases, gross destruction of the enamel-forming tissues may give the appearance of a "ghostlike" shadow of a tooth, often devoid of a normal surrounding follicular space

Differential Diagnosis

Amelogenesis imperfecta
Dental caries
Erosion
Abrasion
Regional odontodysplasia

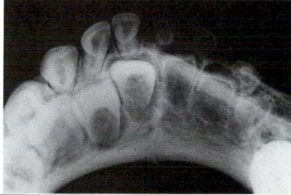

A

Fig. 3-14 A, Ghost teeth in regional odontodysplasia can be compared with normal contralateral dentition. This case affected both dentitions in the region. **B,** Regional odontodysplasia in right mandibular incisor, canine, and premolar region.

REGIONAL ODONTODYSPLASIA

Overview

Definition: Regional odontodysplasia is a localized failure of permanent teeth to form properly.

Pathogenesis: The precise cause of regional odontodysplasia is unknown, although it has been suggested that local vascular abnormalities, genetic mutation, or viral causes may be ultimately responsible.

Clinical Features

Demographics: The condition affects the primary and less commonly the permanent dentition. The anterior teeth are most commonly involved.

Signs and symptoms: Adjacent, unaffected teeth appear perfectly normal, whereas teeth affected by re-

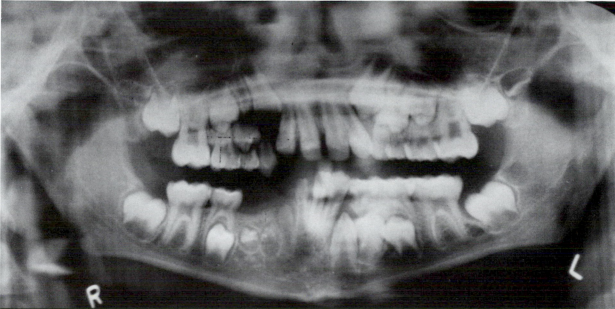

B

gional odontodysplasia may erupt late or not at all. When they do erupt, they may be unable to withstand the forces of mastication. If retained, these teeth exhibit altered crown form and a shriveled appearance like that sometimes seen in environmental enamel hypoplasia.

RADIOLOGIC FEATURES

Cardinal Signs

> In severe cases, diminished radiodensity of one or a few teeth to the point where they appear as ghostlike images of normal teeth
>
> Absence of a well-defined and separate enamel layer and inability to distinguish between enamel and dentinal tissues
>
> Roughened and coarse-appearing outline of crowns
>
> Grossly enlarged pulp chambers and root canal systems
>
> Delayed or absent root formation and apparent small root length for the amount of tooth eruption
>
> Delayed or absent tooth eruption
>
> Pericoronal mixed radiolucency-radiopacity

Differential Diagnosis

> Localized environmental enamel hypoplasia (Turner tooth)

DENTINOGENESIS IMPERFECTA

Overview

Definition: Dentinogenesis imperfecta is an inherited defect of the mesodermal portion of the developing tooth. The disorder may be associated with osteogenesis imperfecta, although not invariably so. There are three forms of dentinogenesis imperfecta according to Shields, Bixler, and El-Kafrawy. Type I is found in association with some cases of osteogenesis imperfecta and may be transmitted in an autosomal dominant or recessive mode. Type II is an autosomal dominant dentinal defect that is not associated with osteogenesis imperfecta. Type III is an autosomal dominant racial isolate found in Brandywine, Maryland, that shares the same clinical features as types I and II.

Clinical Features

Signs and symptoms: The teeth appear smaller than normal and have an opalescent hue. The color of the teeth ranges from normal to brown, and the structure may be altered by fracture of the unsupported enamel and excessive wear of the underlying dentin.

Fig. 3-15 **A,** Patient with dentinogenesis imperfecta showing all of the classic signs of the disease.

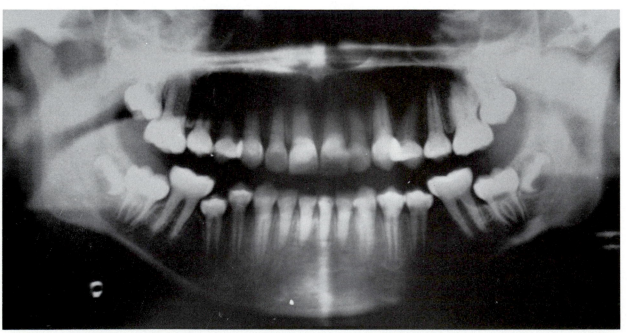

A

Continued.

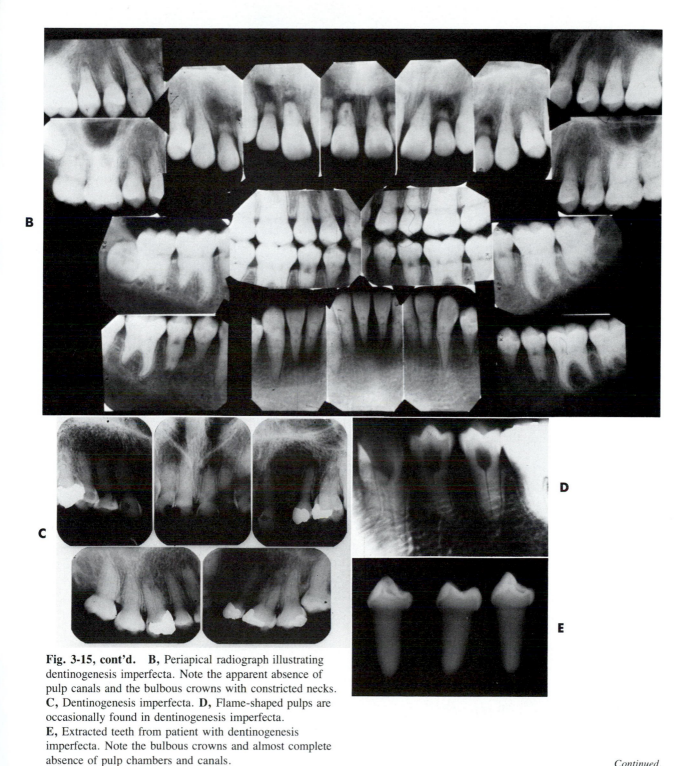

Fig. 3-15, cont'd. **B,** Periapical radiograph illustrating dentinogenesis imperfecta. Note the apparent absence of pulp canals and the bulbous crowns with constricted necks. **C,** Dentinogenesis imperfecta. **D,** Flame-shaped pulps are occasionally found in dentinogenesis imperfecta. **E,** Extracted teeth from patient with dentinogenesis imperfecta. Note the bulbous crowns and almost complete absence of pulp chambers and canals.

Continued.

F

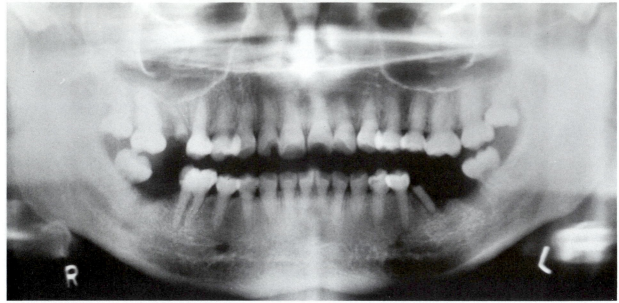

Fig. 3-15, cont'd.   **F,** Panoramic radiograph illustrating dentinogenesis imperfecta.

RADIOLOGIC FEATURES

Clinical Signs

Diminished incisoapical dimension of the teeth

Bulbous or square tooth crowns

Flattened, occasionally featureless occlusal surfaces

Excessive constriction in the region of the cementoenamel junction

Pulp completely calcified, rudimentary, greatly enlarged, or flame shaped

Attrition with or without pulp exposure

Differential Diagnosis

Types may be distinguished by the absence or concurrence of osteogenesis imperfecta.

Dentin dysplasia

DENTIN DYSPLASIA

Overview

Definition and pathogenesis: Dentin dysplasia, also known as rootless teeth, is, according to Witkop and Sauk, two separate conditions. The first, radicular dentin dysplasia type I, is an autosomal dominant disorder characterized by relatively normal coronal appearance and normal eruption pattern, followed by rapid tooth loss as a result of abnormally short roots. Dentin dysplasia type II, also transmitted in an autosomal dominant mode, affects the crowns of both permanent and deciduous teeth.

Clinical Features

Signs and symptoms: The clinical appearance of the deciduous teeth is reminiscent of dentinogenesis imperfecta. They appear opalescent and brown in color, particularly in the deciduous dentition. Although dentinal dysplasia usually affects all the teeth, this is not invariably the case.

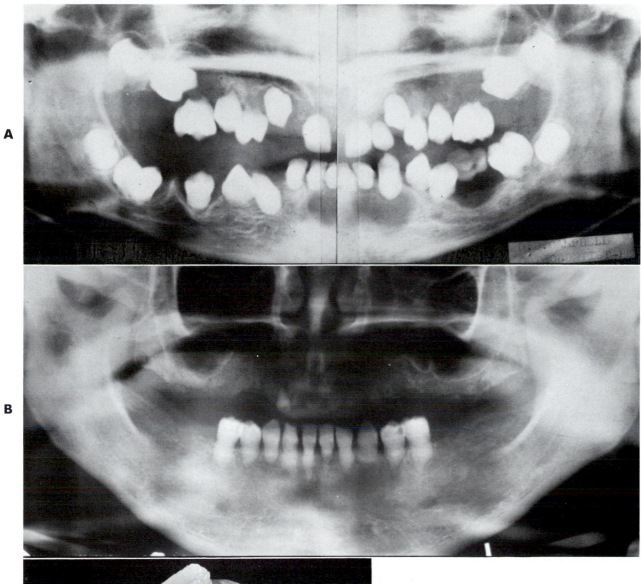

A

B

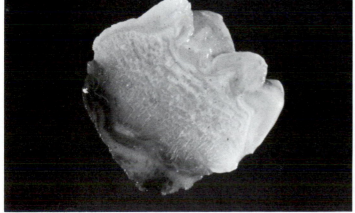

C

Fig. 3-16 **A,** Radicular dentin dysplasia. Note the multiple rootless teeth and periapical rarefactions. **B,** Radicular dentin dysplasia. Only the mandibular premolars and anterior teeth remain in this patient. **C,** Extracted tooth from patient with radicular dentin dysplasia.

RADIOLOGIC FEATURES

Radicular Dentin Dysplasia

Cardinal Signs

Short, blunt roots and rounded, somewhat bulbous crowns

Reduced distance from furcation of roots to root ends in multirooted teeth such that teeth appear "stubby"

Calcification of pulp chambers of teeth and absence of radiographically discernible root canals, often occurring before tooth eruption

Presence of periapical rarefactions in areas with or without apparent cause

Ancillary Signs

Absent teeth in a patient with a few remaining teeth that exhibit short roots

Linear, crescent-shaped radiolucent lines, single or a few in number, that cross the tooth at the region of the crown-root junction

Coronal Dentin Dysplasia

Cardinal Signs

Calcification of pulp chambers of primary but not permanent teeth

Relatively enlarged pulp chambers in permanent teeth with multiple pulpal calcifications reminiscent of pulp stones

No root abnormality and no evidence of periapical rarefactions without discernible cause

Differential Diagnosis

Dentinogenesis imperfecta

Ectodermal dysplasia (missing teeth)

ANOMALIES OF ERUPTION

Overview

Radiography plays an important part in determining the normality of tooth eruption with regard to position and time sequence. This is especially important in patients whose teeth are undetectable by clinical means, such as those with delayed eruption, impaction, or suppression of teeth. In general there is a wide latitude in the time and sequence of normal tooth eruption, which may be influenced by factors such as sex, race, climate and socioeconomic status.

From a radiographic standpoint there are two main areas of interest with respect to anomalies of eruption. The first, time of eruption, is important in planning interceptive orthodontic treatment and in diagnosing conditions that may affect the final number or position of permanent teeth. The second factor, tooth position, may influence treatment options such as surgical approach or orthodontic repositioning. In general, isolated anomalies of eruption are easily detected because the premature or delayed tooth erupts in a manner that is significantly different from the normal side. However, abnormalities in eruption are not so much developmental dental abnormalities as they are radiographic signs of other disorders. The specific radiographic picture accompanying each of the different eruptive abnormalities are listed here.

RADIOLOGIC FEATURES

Transposition

Presence of a disordered sequence of the teeth so that the sequence of teeth from anterior to posterior in the arch is not followed

Ectopia

Radiographic evidence of a tooth or dental follicle at a site where it would not normally be found in a patient without previous surgery or trauma

Suppression

Radiographic evidence of a tooth that is depressed in a superoinferior position into the alveolar process of the jaw

Dilaceration of the root of the involved tooth

Ankylosis of the tooth root to underlying bone

Ankylosis

Loss of demarcation between the tooth root, periodontal ligament space, lamina dura, and alveolar bone such that the tooth root appears to be directly attached to the bone

Occasionally, associated resorption as well as radiographically detectable ingrowth of bone into the root surface

Impaction

Impedance of eruption by either tooth or bone so that eruption of the tooth is rendered unlikely

Text continued on page 98.

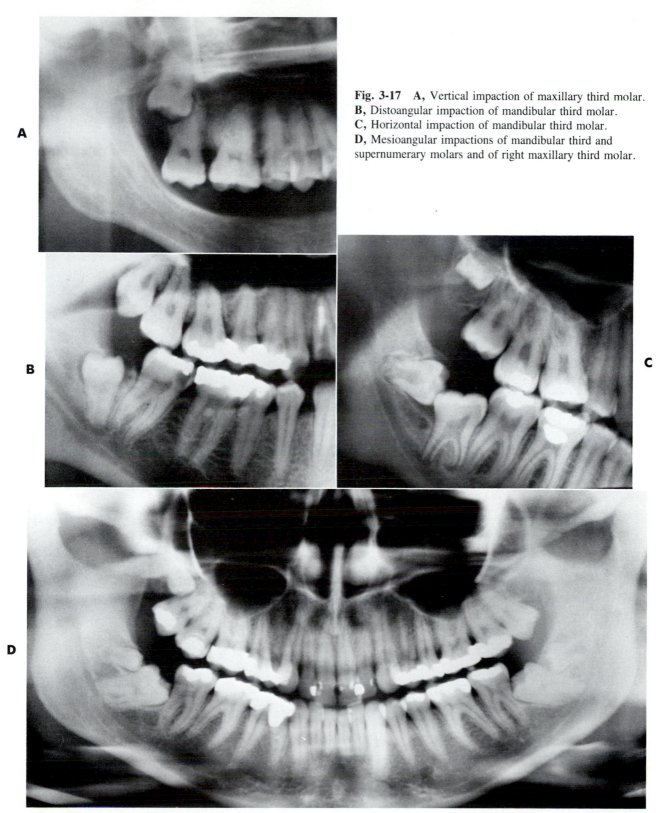

Fig. 3-17 **A,** Vertical impaction of maxillary third molar. **B,** Distoangular impaction of mandibular third molar. **C,** Horizontal impaction of mandibular third molar. **D,** Mesioangular impactions of mandibular third and supernumerary molars and of right maxillary third molar.

Continued.

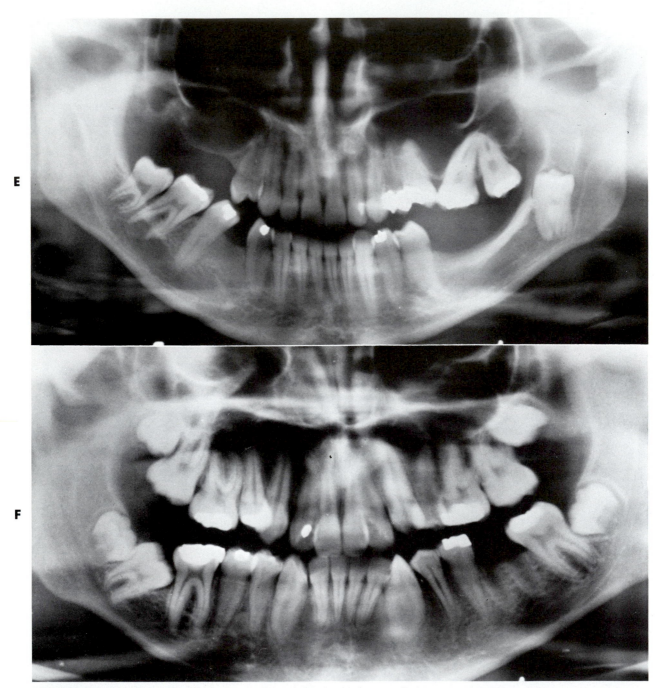

Fig. 3-17, cont'd. **E,** Vertical impaction of left mandibular third molar. **F,** Impacted right mandibular second molar.

G

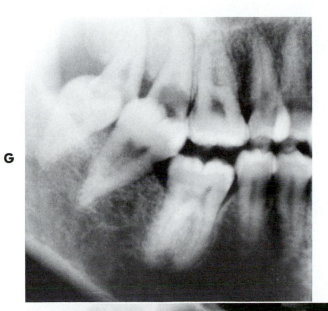

H

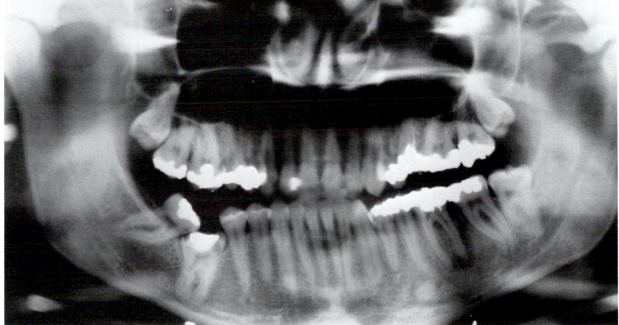

Fig. 3-17, cont'd. **G,** Impacted right mandibular first molar. **H,** Impacted right mandibular first molar.   *Continued.*

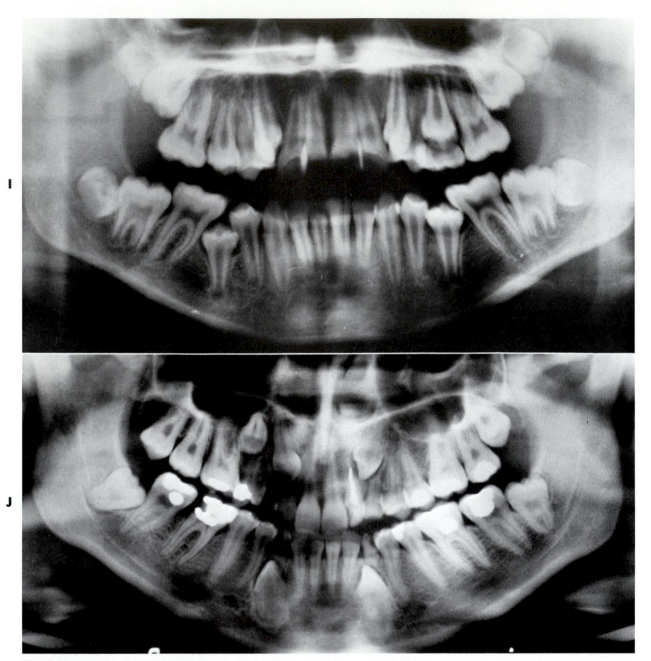

Fig. 3-17, cont'd.   **I,** Bilateral impaction of mandibular second premolars. **J,** Bilateral impaction of canines in both jaws and impaction of right maxillary second premolar.

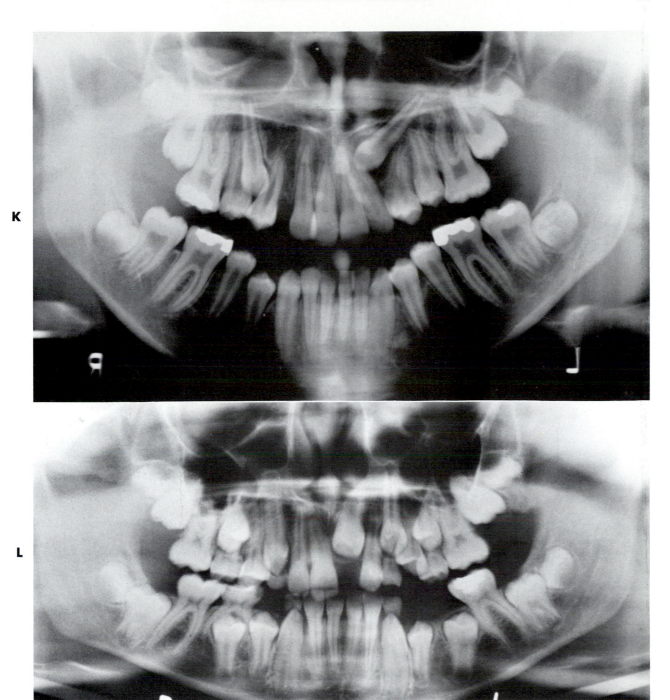

Fig. 3-17, cont'd.   K, Bilateral impaction of maxillary canines. **L,** Impaction of left maxillary central incisor.

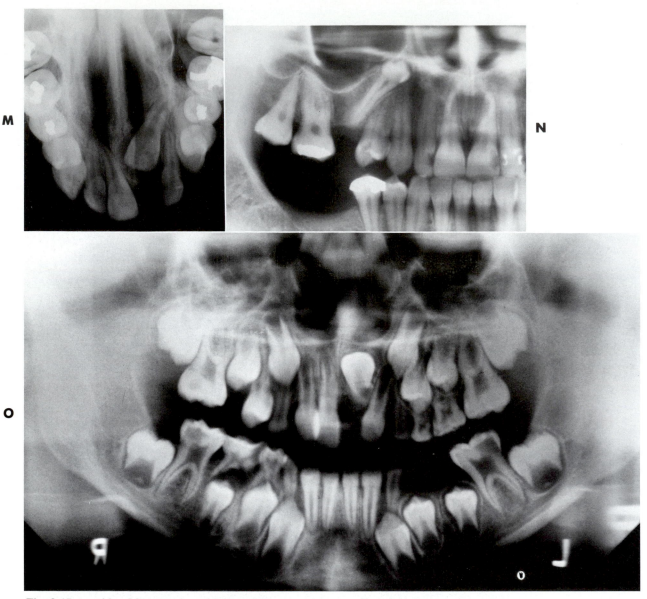

Fig. 3-17, cont'd. **M,** Impaction of left maxillary central incisor. **N,** Ectopic impacted maxillary second premolar. **O,** Ectopic impacted left maxillary central incisor.

Type of impaction (e.g., mesioangular, distoangular), as determined by the position of the long axis of the tooth relative to the occlusal plane

Premature Eruption

Presence of a tooth whose root is less than one-half formed (excess eruption for the amount of root formation)

Associated radiographic evidence for a local cause (e.g., adjacent haemangioma or neurofibroma) or clinical evidence of a systemic condition, such as hyperthyroidism, in cases of generalized premature eruption

Delayed Eruption

Presence of an unerupted tooth not exhibiting any local cause (e.g., ankylosis or suppression) in which the root is fully formed

In localized delayed eruption, affecting one or a few teeth, specific radiographic signs of coronal space-occupying lesions; generalized delayed eruption is more likely to be related to systemic abnormalities

ENAMEL PEARL

Overview

Definition and pathogenesis: Enamel pearls, also known (wrongly) as enamelomas, are classified by Pindborg as being either intradental, i.e., within the confines of the tooth, or extradental, i.e., projecting from the contour of the tooth. Extradental enamel pearls are more common and result from misplaced ameloblasts during tooth formation. Internal enamel pearls presumably result from entrapment of enamel-producing tissue within the expanding mesodermal portion of the tooth germ.

Clinical Features

Demographics and signs and symptoms: Both types of enamel pearls are uncommon but may be found at any point on the surface or within the tooth.

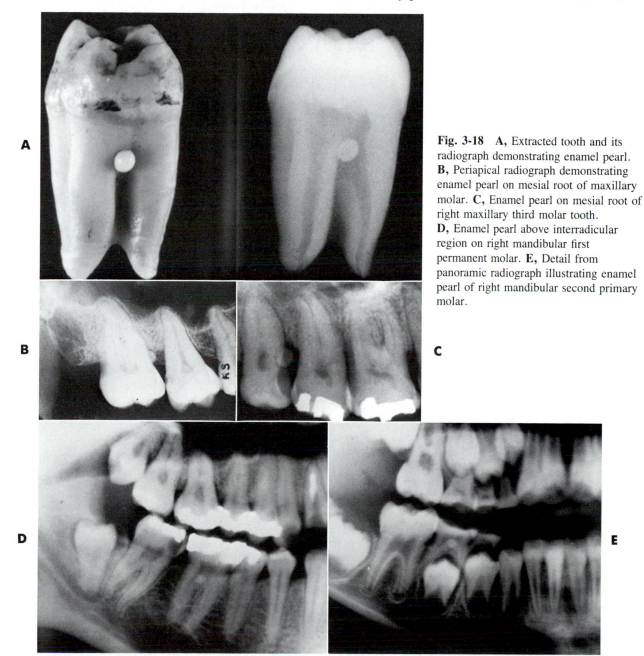

Fig. 3-18 A, Extracted tooth and its radiograph demonstrating enamel pearl. **B,** Periapical radiograph demonstrating enamel pearl on mesial root of maxillary molar. **C,** Enamel pearl on mesial root of right maxillary third molar tooth. **D,** Enamel pearl above interradicular region on right mandibular first permanent molar. **E,** Detail from panoramic radiograph illustrating enamel pearl of right mandibular second primary molar.

The most common site is at the cementoenamel junction of a multirooted maxillary tooth. When enamel pearls occur on multirooted teeth, they commonly do so on the mesial and distal surfaces of maxillary teeth and the buccal or lingual surfaces of mandibular teeth. Bilateral cases are common. Enamel pearls often occur singly and may be composed exclusively of enamel. They may include dentin and/or pulpal tissue also, in which case their radiographic shadow is changed. They vary in size from microscopic to a few millimeters in diameter.

RADIOLOGIC FEATURES

Cardinal Signs

> Dense, smooth globular radiopacity projecting from the normal root contour of an otherwise unaffected tooth
> Dense, smooth globular radiopacity overlying any portion of the crown or root of an otherwise unaffected tooth
> Dense, globular radiopacity within the confines of an otherwise normal tooth

Ancillary Signs

> Rarely, a radiolucent round lesion within the confines of the tooth, representing an uncalcified internal enamel pearl
> Lack of a homogeneous radiopacity does not rule out enamel pearls because many of them have dentinal and pulpal components

Differential Diagnosis

> Overlap of root contours in multirooted teeth
> Pulpal calcifications
> Radiopaque composite resin restorative materials

TALON CUSP

Overview

Definition: A tooth with a talon cusp appears to be T-shaped when viewed from the incisal edge. The condition involves incisor teeth in which a straight projection meets the lingual aspect of the incisal edge at a right angle. The incisal aspect of this projection blends smoothly with the normal incisor contour.

Pathogenesis: Talon cusp may be more common in patients with Rubinstein-Taybi syndrome.

Clinical Features

Signs and symptoms: From a clinical point of view, talon cusp is innocuous unless the tooth compromises appearance or fractures, in which case pulp exposure is likely. If the tooth is removed, the pulp is invariably exposed, in which case endodontic therapy is required.

RADIOLOGIC FEATURES

Cardinal Signs

> Crown shape with accentuation of the mesial and distal marginal ridges and mild notching of the incisal edge

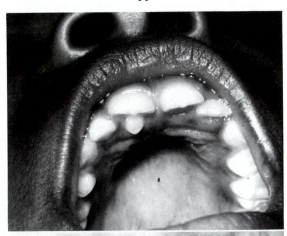

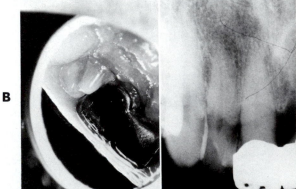

Fig. 3-19　A, Talon cusp on right maxillary central incisor. B, Talon cusp on right maxillary lateral incisor. C, Same patient as in B. Talon cusp on lateral incisor.

Dense radiopaque linear shadow extending from the incisal edge to the cingulum

Ancillary Signs
Pulpal extension into the incisolingual projection

Differential Diagnosis
No other condition results in precisely the same radiographic picture as talon cusp.

PULP STONES

Overview

Pulp stones are not so much a developmental dental anomaly as a variant of normal. In reality, freestanding pulp stones are uncommon. Radiographically, visible pulpal calcification extending from one of the dentinal walls may give the appearance of pulp stones.

Pathogenesis: The presence of pulp stones may be a function of age and is not related to systemic disease, infection, or restorative treatment of the teeth.

Clinical Features

Signs and symptoms: Clinically, the teeth appear perfectly normal and exhibit no increased incidence of pain. They require no special treatment, although endodontic therapy may be be difficult in patients with large pulp stones.

RADIOLOGIC FEATURES

Cardinal Signs
Radiopacity, with the density of tooth material in the pulp chamber (and, more rarely, the root canal system)

Ancillary Signs
Widening of the pulp chamber as it encompasses the pulpal calcification.

Differential Diagnosis
Enamel pearl
Overlapped radicular structures

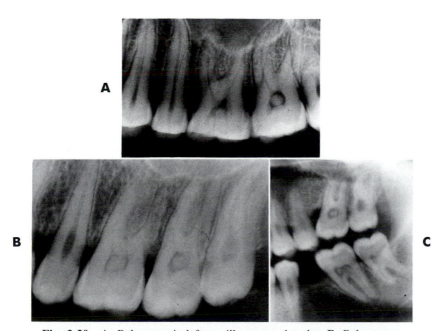

Fig. 3-20   A, Pulp stone in left maxillary second molar. **B,** Pulp stones in maxillary first and second molars. **C,** Pulp stones of maxillary and mandibular second molars. (First molars missing, presumed extracted.)

BIBLIOGRAPHY

Hypodontia

Cullen CL, Wesley RK: Russell-Silver syndrome associated with missing teeth, *ASDC J Dent Child* 54:201, 1987.

Dermaut LR, Goeffers KR, DeSmit AA: Prevalence of tooth agenesis correlated with jaw relationship and dental crowding, *Am J Orthod Dentofacial Orthop* 90:204, 1986.

Dorland's illustrated medical dictionary, ed 27, Philadelphia, 1985, W.B. Saunders, pp 92, 804.

Eidelman E, Chosack A, Wagner ML: Orodigitofacial dysostosis and oculodentodigital dysplasia, *Oral Surg Oral Med Oral Pathol* 23:311, 1967.

Gibson ACL: Concomitant hypo-hyperodontia, *Br J Orthod* 5:101, 1979.

Hellman M: Our third molar teeth: their eruption, presence and absence, *Dent Cosmos* 78:750, 1936.

Jarvinen S, Vaataja PH: Congenitally missing maxillary permanent cuspids, *Proc Finn Dent Soc* 2:11, 1979.

Lavelle CLB, Ashton EH, Flinn RM: Cusp pattern, tooth size and third molar agenesis in the human mandibular dentition, *Arch Oral Biol* 15:227, 1970.

Le Bot P, Salmon D: Congenital defects of the upper lateral incisors: condition and measurements of other teeth, measurements of superior arch, head and face, *Am J Phys Anthropol* 46:231, 1977.

Maklin M, Dummett O, Weinbergh R: A study of oligodontia in a sample of New Orleans children, *J Dent Child* 46:478, 1979.

Niswander JD, Sujaku C: Congenital anomalies of teeth in Japanese children, *Am J Phys Anthropol* 21:569, 1963.

Nortje CJ, et al: X-linked hypohydrotic ectodermal dysplasia—an unusual prosthetic problem, *J Prosthet Dent* 40:137, 1978.

Rappaport EB, Ultstrom R, Gorlin RJ: Monosuperocentroincisivodontic dwarfism, *Birth Defects* 12:243, 1976.

Rolling S: Hypodontia of permanent teeth in Danish school children, *Scand J Dent Res* 88:365, 1980.

Rose JS: A survey of congenitally missing teeth, excluding third molars, in 6,000 orthodontic patients, *Dent Practit Dent Rec* 17:107, 1966.

Ruprecht A, Batniji S, El-Neweihi E: Incidence of oligodontia (hypodontia), *J Oral Med* 41:143, 1986.

Sarnat H, Amir E, Legum CP: Developmental dental anomalies in chondroectodermal dysplasia (Ellis-van Crevald syndrome), *J Dent Child* 47:28, 1980.

Spitzer R: Observations on congenital dentofacial disorders in Mongolism and microcephaly, *Oral Surg Oral Med Oral Pathol* 24:325, 1967.

Werther R, Rothenberg F: Anodontia, *Am J Orthod* 25:61, 1939.

Worth HM: *Principles and practice of oral radiologic interpretation,* Chicago, 1963, Year Book Medical, p 101.

Supernumerary Teeth

Duncan BR, Dohner VA, Priest JH: The Gardner syndrome: need for early diagnosis, *J Pediatr* 72:497, 1968.

Fader M, et al: Gardner's syndrome (intestinal polyposis, osteomas, sebaceous cysts) and a new dental discovery, *Oral Surg Oral Med Oral Pathol* 15:153, 1962.

Farman AG, Nortje CJ, Joubert JJ: Missing central incisors, *Rhodesian Dent J* 3:4, 1979.

Pindborg JJ: *Pathology of the dental hard tissues,* Copenhagen, 1970, Munksgaard, pp 26-29.

Shafer WG, et al: *A textbook of oral pathology,* ed 4, Philadelphia, 1983, W.B. Saunders, p 47.

Wood RE, et al: *Handbook of signs in dental and maxillofacial radiology,* Toronto, 1988, Warthog Press.

Worth HM: *Principles and practice of oral radiologic interpretation,* Chicago, 1963, Year Book Medical, p 101.

Macrodontia

Dorland's illustrated medical dictionary, ed 27, Philadelphia, 1985, W.B. Saunders, p 969.

Rappaport EB, Ultstrom R, Gorlin RJ: Monosuperocentroincisivodontic dwarfism, *Birth Defects* 12:243, 1976.

Worth HM: *Principles and practice of oral radiologic interpretation,* Chicago, 1963, Year Book Medical, p 80.

Microdontia

Dorland's illustrated medical dictionary, ed 27, Philadelphia, 1985, W.B. Saunders, p 1033.

McGinnis JP, et al: Microdontia after mantle radiation, *Oral Surg Oral Med Oral Pathol* 63:630, 1987.

Shafer WG, et al: *Textbook of oral pathology,* ed 4, Philadelphia, 1983, W.B. Saunders, p 37.

Worth HM: *Principles and practice of oral radiologic interpretation,* Chicago, 1963, Year Book Medical, p 80.

Concrescence

Pindborg JJ: *Pathology of the dental hard tissues,* Copenhagen, 1970, Munksgaard, p 48.

Shafer WG, Hine MK, Levy BM: *Textbook of oral pathology,* ed 4, Philadelphia, 1983, W.B. Saunders, p 37.

Worth HM: *Principles and practice of oral radiologic interpretation,* Chicago, 1963, Year Book Medical, p 176.

Fusion

Lowell RJ, Soloman AL: Fused teeth, *J Am Dent Assoc* 68:762, 1964.

Mader CL: Fusion of the teeth, *J Am Dent Assoc* 98:62, 1979.

Pindborg JJ: *Pathology of the dental hard tissues,* Copenhagen, 1970, Munksgaard, p 48.

Shafer WG, et al: *Textbook of oral pathology,* ed 4, Philadelphia, 1983, W.B. Saunders, p 37.

Spouge JD: *Oral pathology,* St Louis, 1973, CV Mosby, p 134.

Gemination

Clayton JM: Congenital dental anomalies occurring in 3,557 children, *ASDC J Dent Child* 26:206, 1956.

von Hollaender K: Klinisch-roentgenologiische Untersuchung von drei Geschwistern mit Doppelbildung von Milchfrontzaehnen. *Dtsch Zahnartzl Z* 35:831, 1980.

Levitas TC: Gemination, fusion, twinning and concrescence, *ASDC J Dent Child* 32:93, 1965.

Ruprecht A, Batniji S, El-Neweihi E: Double teeth: the incidence of gemination and fusion, *J Pedod* 9:332, 1985.

Dens in Dente

Amos ER: Incidence of the small dens in dente, *J Am Dent Assoc* 51:31, 1955.

Atkinson SR: Permanent maxillary lateral incisors, *Am J Orthod Oral Surg* 29:685, 1943.

De Smit A, Jansen HWB, Dermaut L: An histological investigation of invaginated human incisors. *J Biol Buccale* 12:201, 1984.

Hallett GEM: The incidence, nature, and clinical significance of palatal invaginations in the maxillary incisor teeth, *Proc R Soc Med* 46:491, 1953.

Omnell KA, Swanbeck G, Lindahl B: Dens invaginatus II: a microradiographical, histological, micro x-ray diffraction study, *Acta Odontol Scand* 18:303, 1960.

Worth HM: *Principles and practice of oral radiologic interpretation,* Chicago, 1963, Year Book Medical, p 84.

Dens Evaginatus

Merrill RG: Occlusal anomalous tubercles on premolars of Alaskan Eskimos and Indians, *Oral Surg Oral Med Oral Pathol* 17:484, 1964.

Palmer ME: Case reports of evaginated odontomes in Caucasians, *Oral Surg Oral Med Oral Pathol* 35:772, 1973.

Pindborg JJ: *Pathology of the dental hard tissues,* Copenhagen, 1970, Munksgaard, p 65.

Yip WK: The prevalence of dens evaginatus, *Oral Surg Oral Med Oral Pathol* 38:80, 1974.

Taurodontism

Mangion JJ: Two cases of taurodontism in modern human jaws, *Br Dent J* 113:309, 1962.

Shafer WG, et al: *Textbook of oral pathology,* ed 4, Philadelphia, 1983, W.B. Saunders, p 43.

Dilaceration

Pindborg JJ: *Pathology of the dental hard tissues,* Copenhagen, 1970, Munksgaard, p 128.

Worth HM: *Principles and practice of oral radiologic interpretation,* Chicago, 1963, Year Book Medical, p 96.

Amelogenesis Imperfecta

Gibilisco JA: *Stafne's oral radiographic diagnosis,* Philadelphia, 1985, W.B. Saunders, p 35.

Witkop CJ, Sauk JJ: *Heritable defects in enamel.* In Stewart RE, Prescott GH, editors: *Oral facial genetics,* St Louis, 1976, Mosby–Year Book.

Worth HM: *Principles and practice of oral radiologic interpretation,* Chicago, 1963, Year Book Medical, p 86.

Environmental Enamel Hypoplasia

Fiumara NJ, Lessell S: Manifestations of late congenital syphilis, *Arch Dermatol* 102:78, 1970.

Miller J, Forrester RM: Neonatal enamel hypoplasia associated with hemolytic disease and with prematurity, *Br Dent J* 106:93, 1959.

Schour I: The neonatal line in the enamel and dentin of the human deciduous teeth and the first permanent molar, *J Am Dent Assoc* 23:1946, 1936.

Shafer WG, et al: *Textbook of oral pathology,* ed 4, Philadelphia, 1983, W.B. Saunders, p 53.

Shelling DH, Anderson GM: Relation of rickets and vitamin D to the incidence of dental caries, enamel hypoplasia, and malocclusion in children, *J Am Dent Assoc* 23:840, 1936.

Regional Odontodysplasia

Bergman G, Lysell L, Pindborg JJ: Unilateral dental malformation, *Oral Surg Oral Med Oral Pathol* 16:48, 1963.

Gould AR, Farman AG: Pericoronal features of regional odontodysplasia, *J Oral Med* 39:236, 1984.

Pindborg JJ: *Pathology of the dental hard tissues,* Copenhagen, 1970, Munksgaard, p 120.

Rushton MA: Odontodysplasia: "ghost teeth," *Br Dent J* 119:109, 1965.

Shafer WG, Hine MK, Levy BM: *Textbook of oral pathology,* ed 4, Philadelphia, 1983, W.B. Saunders, p 63.

Walton JL, Witkop CJ, Walker PO: Odontodysplasia, *Oral Surg Oral Med Oral Pathol* 46:676, 1978.

Dentinogenesis Imperfecta

Gibilisco JA: *Stafne's oral radiographic diagnosis,* Philadelphia, 1985, W.B. Saunders, p 34

Mendel R, Shawkat AH, Farman AG: Management of opalescent dentin, *J Am Dent Assoc* 102:53, 1981.

Perl T, Farman AG: Radicular dentin dysplasia, *Oral Surg Oral Med Oral Pathol* 43:746, 1977.

Shields ED, Bixler D, El-Kafrawy AM: A proposed classification for heritable human dentin defects with a description of a new entity, *Arch Oral Biol* 18:543, 1973.

Dentin Dysplasia

Logan J, et al: Dentinal dysplasia, *Oral Surg Oral Med Oral Pathol* 15:317, 1962.

Stafne EC, Gibilisco JA: Calcifications of the dentinal papilla that may cause anomalies of the roots of teeth, *Oral Surg Oral Med Oral Pathol* 14:683, 1961.

Witkop CJ, Sauk JJ: *Heritable defects of enamel*. In Stewart RE, Prescott GH, editors: *Oral facial genetics*, St Louis, 1976, Mosby–Year Book.

Anomalies of Eruption

Pindborg JJ: *Pathology of the dental hard tissues*, Copenhagen, 1970, Munksgaard, p 321.

Wood RE, et al: *Handbook of signs in dental and maxillofacial radiology*, Toronto, 1988, Warthog Press.

Enamel Pearl

Pindborg JJ: *Pathology of the dental hard tissues*, Copenhagen, 1970, Munksgaard, p 46.

Shafer WG, Hine MK, Levy BM: *Textbook of oral pathology*, ed 4, Philadelphia, 1983, W.B. Saunders, p 276.

Talon Cusp

Gardner DG, Girgis SS: Talon cusps: a dental anomaly in the Rubinstein-Taybi syndrome, *Oral Surg Oral Med Oral Pathol* 44:549, 1977.

Pulp Stone

Krestchner OS, Seybold JW: The bacteriology of dental pulp stones, *Dent Cosmos* 78:292, 1936.

Pindborg JJ: *Pathology of the dental hard tissues*, Copenhagen, 1970, Munksgaard, p 189.

Shafer WG, Hine MK, Levy BM: *Textbook of oral pathology*, ed 4, Philadelphia, 1983, W.B. Saunders, p 325.

Stafne EC, Szabo SE: The significance of pulp nodules, *Dent Cosmos* 75:160, 1933.

4

DEVELOPMENTAL ANOMALIES OF THE SKULL AND JAWS

ACHONDROPLASIA

Overview

Definition: Achondroplasia is a skeletal condition involving disordered growth of cartilage.

Pathogenesis: Achondroplasia may be familial in origin or result from nutritional deficiency. Familial achondroplasia is inherited as a mendelian dominant trait, with about half of the offspring of an affected parent being affected.

Clinical Features

Symptoms and signs: In familial achondroplasia there is disordered growth of epiphyseal cartilage in the long bones. The ribs and sphenoethmoidal synchondrosis in the base of the skull also show premature ossification. The primary defect is retardation, or even aplasia, of the zone of provisional calcification of endochondral growth.

Premature ossification in familial achondroplasia permanently limits skeletal development. Achondroplastic dwarves, the most common type of dwarf, have disproportionately short, thick arms and bowed legs with prominent buttocks; a normal-sized trunk with protruding abdomen; lumbar lordosis; a large, brachycephalic head with a protruding forehead; a small face with depressed nasal bridge; and small trident hands with stubby fingers. Because growth of the base of the skull is restricted, the maxilla is often retruded and hypoplastic; this leads to a relative man-

dibular prognathism with concomitant malocclusion and anterior open bite. The dentition is usually normal, though minor dental anomalies such as supernumerary teeth, oligodontia, embedded permanent teeth, and morphologic variations (all perhaps incidental findings) have occasionally been documented. There is usually no involvement of the central nervous system, and intelligence is unaffected.

RADIOLOGIC FEATURES

Cardinal Signs

Short appendicular bones
Thickening and mild clubbing at ends of long bones
Shortened base of skull
Narrowed foramen magnum
Maxillary hypoplasia

Ancillary Signs

Malocclusion; crowding of teeth
Relative mandibular prognathism
Depressed nasal bridge
Frontal bossing
Multiple supplemental teeth
Wormian bones in calvarium
Lumbar lordosis

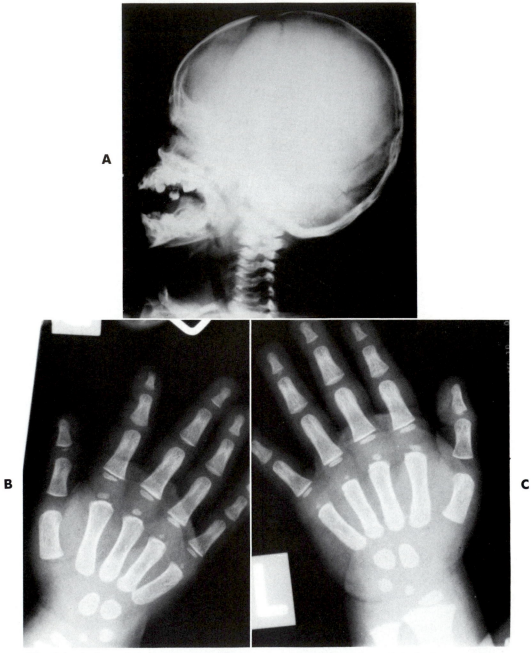

Fig. 4-1 **A,** Lateral skull radiograph illustrating achondroplasia. Note relatively depressed nasal bridge, frontal bossing, and short cranial base. Wormian bones are evident in the base of the skull. **B** and **C,** Hand-wrist films of patient in **A.** Note phalanges are relatively short with terminal clubbing.

Differential Diagnosis

Achondrogenesis
Thanatrophic dwarfism
Ellis-van Creveld syndrome
Metatrophic dwarfism
Diastrophic dwarfism
Hypochondroplasia
Pseudoachondroplasia

APERT SYNDROME (ACROCEPHALOSYNDACTYLY TYPE I)

Overview

Definition: Apert syndrome is a rare developmental condition characterized by premature cranial synostosis and resultant growth disturbances. Syndactyly is also present.

Clinical Features

Symptoms and signs: Signs of Apert syndrome include a peaked and vertically elongated head, widespread bulging eyes, and a protuberant frontal region with an anteroposterior ridge overhanging the frontal eminence. There is hypoplasia of the maxilla with relative mandibular prognathism. The palate is high, arched, and occasionally cleft. Dental malocclusion with crowding and delayed dental eruption in the maxilla are common. The facial angle is exaggerated; the nose is small and has been compared to a parrot's beak in appearance. Hypertelorism, exophthalmos, and divergent strabismus are often present, sometimes with blindness. Spina bifida has been recorded in some patients. Syndactyly of the hands and feet varies greatly and can be complete with apparent fusion of all digits externally. The patient may be retarded or of normal intelligence. Apert syndrome may be associated with advanced paternal age.

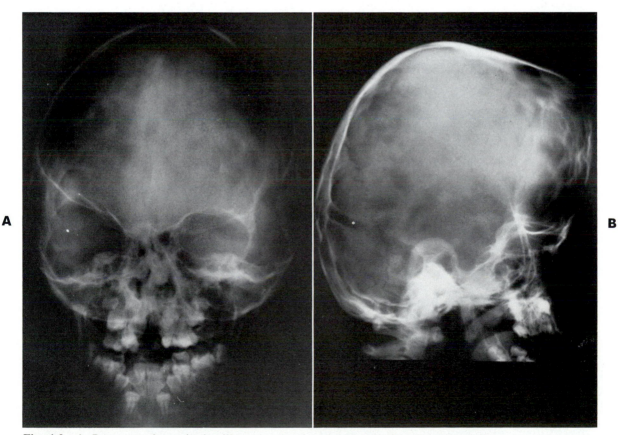

A   **B**

Fig. 4-2   A, Posteroanterior projection illustrating Apert syndrome. Note the tall (turricephalic) skull, open metopic suture, and faint beaten-silver appearance of the calvarium. **B,** Lateral skull radiograph of patient in **A.** The patient has turribrachycephaly. Skull base and roof of the calvarium are flattened, with a noticeable beaten-silver appearance in this projection. Note the hypoplastic maxilla.

Continued.

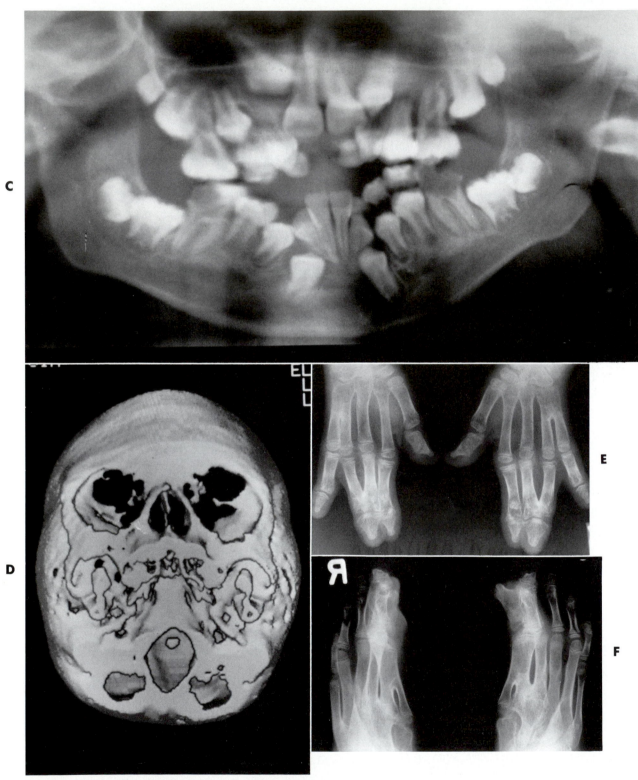

Fig. 4-2, cont'd.   For legends see opposite page.

RADIOLOGIC FEATURES

Cardinal Signs

Brachycephaly
Turricephaly/Oxycephaly
Beaten-silver appearance of calvarium
Absence of demonstrable cranial sutures in coronal
    dimension in young patients
Hypoplastic maxilla
Syndactyly of hands and feet

Ancillary Signs

Posterior flattening of skull
Lateral bulging of skull
Open anterior fontanelle
Late closure of metopic suture
Posterior cleft palate
Relative mandibular prognathism
Overcrowding of dentition
Retarded dental eruption

Differential Diagnosis

Craniofacial dysostosis (Crouzon disease)
Pfeiffer syndrome
Carpenter syndrome
Summitt syndrome

CAFFEY DISEASE (INFANTILE CORTICAL HYPEROSTOSIS)

Overview

Definition: Caffey disease is an unusual cortical thickening of uncertain etiology occurring in the bones of infants.

Pathogenesis: Caffey disease may result from an embryonal osteodysgenesis following a local disrup-

tion to the blood supply in the area. Alternatively, it may be an inherited arteriolar defect causing hypoxia and subsequent focal necrosis of overlying soft tissues with periosteal proliferation. The occurrence of multiple cases in several generations of single families supports a hereditary pattern, possibly autosomal dominant with incomplete penetrance. Sporadic cases have also been noted.

Clinical Features

Demographics: Caffey disease usually arises during the first 3 months of life, but may not appear until as late as the second year. About one in four cases is present at birth. Boys are affected more frequently than girls.

Symptoms and signs: The disease is characterized by tender, deeply placed soft tissue swelling with subjacent cortical thickening or hyperostosis. In sporadic cases, the mandible, ulna, and clavicle are most commonly affected. When the mandible is affected, there is associated facial swelling; a residual asymmetric deformity may be present even years after the disease has subsided. In familial cases, however, the lower limbs are most frequently affected. Other bones reported as being involved include the calvarium, ribs, scapula, and metatarsals. Sometimes Caffey disease is associated with such signs and symptoms as pyrexia, hyperirritability, pseudoparalysis, dysphagia, pleurisy, anemia, leukocytosis, monocytosis, elevated erythrocyte sedimentation rate, and raised serum alkaline phosphatase level. Usually the disease subsides in a few days with no aftereffects.

RADIOLOGIC FEATURES

Cardinal Signs

Hyperostosis
"Reduplication" of cortex (so-called onion-skin appearance) with persistence of original outline of
    the jaw
Gross thickening and sclerosis of cortex

Ancillary Signs

Often bilateral
Granular appearance of new bone
Dental malocclusion
Adjacent soft tissue swelling
Mandibular asymmetry
Opacification of bone on periapical views because
    of increased girth of bone

Fig. 4-2, cont'd. **C,** Panoramic radiograph of patient in **A.** There is crowding of the dental arches. **D,** 3-D CT reconstruction of patient with Apert syndrome. Note the hypoplastic maxilla with posterior cleft. **E,** Hand films in Apert syndrome showing syndactyly with fusion of three fingers in both hands and webbing. **F,** Syndactyly of feet in same patient as in **E.**

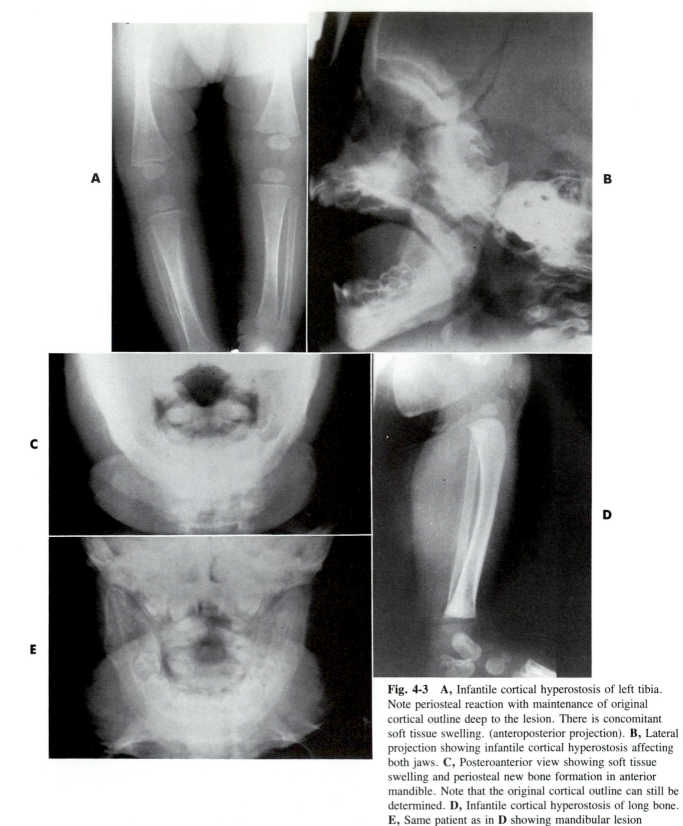

Fig. 4-3 **A,** Infantile cortical hyperostosis of left tibia. Note periosteal reaction with maintenance of original cortical outline deep to the lesion. There is concomitant soft tissue swelling. (anteroposterior projection). **B,** Lateral projection showing infantile cortical hyperostosis affecting both jaws. **C,** Posteroanterior view showing soft tissue swelling and periosteal new bone formation in anterior mandible. Note that the original cortical outline can still be determined. **D,** Infantile cortical hyperostosis of long bone. **E,** Same patient as in **D** showing mandibular lesion (posteroanterior projection).

Differential Diagnosis

Scurvy
Rickets
Syphilis
Bacterial osteitis
Neoplasia including osteogenic sarcoma
Traumatic injury with callus
Hypervitaminosis A
Fibrous dysplasia
Diffuse idiopathic sclerosis of dysproteinemia

CHERUBISM

Overview

Definition: Cherubism is a hereditary condition characterized by progressive bilateral swelling at the mandibular angle during childhood.

Pathogenesis: Inheritance is probably autosomal dominant with variable expressivity; however, sporadic cases also have been reported.

Clinical Features

Symptoms and signs: Cherubism becomes apparent during early childhood, generally by 4 years of age. There is progressive, painless, and usually symmetric firm swelling of the jaws. In most cases only the mandible is involved but occasionally the maxilla is affected, and there may be palatal enlargement. No other elements of the skeleton are involved. Oral man-

Text continued on page 113.

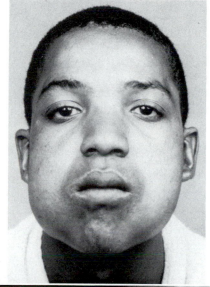

A

Fig. 4-4   A, Clinical features of cherubism include vertical and horizontal enlargement of the lower jaw. **B,** Panoramic radiograph of same patient as in **A.** Note bilateral multilocular radiolucencies at angles of mandible, occupying much of the rami but sparing the condyles. The right first and left second molars are displaced.

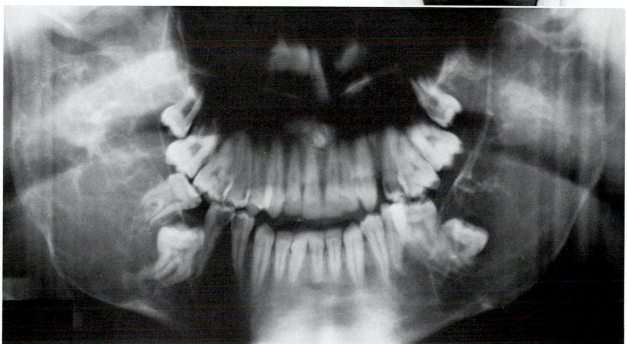

B

Continued.

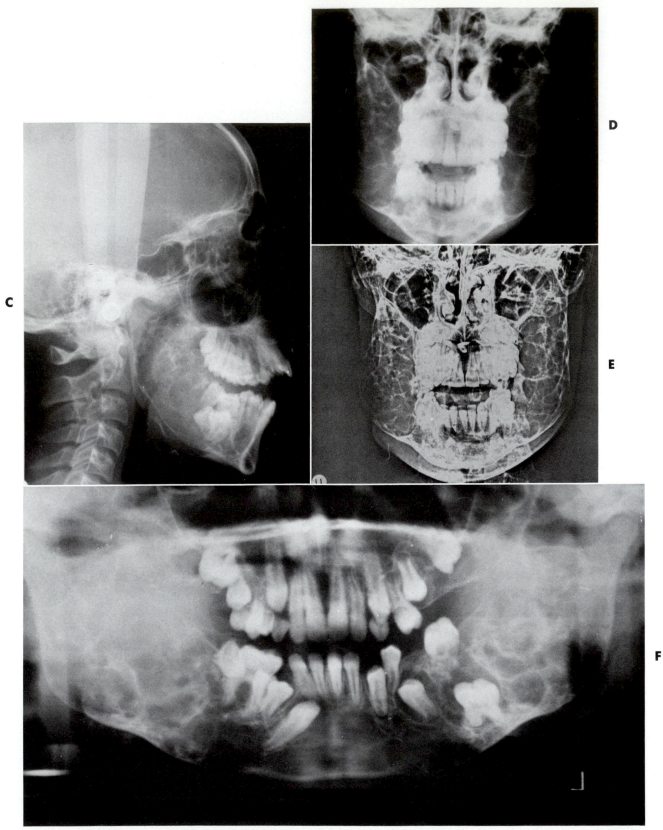

Fig. 4-4, cont'd. For legends see opposite page.

ifestations sometimes include premature shedding of primary teeth and displacement and lack of eruption of involved permanent teeth. The covering mucosa is normal in color and consistency. Diagnosis is made by clinical and radiographic findings as well as the family history. Serologic evaluations for calcium, phosphorus, and alkaline phosphatase are within normal limits. Histologic evaluation is only necessary in the rare unilateral cases.

RADIOLOGIC FEATURES

Cardinal Signs

Bilateral multilocular radiolucencies at angles of mandible

Displaced permanent teeth and toothbuds, especially mandibular first permanent molars, which are almost always displaced mesially

Mandibular enlargement in both vertical and lateral directions

Ancillary Signs

Sparing of the mandibular condyles

Opacification on maturation in fourth decade

Cystlike radiolucencies in maxillary tuberosities

Impacted permanent teeth

Displacement of mandibular canals

Resorption of roots of adjacent teeth

Premature exfoliation of primary teeth

Rarely, unilateral distribution

Differential Diagnosis

Odontogenic keratocyst – basal cell nevus (Gorlin-Goltz) syndrome

Central giant cell granuloma

Ameloblastoma

Ameloblastic fibroma

Fig. 4-4, cont'd. **C,** Lateral skull radiograph demonstrating multilocular radiolucencies of mandibular rami and radiolucency of maxillary tuberosity region. Note displacement of permanent molars. **D,** Posteroanterior radiograph showing bilateral multilocular radiolucencies in cherubism. **E,** Xeroradiograph of patient in **D** defines the locularity of the lesions with better edge detail. **F,** Panoramic radiograph demonstrating extensive lesions of cherubism. Tooth displacement is marked, and there is some external tooth root resorption. Radiolucencies are also seen in the maxillary tuberosities. Again, the mandibular condyles are spared.

Odontogenic myxoma

Odontogenic keratocyst

Aneurysmal bone cyst

Fibrous dysplasia

CLEFT PALATE

Overview

Definition: Cleft palate is a defect in the continuity of the palate resulting from development or maturation of embryonal processes. It is often but not invariably accompanied by cleft lip.

Pathogenesis: Cleft palate may be an isolated occurrence or may be part of various specific syndromes.

Clinical Features

Demographics: Cleft palate occurs in about 1 in 1,000 live births. It is reportedly most common in the Japanese and least common in blacks.

Symptoms and signs: Cleft palate varies greatly in severity and tissue involvement. The hard or soft palate, or a combination of both, can be affected. Frequently, clefts of the hard palate extend anteriorly through the alveolar ridge and lip, deviating to the right or left in the premaxilla. Sometimes, although much less often, the premaxillary defect is bilateral. On occasion only the soft palate or a bifid uvula is involved. When the alveolar ridge is affected, teeth in the region can be missing, deformed, or displaced, or supernumerary teeth can be present. In about half of cases, other developmental abnormalities are present. These include a variety of specific syndromes, congenital heart defects, polydactyly or syndactyly, hydrocephalus, spina bifida, and mental deficiency.

RADIOLOGIC FEATURES
Cardinal Signs

Elongated radiolucency with clearly corticated margins

Loss of continuity in floor of nose.

Ancillary Signs

Maxillary hypoplasia apparent in lateral skull views as retrognathic maxilla

Missing, deformed, or supernumerary teeth adjacent to the cleft site

Differential Diagnosis

Various syndromes with clefting

Trauma or surgical defect

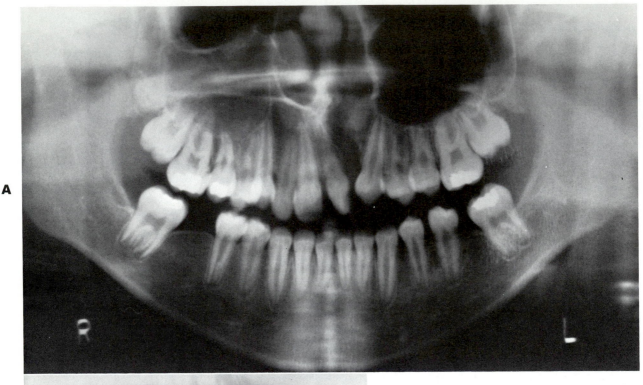

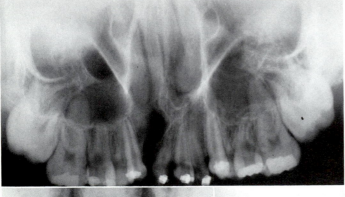

Fig. 4-5   A, Panoramic radiograph showing unilateral cleft palate on left side. The lateral incisor normally present in that site is missing, and the adjacent central incisor is rotated. **B,** Status-X intraoral source panoramic radiograph of maxilla showing unilateral cleft in anterior palate. **C,** Topographic occlusal radiograph showing bilateral cleft palate. The lateral incisors are displaced and impacted. **D,** Bilateral cleft palate resulting in maxillary hypoplasia with retrognathia seen on lateral cephalometric radiograph of young infant.

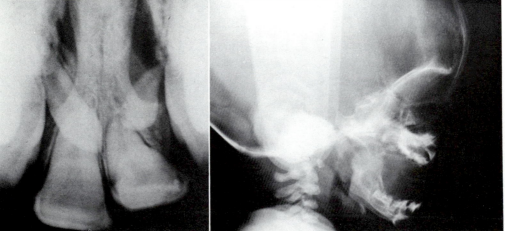

CLEIDOCRANIAL DYSPLASIA

Overview

Definition: Cleidocranial dysplasia (or dysostosis) is characterized by defective ossification of the cranial bones and complete or partial absence of the clavicles.

Pathogenesis: Cleidocranial dysplasia is usually, but not invariably, transmitted as an autosomal dominant trait.

Clinical Features

Demographics: Men and women are affected with equal frequency.

Symptoms and signs: Defective ossification of the cranial bones delays closure of the cranial sutures, resulting in fontanelles remaining open or showing delayed closure. Hence the fontanelles tend to be large. A characteristically sunken sagittal suture gives the skull a flat appearance. The skull is also brachycephalic with prominent frontal, occipital, and parietal bones. The paranasal sinuses are underdeveloped and narrow. The clavicles are usually hypoplastic, especially at their medial ends, and are completely absent in 10% of patients. This allows an unusual mobility of the shoulders, with affected individuals often being able to bring their shoulders forward until they meet in the midline. Cleidocranial dysplasia was once thought to involve only membrane bones but now is recognized to affect other parts of the skeleton. Defects have been found quite frequently in the vertebral column, digits, and long bones of affected persons.

Intraoral examination characteristically reveals a narrow, high-arched palate. Clefts are not infrequent, and mandibular prognathism is usually present. The most evident orodental findings, however, involve the dentitions. There is prolonged retention of deciduous teeth and numerous unerupted regular permanent and supernumerary teeth. Associated supernumerary teeth are more prevalent in the incisor and mandibular premolar regions.

RADIOLOGIC FEATURES

Cardinal Signs

Multiple supernumerary teeth in jaws anterior to first permanent molar

Supplementary supernumerary teeth resembling regular premolars in posterior segments

Conical supernumerary teeth in anterior segments

Retained primary teeth

Unerupted permanent teeth or delayed eruption

Fig. 4-6 **A,** Clinical features of child with cleidocranial dysplasia. The child can bring the shoulders together towards the midline because of the absence of clavicles. **B,** Chest radiograph of patient in **A.** Note absence of clavicles.

A
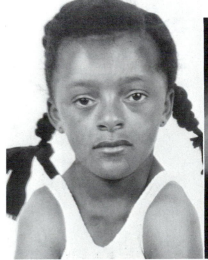

B
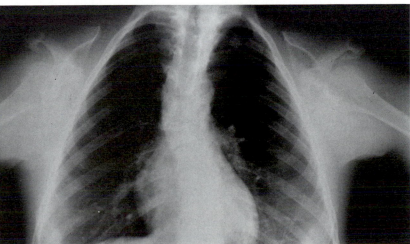

Continued.

Fig. 4-6, cont'd. **C,** Posteroanterior radiograph of patient in **A.** Note the multiple unerupted teeth in both arches, the "light bulb" shape of the skull, the open anterior fontanelle, and the depressed vault of the skull. **D,** Lateral skull radiograph of patient in **A.** The maxilla and maxillary sinuses are hypoplastic and there is a relative mandibular prognathism. **E,** Panoramic radiograph of patient in **A.** There are multiple supplemental premolars in both dental arches, delayed eruption of permanent teeth, and prolonged retention of primary teeth. Note the persistence of a median mandibular suture.

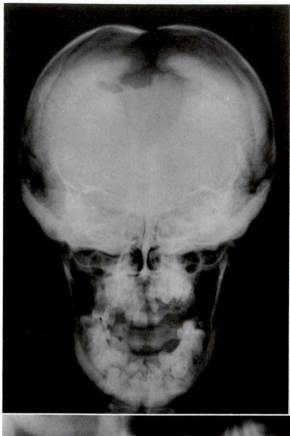

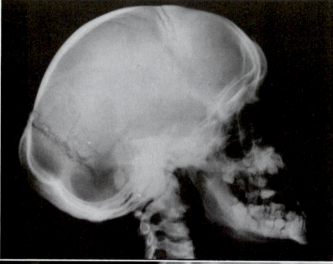

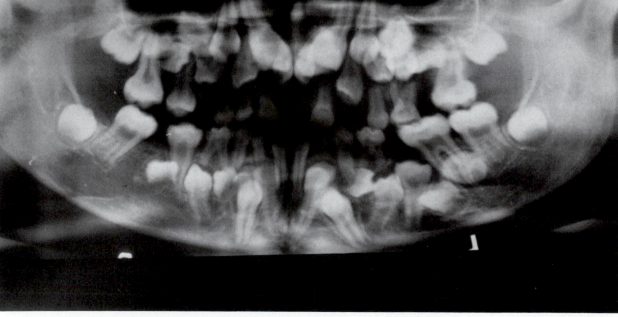

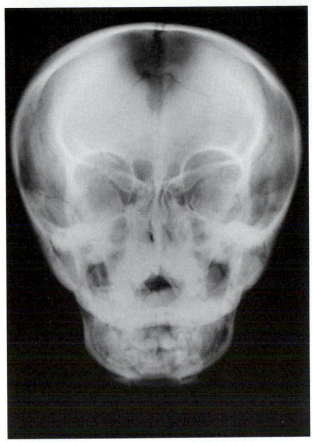

Fig. 4-6, cont'd.   F, Posteroanterior radiograph of mother of patient in **A.** Note persistence of the anterior fontanelle and the metopic suture. Wormian bones are evident in the skull.

Delayed closure of fontanelles
Hypoplasia or aplasia of clavicles
"Light bulb" head on posteroanterior skull view

Ancillary Signs
   Lateral splaying of coronoid processes when viewed posteroanteriorly
   Brachycephaly
   Vertebral abnormalities
   Long bone abnormalities
   Digital abnormalities
   Cleft palate
   Mandibular prognathism
   Wormian cranial bones
   Persistent metopic suture
   Small paranasal sinuses

Small maxilla with retrognathism
Delayed or failed closure of median mandibular suture
Basilar invagination
Depressed nasal bridge
Cyst formation around unerupted teeth
Gemination of teeth
Dilaceration of teeth

Differential Diagnosis
   Gardner syndrome

CRANIOFACIAL DYSOSTOSIS (CROUZON DISEASE)

Overview
   Definition: Craniofacial dysostosis is the most common genetic disease involving premature craniosynostosis without syndactyly.
   Pathogenesis: Most cases of craniofacial dysostosis, but not all, are transmitted in an autosomal dominant manner.

Clinical Features
   Symptoms and signs: Patients have a protuberant frontal bone with an anteroposterior ridge overhanging the frontal eminence, brachyturricephaly, and maxillary hypoplasia with mandibular prognathism. The palate is narrow and higharched with clefting in some instances. The nose is small and shaped like a parrot's beak. Ocular changes include hypertelorism, exophthalmos, and divergent strabismus. Optic neuritis and choked disks can result in blindness. Patients may have normal intelligence or mental retardation. Other anomalies, such as spina bifida, have occasionally been reported.

RADIOLOGIC FEATURES

Cardinal Signs
   Brachyturricephaly
   Hypertelorism
   Maxillary hypoplasia
   Beaten-silver appearance of skull
   Absence of cranial sutures (premature synostosis)
   Thin cranial walls
   Small maxillary sinuses
   Mandibular prognathism
   Cleft palate

Text continued on page 119.

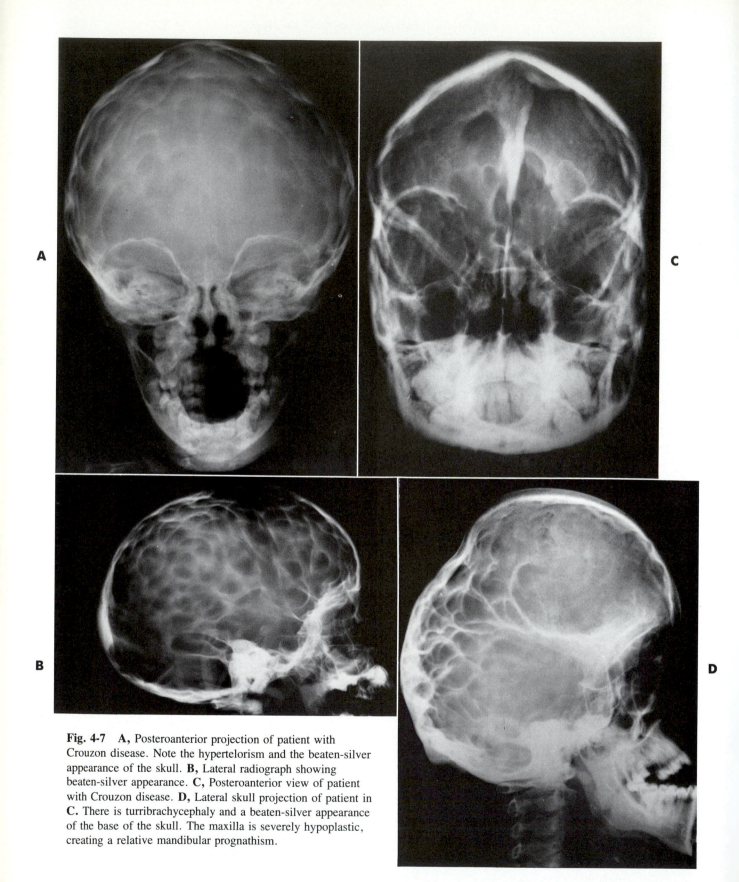

Fig. 4-7 **A,** Posteroanterior projection of patient with Crouzon disease. Note the hypertelorism and the beaten-silver appearance of the skull. **B,** Lateral radiograph showing beaten-silver appearance. **C,** Posteroanterior view of patient with Crouzon disease. **D,** Lateral skull projection of patient in **C.** There is turribrachycephaly and a beaten-silver appearance of the base of the skull. The maxilla is severely hypoplastic, creating a relative mandibular prognathism.

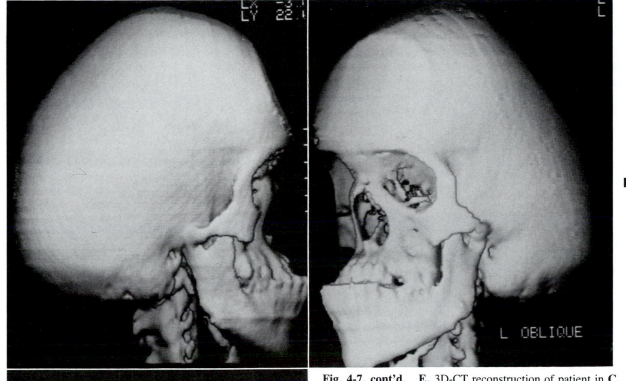

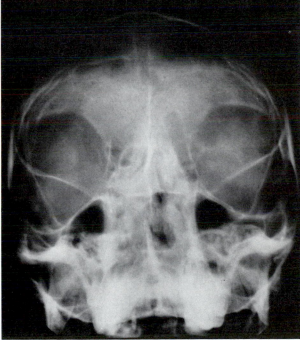

Fig. 4-7, cont'd. E, 3D-CT reconstruction of patient in **C.** Note turribrachycephaly and maxillary hypoplasia with relative mandibular prognathism. **F,** 3D-CT reconstruction of patient in **C,** further demonstrating hypoplasia of the midface, relative mandibular prognathism, and turribrachycephaly. **G,** Posteroanterior projection with Waters correction. This illustrates the extreme hypertelorism found in some cases of Crouzon disease.

Ancillary Signs

    Oligodontia

    Macrodontia

    Widely spaced teeth

    Flattened or shallow orbit on lateral view

Differential Diagnosis

    Simple craniostenosis

    Apert syndrome

    Pyknodysostosis

    Pfeiffer syndrome

    Saerthre-Chotzen syndrome

ECTODERMAL DYSPLASIAS

Overview

Definition: Ectodermal dysplasias are developmental abnormalities affecting tissues of ectodermal origin, including the skin, dermal appendages, and dentition.

Pathogenesis: There are at least 40 ectodermal dysplasias with various inheritance patterns. The most common is X-linked recessive, which is carried as a trait by the mother and has full expression in 1 in 2 sons.

Clinical Features

Symptoms and signs: Dysplasia of ectodermal tissues can cause abnormal hair (trichodysplasia), abnormal teeth (microdontia) or missing teeth (oligodontia or anodontia), and abnormal or missing sweat glands (hypohidrosis or anhidrosis). At least two of these components must be present to diagnose the condition as an ectodermal dysplasia. Patients with hypohidrotic, X-linked recessive ectodermal dysplasia have thin, dry skin with partial or complete absence of the sweat glands, which inhibits perspiration. Such individuals suffer from hyperpyrexia with an inability to endure warm climates. Sebaceous glands, hair follicles, and salivary glands may also be defective. Mucous gland hypoplasia can result in xerostomia, chronic rhinitis, and pharyngitis with hoarseness. The hair of the scalp and eyebrows is generally scant, fine, and blond. The bridge of the nose is depressed and there is frontal bossing and prominent lips resulting from a reduced vertical dimension of the face. The latter is a consequence of oligodontia and the absence of alveolar bone. The lips may be dry and cracked with pseudorhagades.

RADIOLOGIC FEATURES

Cardinal Signs
Oligodontia or anodontia
Diminutive and conical or peg-shaped teeth
Frontal bossing

Ancillary Signs
Diminished or absent alveolar support bone
Disproportionately large calvarium compared with facial complex
Retarded dental eruption

Differential Diagnosis
Sporadic oligodontia
Radiation therapy in childhood
Chondroectodermal dysplasia
Cleidocranial dysplasia

Text continued on page 122.

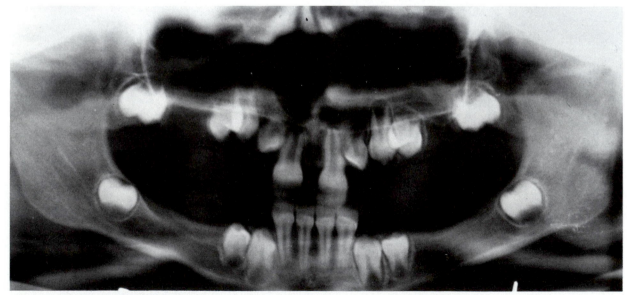

A

Fig. 4-8 A, Panoramic radiograph of patient with ectodermal dysplasia. Note oligodontia and diminutive lateral incisors.

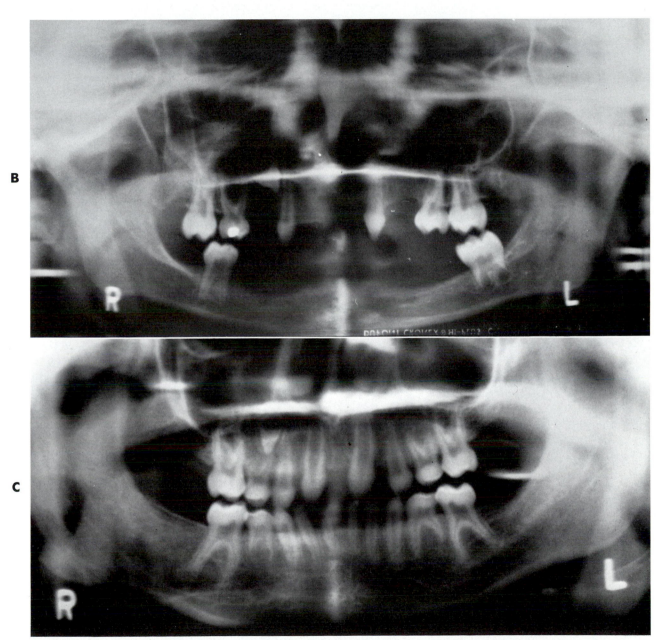

Fig. 4-8, cont'd.   B, Panoramic radiograph showing oligodontia and conical maxillary anterior teeth in patient with ectodermal dysplasia. **C,** Oligodontia and conical anterior teeth in patient with ectodermal dysplasia (panoramic radiograph).   *Continued.*

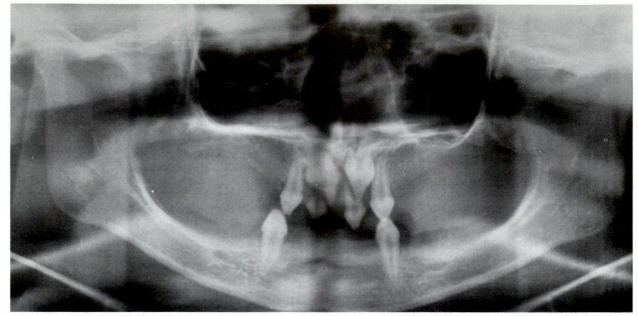

D

Fig. 4-8, cont'd.   D, Panoramic radiograph showing almost complete absence of teeth in patient with ectodermal dysplasia.

FRONTONASAL MALFORMATION

Overview

Definition: Frontonasal malformation refers to a variety of developmental conditions leading to a triangular defect in the frontal bone, with marked hypertelorism and partial or complete division of the nose.

Pathogenesis: The condition is a developmental field defect, probably occurring between 21 and 70 days of uterine life, rather than an individual syndrome. As such the etiology and pathogenesis are probably heterogeneous.

Clinical Features

Symptoms and signs: Frontonasal malformation has been defined as a combination of two or more of the following characteristics: (a) hypertelorism, (b) broadened nasal bridge, (c) median facial cleft affecting the nose or both the nose and upper lip and sometimes the palate, (d) unilateral or bilateral clefting of the nasal alae, (e) lack of formation of the nasal tip, (f) anterior cranium bifidum occultum, and (g) V-shaped hairline prolongation onto the middle of the forehead. The phenotype can be associated with frontal encephalocele, frontal teratoma, frontal lipoma, early ossification of the lesser wings of the sphenoid,

craniosynostosis, enlarged ethmoidal sinuses, and primary deformity of the nasal capsule. Most cases occur sporadically, but some, as part of the syndromes of craniofrontonasal dysplasia, ophthalmofrontonasal dysplasia, and Greig cephalopolysyndactyly, exhibit a familial pattern.

RADIOLOGIC FEATURES

Cardinal Signs

   Hypertelorism
   Frontal bossing
   Delayed closure of metopic suture
   Broad nasal bridge

Ancillary Signs

   Asymmetric coronal synostosis
   Hypoplastic paranasal sinuses
   Hypoplastic nasal bones
   Palatal cleft
   Broad halluces
   Thoracolumbar scoliosis
   Asymmetric sacrum and pubic bones
   Small iliac bones

Differential Diagnosis

   Oculodentoosseous dysplasia
   Mucopolysaccharoidoses

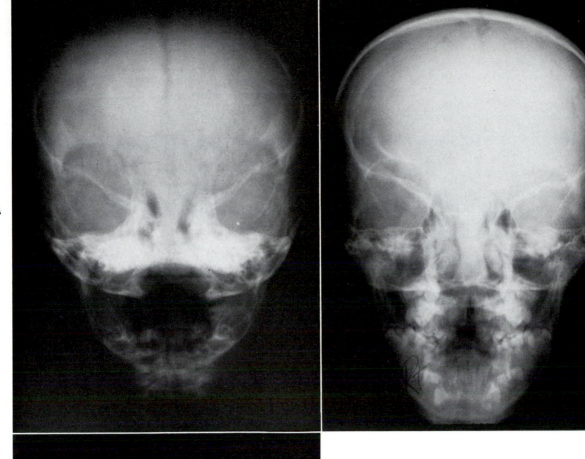

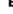

B

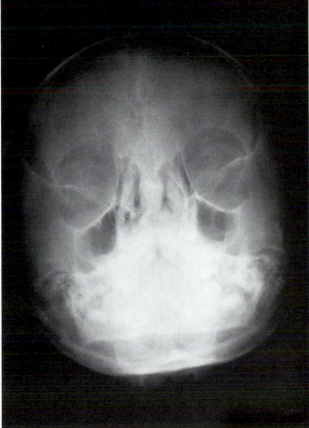

Fig. 4-9 A, Posteroanterior view of frontonasal malformation showing hypertelorism, widened nasal bridge, and persistence of the metopic suture.
B, Posteroanterior view of frontonasal malformation. Note persistence of anterior fontanelle and widened nasal bridge, with concomitant hypertelorism. **C,** Waters view of patient with frontonasal malformation. The maxillary sinuses are hypoplastic. There is marked hypertelorism and a widened nasal bridge.

GARDNER SYNDROME INTESTINAL POLYPOSIS TYPE II

Overview

Pathogenesis: Gardner syndrome is a disease complex caused by a single pleiotropic gene with autosomal dominant inheritance, complete penetrance, and variable expressivity.

Clinical Features

Symptoms and signs: Gardner syndrome consists of multiple polyposis of the large intestines; osteomas of bones including the limbs, skull, and jaws; multiple epidermoid or sebaceous cysts of skin, especially on the back; occasional desmoid tumors; and occasional multiple supernumerary teeth with consequent dental impactions. The intestinal polyps, which are present in 85% of patients, are premalignant. Because the first features of the disease may be osteomas of the jaws or supernumerary teeth, the dentist may be the first to make the tentative diagnosis. Through appropriate referral, the patient's prognosis can be improved by early detection of the premalignant intestinal polyps.

RADIOLOGIC FEATURES

Cardinal Signs

Multiple osteomas
Intestinal polyposis demonstrated by lower gastrointestinal tract radiographic series

Ancillary Signs

Multiple supernumerary teeth
Pericoronal radiolucency/dentigerous cysts
Dental impactions (usually multiple)
Hypercementosis
Compound odontomas

Differential Diagnosis

Florid osseous dysplasia
Paget disease of bone
Craniofacial fibrous dysplasia
Cleidocranial dysplasia

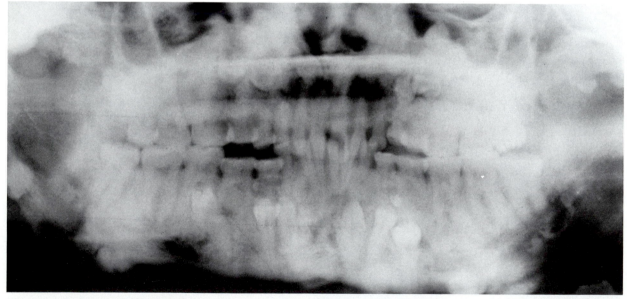

Fig. 4-10 A, Panoramic radiograph of patient with Gardner syndrome, showing multiple osteomas in both jaws, retained primary teeth, and multiple impacted permanent teeth.

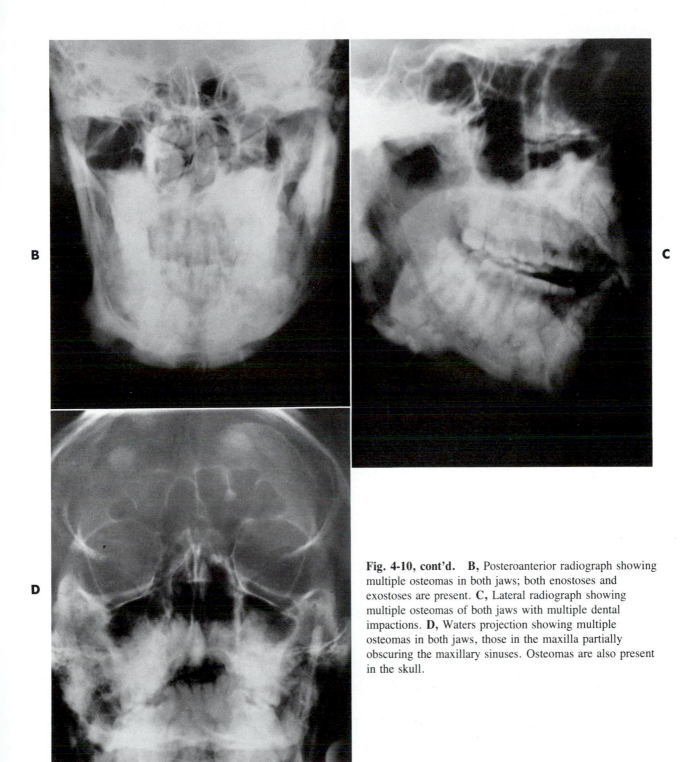

Fig. 4-10, cont'd.   B, Posteroanterior radiograph showing multiple osteomas in both jaws; both enostoses and exostoses are present. **C,** Lateral radiograph showing multiple osteomas of both jaws with multiple dental impactions. **D,** Waters projection showing multiple osteomas in both jaws, those in the maxilla partially obscuring the maxillary sinuses. Osteomas are also present in the skull.

GOLDENHAR SYNDROME (HEMIFACIAL MICROSOMIA)

Overview

Definition: Goldenhar syndrome is a generally sporadic congenital condition with unilateral mandibular hypoplasia.

Pathogenesis: The condition probably results from a vascular supply deficiency during development.

Clinical Features

Symptoms and signs: Patients with Goldenhar syndrome have asymmetry of the face with a shortened mandible and ipsilateral defects in adjacent structures such as the ear. Affected individuals may be partially or fully deaf and have temporomandibular joint hypoplasia.

RADIOLOGIC FEATURES

Cardinal Signs

Unilateral mandibular, maxillary, and malar hypoplasia.

Absence of glenoid fossa of skull (unilateral)

Ancillary Signs

Cleft lip or palate

Micrognathia

Microtia

Differential Diagnosis

Pierre Robin syndrome

Mandibulofacial dysostosis (Treacher Collins syndrome)

Weyers mandibulofacial dysostosis

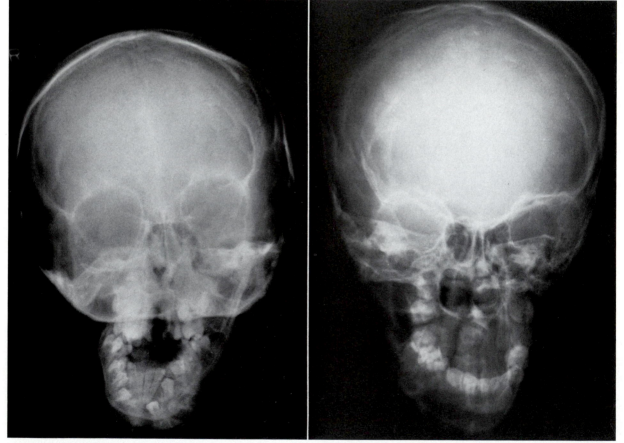

Fig. 4-11   A, Posteroanterior radiograph of patient with Goldenhar syndrome, showing unilateral maxillary, mandibular, and malar hypoplasia. **B,** Posteroanterior radiograph showing unilateral maxillary, mandibular, and malar hypoplasia.

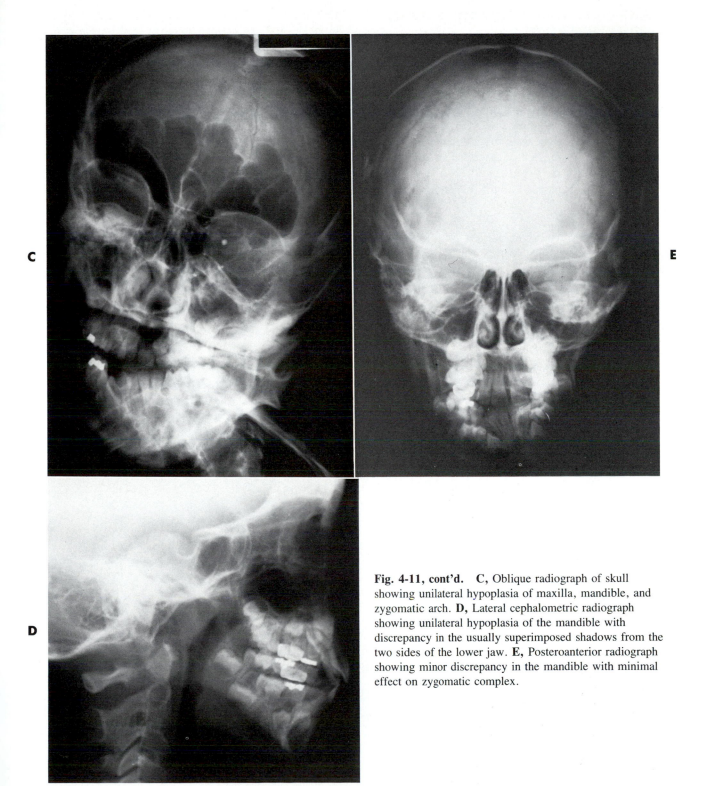

Fig. 4-11, cont'd. **C,** Oblique radiograph of skull showing unilateral hypoplasia of maxilla, mandible, and zygomatic arch. **D,** Lateral cephalometric radiograph showing unilateral hypoplasia of the mandible with discrepancy in the usually superimposed shadows from the two sides of the lower jaw. **E,** Posteroanterior radiograph showing minor discrepancy in the mandible with minimal effect on zygomatic complex.

HEMIFACIAL HYPERTROPHY (FACIAL HEMIHYPERTROPHY)

Overview

Definition: Nearly everybody has mild facial asymmetry. In hemifacial hypertrophy, however, this asymmetry causes obvious disfigurement. This hypertrophy—or perhaps more accurately "hyperplasia" because it is the number of cells and not their size that is involved—may be limited to the head or may even involve one half of the body.

Pathogenesis: The condition is idiopathic.

Clinical Features

Demographics: The right and left sides are almost equally involved. About two thirds of reported cases are in females.

Symptoms and signs: Affected patients have enlargement of one half of the head, which may be present at birth or develop later. The disproportion remains and can worsen during growth. A relationship has been reported between hemifacial hypertrophy and childhood neoplasia including Wilms tumor, hepatoblastoma, and tumors of the suprarenal gland cortex.

Oral manifestations sometimes include developmental anomalies of the dentition on the affected side. Permanent teeth may show macrodontia, being up to 50% larger than those on the unaffected side. Canine, premolar, and first permanent molar teeth appear to be the most commonly enlarged. Teeth on the affected side may develop more rapidly and erupt before those on the contralateral side. The jaws and tongue are often involved in hemihypertrophy.

RADIOLOGIC FEATURES

Cardinal Signs
Unilaterally enlarged jaws
Unilateral macrodontia
Progressive asymmetry
Enlargement of soft tissue shadows

Ancillary Signs
Increased coarseness of bony trabeculations
Advanced eruption of dentition on affected side

Differential Diagnosis
Hypoplastic condyle
Neurofibromatosis
Vascular hamartoma, especially cystic hygroma
Lymphedema
Russell-Silver syndrome
McCune-Albright syndrome

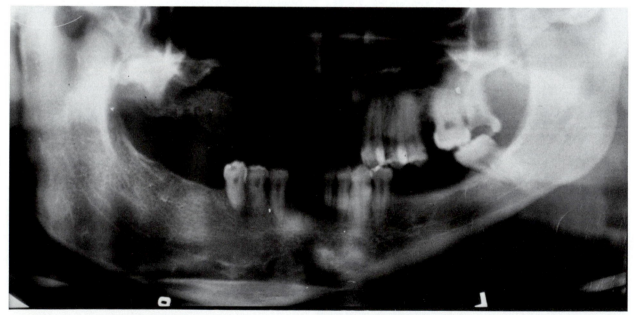

A

Fig. 4-12   A, Panoramic radiograph of patient with hemifacial hypertrophy, showing marked "hypertrophy" of the right side of the mandible.

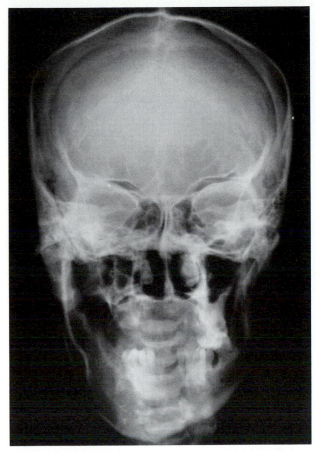

Fig. 4-12, cont'd.   B, Posteroanterior projection of patient in **A.**

MANDIBULOFACIAL DYSOSTOSIS (TREACHER COLLINS SYNDROME)

Overview

Definition and pathogenesis: Mandibulofacial dysostosis is a group of head and face malformations, most often hereditary in pattern and generally dominant in transmission. The condition is thought to result from failure in differentiation of maxillary mesoderm at the 50 mm stage of intrauterine development (i.e., at about 2 months).

Clinical Features

Symptoms and signs: There is a wide variability in the presentation of mandibulofacial dysostosis. However, the full manifestation includes antimongoloid palpebral fissures with coloboma of the outer part of the lower lid; deficiency of the eyelashes; hypoplasia or agenesis of the malar bone; malformation of the external ear (and occasionally of the middle or inner ear); macrostomia; narrow, high-arched (and occasionally cleft) palate; mandibular hypoplasia (or rarely agenesis); dental malocclusion; blind fistulae between the angles of the ears and the commissures of the lips; and arid, atypical tongue-shaped processes of the hairline extending toward the cheeks. The characteristic facial appearance is described as "birdlike" or "fishlike." The cranial vault is normal, and most patients have normal longevity.

RADIOGRAPHIC FEATURES

Cardinal Signs
Hypoplasia of malar bones
Nonfusion of zygomatic arches
Absent palatine bones
Concavity of inferior surface of mandible
Mandibular hypoplasia
Underdeveloped paranasal sinuses
Disproportionately small facial bones

Ancillary Signs
Obtuse gonial angles
Mandibular agenesis
Cleft palate
Small sclerotic mastoids
Malar bone agenesis
Auditory ossicle deficiency
Spacing of teeth
Occasional macrostomia
Occasional anterior open bite

Differential Diagnosis
Goldenhar syndrome (hemifacial microsomia)
Apert syndrome (acrocephalosyndactyly type I)

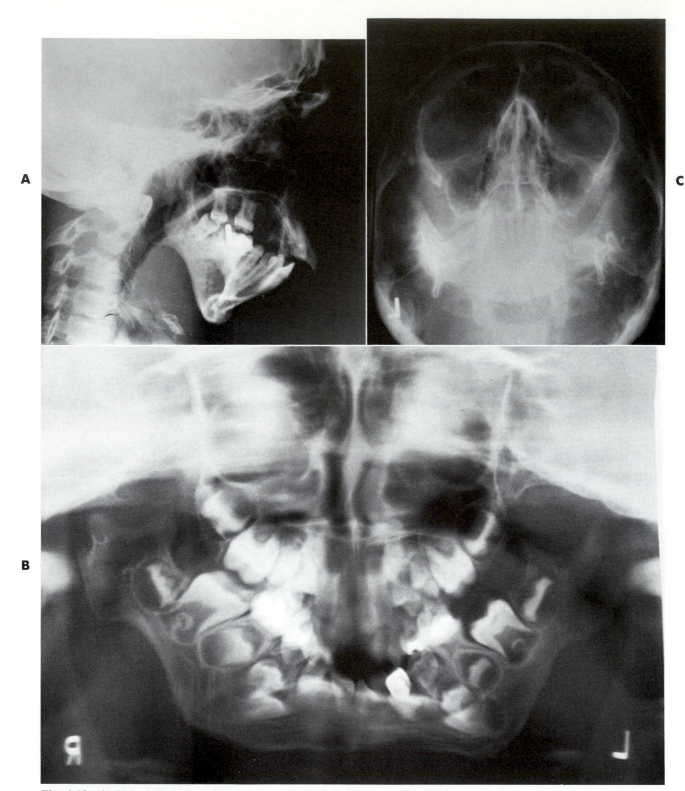

Fig. 4-13 A, Lateral projection of patient with mandibulofacial dysostosis, showing mandibular hypoplasia with concavity in lower border, anterior open bite, and sclerotic mastoids. **B,** Panoramic radiograph showing bilateral mandibular hypoplasia with very short rami and concavities in the posterior regions bilaterally. **C,** Waters projection showing severe hypoplasia of the zygomatic arches bilaterally.

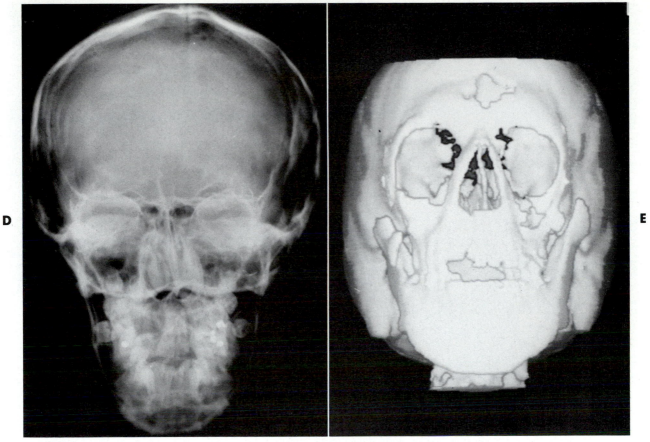

D

E

Fig. 4-13, cont'd. **D,** Posteroanterior radiograph showing incomplete fusion in the zygomatic arches. **E,** 3D-CT reconstruction of same patient as in **D.** Note defects in the zygomatic arches.

MARFAN SYNDROME (ARACHNODACTYLY)

Overview

Definition: Marfan syndrome is a connective tissue disease that is inherited as an autosomal dominant trait and results in defective organization of collagen.

Clinical Features

Symptoms and signs: The head is characteristically long and narrow, the forehead receding, and the chin prominent. There is a narrow, high-arched palate with consequent dental crowding. Temporomandibular joint dysarthrosis, bifid uvula, and multiple odonto-genic cysts have also been reported. The tubular bones of the fingers and legs are very long. The fingers are described as "spiderlike" (arachnodactyly). Myopia is usually present. The eyes are deeply set, sometimes with displacement of the optic lens resulting from weakening or rupture of the suspensory ligaments. Congenital heart disease may be present, and specific reported cardiovascular complications have included aortic aneurysm, aortic regurgitation, valvular defects, and cardiomegaly. Other features include joint hyper-extensibility and dislocation, kyphoscoliosis, and flat-foot.

Fig. 4-14 **A,** Lateral cephalometric radiograph of patient with Marfan syndrome, showing mandibular prognathism with proportionately short rami, large maxillary sinuses, and a characteristic long narrow head. **B,** Posteroanterior view of same patient as in **A.** Note large maxillary sinuses.

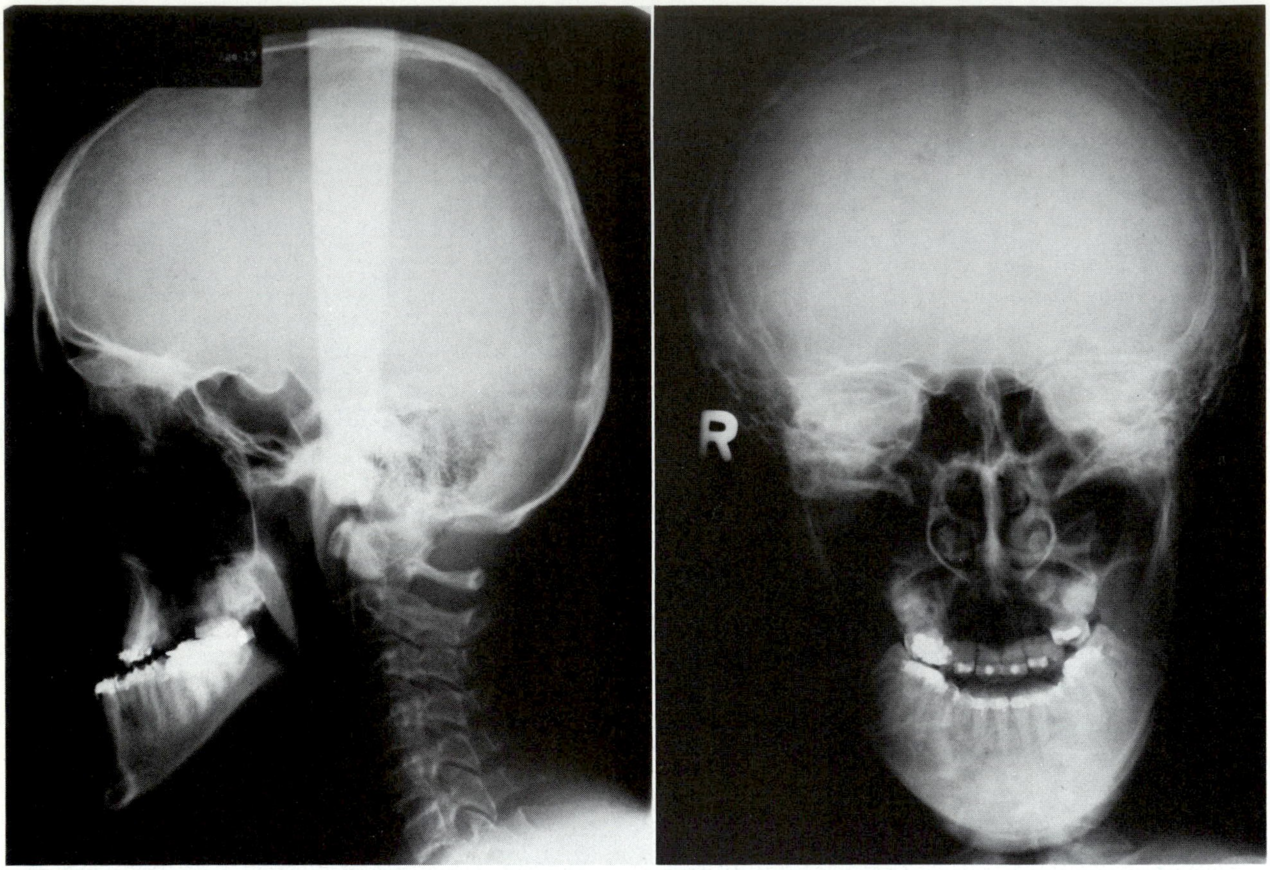

RADIOLOGIC FEATURES
Cardinal Signs
Dolichostenomelia
Dolichocephaly
Receding forehead
Prominent chin
Long fingers
Legs proportionately longer than trunk
Ancillary Signs
Narrow, high palate
Dental crowding
Vertebral anomalies
Proportionately short mandibular rami
Multiple odontogenic cysts
Cleft palate
Long, narrow teeth
Enlarged maxillary sinuses
Mandibular prognathism
Differential Diagnosis
Acromegaly
Crouzon disease
Apert syndrome
Hurler syndrome

MUCOPOLYSACCHAROIDOSES

Overview

Definition: The mucopolysaccharoidoses are a group of conditions in which there is abnormal metabolism or storage of hexamine-containing polysaccharides, which are found in connective tissue ground substance and epithelial mucins. An example is the autosomal recessive disorder Hurler syndrome (mucopolysaccharoidosis IH or gargoylism).

Clinical Features

Symptoms and signs: Hurler syndrome is associated with elevated mucopolysaccharide excretion in urine and excessive intracellular accumulation of chondroitin sulfate B and heparin sulfate resulting from a deficiency of α-L-iduronidase. The disease is generally detected during the first 2 years of life and results in death, usually before puberty. Affected individuals are mentally retarded dwarfs with a large head and prominent forehead, broad saddle-nose with wide nostrils, hypertelorism, swollen eyelids and coarse bushy eyebrows, thick lips, and large tongue. The mandible is shortened and broadened with prominent gonions. Localized bone destruction may result from deposition of mucopolysaccharide. Dental anomalies (e.g., microdontia) and gingival hyperplasia may or may not be present. Progressive corneal clouding and hepatosplenomegaly are classically present. Spinal anomalies are frequent, and flexion contractures may lead to "clawhand."

Laboratory findings

Elevated mucopolysaccharide level in urine
Metachromatic Reilly bodies in circulating lymphocytes

RADIOLOGIC FEATURES

Cardinal Signs

Widened mandible
Short rami
Enlarged follicular spaces simulating dentigerous cysts
Widened temporomandibular joint space and flattening of mandibular condylar heads

Ancillary Signs

Dolichocephaly
Enlarged pituitary fossa

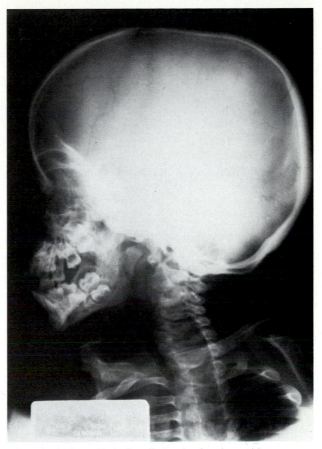

Fig. 4-15 Lateral skull radiograph of patient with mucopolysaccharoidosis. Note short rami, flattened superior surface of mandibular condyle, widened temporomandibular joint space, and widened dental follicle spaces.

Obtuse gonial angle
Concave superior surface of mandibular condyles
Limited translational movement of mandibular condyles
Lytic lesions in jaws
Hypertelorism
Broad nasal fossa
Conical teeth
Delayed or ectopic eruption of teeth
Spacing of teeth
Hypoplastic alveolar ridges

Differential Diagnosis

Frontonasal malformation
Histiocytosis X

NEUROFIBROMATOSIS (VON RECKLINGHAUSEN DISEASE)

Overview

Definition: Neurofibromatosis is one of the phako-matoses, a group of congenital and hereditary developmental anomalies characterized by tumorlike malformations with blastomatous tendencies and pigmented patches.

Pathogenesis: Neurofibromatosis is inherited as a simple dominant trait with variable penetrance and a 50% mutation rate.

Clinical Features

Demographics: Neurofibromatosis occurs in all races and is found in about 1 in 3,000 births in the general population.

Symptoms and signs: Affected patients develop multiple neurofibromas. Superficial lesions are sessile or pedunculated, frequently consisting of numerous smooth-surfaced nodules that are widely distributed in the skin. Deeper, more diffuse lesions, or "elephantiasis neuromatosa," are often large in dimension. Moreover, most affected individuals have asymmetric areas of melanin pigmentation of the skin, termed *café au lait spots.* Hirsutism is sometimes present. Intraoral neurofibromas occur in up to 20% of cases. When neurofibromas are present within the jaws, they are usually associated with the mandibular nerve, resulting in a fusiform enlargement of the canal with pain or paresthesia. In the early literature, malignant transformation of neurofibromas occurred in 15% of patients.

RADIOLOGIC FEATURES

Cardinal Signs

Fusiform enlargement of mandibular canal

Sharply defined, and occasionally corticated, radiolucency

Subperiosteal "blister" lesion

Enlargement of jaw adjacent to a soft tissue tumor

Ancillary Signs

Coarseness of trabeculation adjacent to a soft tissue tumor

Enlarged mandibular or sigmoid notch with elongated condylar neck

Maldevelopment of facial bones

Differential Diagnosis

Mucopolysaccharoidoses

Histiocytosis X

Multiple basal cell carcinoma syndrome

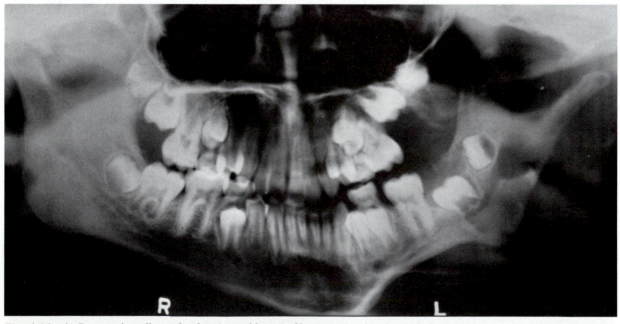

Fig. 4-16   A, Panoramic radiograph of patient with neurofibromatosis, showing lytic lesion above mandibular foramen on left side. Note displacement of lower border of left mandibular body adjacent to soft tissue lesion.

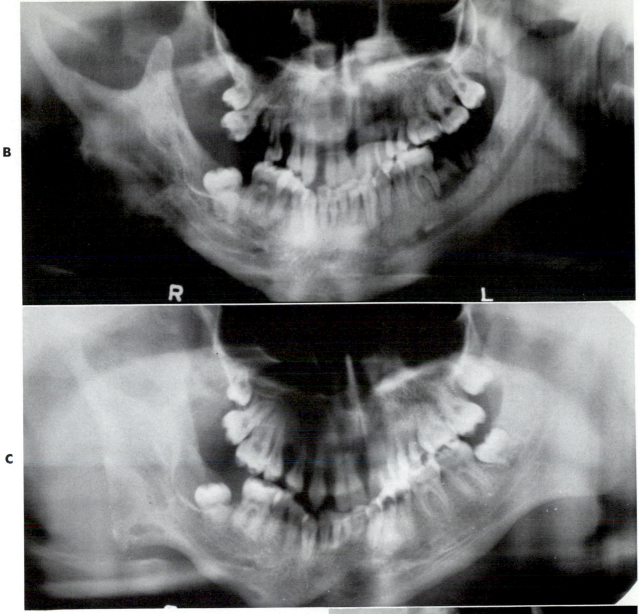

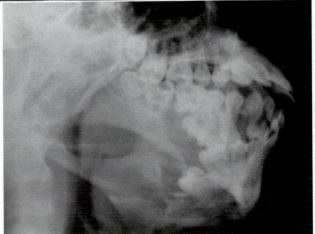

Fig. 4-16, cont'd.   B, Panoramic radiograph showing
subperiosteal "blister" lesion at right mandibular angle and
fusiform enlargement of right mandibular canal.
C, Panoramic radiograph showing sharply demarcated lytic
lesions of right mandibular ramus and angle, enlarged
mandibular notch, and "elongated" right condyle.
D, Lateral-oblique projection of patient in C. Note
widening of mandibular foramen and deepening of
mandibular notch.

Continued.

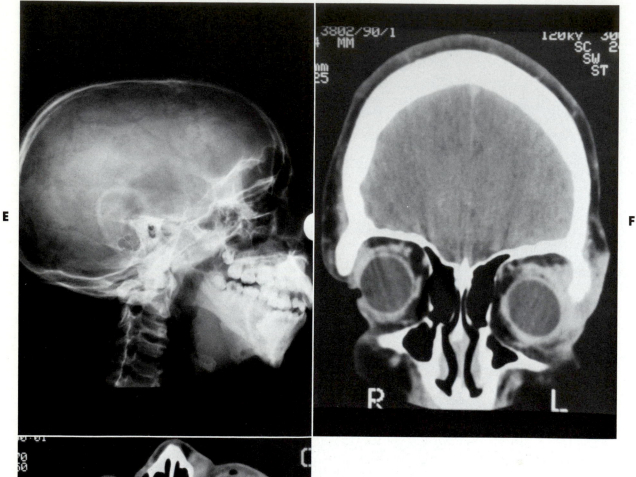

Fig. 4-16, cont'd.   **E,** Lateral skull radiograph demonstrating neurofibroma subjacent to mandible. **F,** Coronal CT scan showing soft tissue mass affecting left orbit. **G,** Axial CT scan of patient in **F.**

OCULODENTOOSSEOUS DYSPLASIA

Overview

Definition: Oculodentoosseous dysplasia is an unusual syndrome characterized by typical facies and certain anomalies of the eyes, teeth, and digits.

Clinical Features

Demographics: There is no sex predilection; reported cases have been in whites.

Symptoms and signs: The syndrome is characterized by severe hypoplasia of dental enamel affecting both dentitions, microphthalmia, hypotelorism, digital anomalies including camptodactyly and syndactyly, and a thin nose with hypoplastic alae and antiverted nostrils. There is a generalized relative sclerosis of the skeleton. Other defects occasionally described include thickening of the mandibular alveolar ridge, cleft lip and palate, and thin lusterless hair.

RADIOLOGIC FEATURES

Cardinal Signs

Sclerosis and thickening of all bones
Enamel hypoplasia
Hypotelorism
Oligodontia
Cleft palate

Ancillary Signs

Widened mandibular alveolar ridges

Differential Diagnosis

Hallermann-Streiff syndrome
Rieger syndrome
Trisomy D

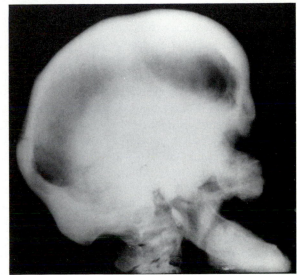

A

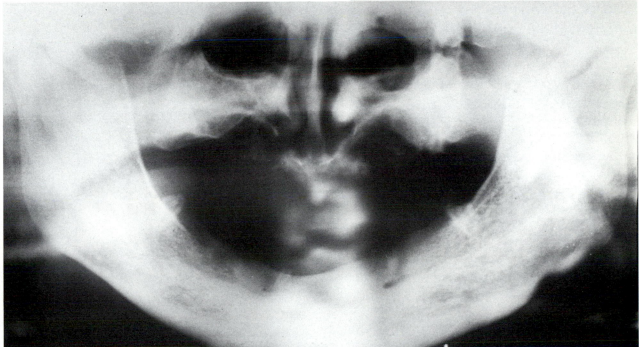

B

Fig. 4-17 A, Lateral skull radiograph showing generalized increased mineralization of the skull and jaws in oculodentoosseous dysplasia. **B,** Panoramic radiograph showing generalized increased bone density and oligodontia.

ODONTOGENIC KERATOCYST–BASAL CELL NEVUS (GORLIN-GOLTZ) SYNDROME

Overview

Definition and pathogenesis: Odontogenic keratocyst–basal cell nevus syndrome is a hereditary condition, transmitted as an autosomal dominant trait with high penetrance and variable expressivity. The principal defects are basal cell nevi or basal cell carcinomas of the skin and multiple jaw cysts.

Clinical Features

Symptoms and signs: The syndrome has numerous and variable manifestations. Cutaneous anomalies include basal cell carcinomas at a young age, occasional benign dermal cysts, palmar and plantar keratosis, and dermal calcinosis. Osseous anomalies include multiple odontogenic keratocysts, frontal bossing, occasionally bifid ribs, vertebral anomalies, and brachymetacarpalism. Keratocysts are most commonly found in the mandibular molar region. Other findings include mild hypertelorism with a relatively wide nasal bridge, infrequent ocular defects, and neurologic anomalies. Laminar calcification of the falx cerebri is common. Odontogenic keratocysts may cause displacement or impaction of teeth. Rarely, mental retardation, agene-sis of the corpus callosum, congenital hydrocephalus, medulloblastoma, hypogonadism in males, and ovarian tumors in females are noted.

RADIOLOGIC FEATURES

Cardinal Signs

Multiple well-defined, well-corticated, unilocular, crenulated, or multilocular radiolucencies in jaws

Minimal jaw expansion with tendency for cysts to grow along the bone

Calcified falx celebri (laminar on posteroanterior view)

Frontal bossing

Ancillary Signs

Bifid ribs
Dental impactions
Bridging of sella turcica
Broadened nasal root
Hypertelorism

Differential Diagnosis

Cherubism
Ameloblastoma
Central giant cell granuloma

Text continued on page 140.

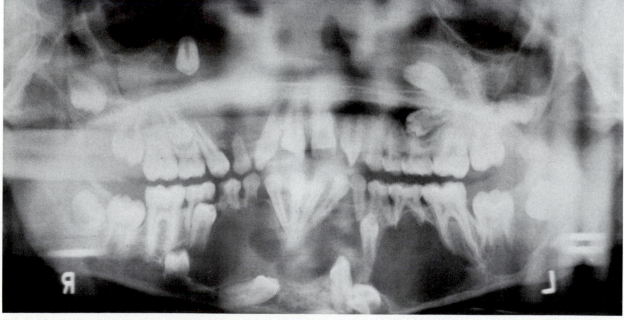

Fig. 4-18 **A,** For legend see opposite page.

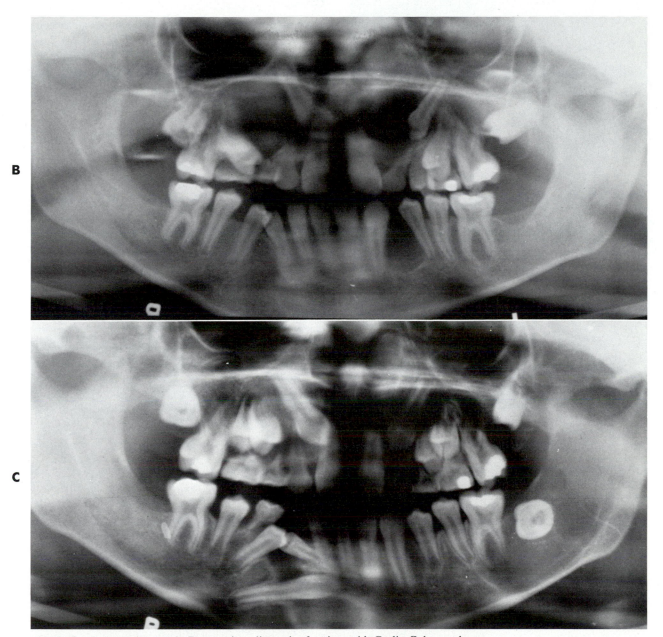

Fig. 4-18 **A (opposite page),** Panoramic radiograph of patient with Gorlin-Goltz syndrome, showing multiple radiolucent lesions in both jaws. Both unilocular and multilocular lesions are present. Proportionate to the size of the lesions, there is very little jawbone expansion. Multiple permanent teeth have been displaced and are impacted. **B (above),** Multiple envelopmental, unilocular radiolucencies are present in the maxilla. A solitary unilocular lesion is present in the left mandible between the canine and first premolar teeth. **C,** Panoramic radiograph showing multiple radiolucencies in both jaws with very little osseous cortical expansion.

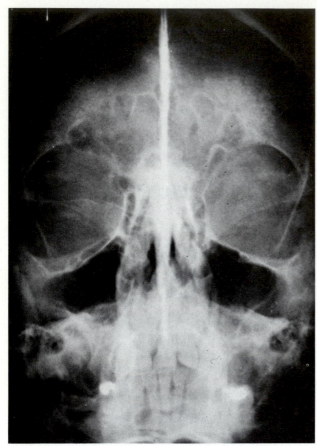

Fig. 4-18, cont'd.   D, Posteroanterior projection showing calcified falx cerebri in Odontogenic Keratocyst-Basal cell nevus syndrome.

OSTEOGENESIS IMPERFECTA

Overview

Definition: Osteogenesis imperfecta is a disease of mesenchymal tissues that is generally present at birth but sometimes not recognized until later in childhood.

Pathogenesis: Osteogenesis imperfecta is generally transmitted as an autosomal dominant trait.

Clinical Features

Symptoms and signs: Affected individuals have extremely fragile bones that are prone to fracture. The fractures heal readily, but the new bone is also of imperfect quality. Multiple fractures can lead to gross deformity. The sclerae are blue in color in about 70% of patients; however, blue sclerae are present in all normal infants up to about 6 months of age and have been reported in fetal rickets, osteopetrosis, Marfan syndrome, and Ehlers-Danlos syndrome. Other findings in osteogenesis imperfecta include deafness resulting from otosclerosis, and, in 80% of patients, teeth resembling dentinogenesis imperfecta. A tendency to capillary bleeding has been mentioned, but no specific defect has been demonstrated. Lax ligaments, an abnormal electrical reaction of the muscles, and skull deformity have also been reported.

RADIOLOGIC FEATURES

Cardinal Signs

> Thinned diploë
> Relative generalized porosity/radiolucency of bone with reduced number of trabeculae
> Thinned mandibular cortex
> Teeth similar to dentinogenesis imperfecta

Ancillary Signs

> Bone deformity following fracture healing
> Hyperplastic callus, sometimes exuberant to the point of mimicking osteogenic sarcoma
> Wormian bones in skull

Differential Diagnosis

> Osteoporosis
> Hyperparathyroidism
> Dentinogenesis imperfecta

Text continued on page 142.

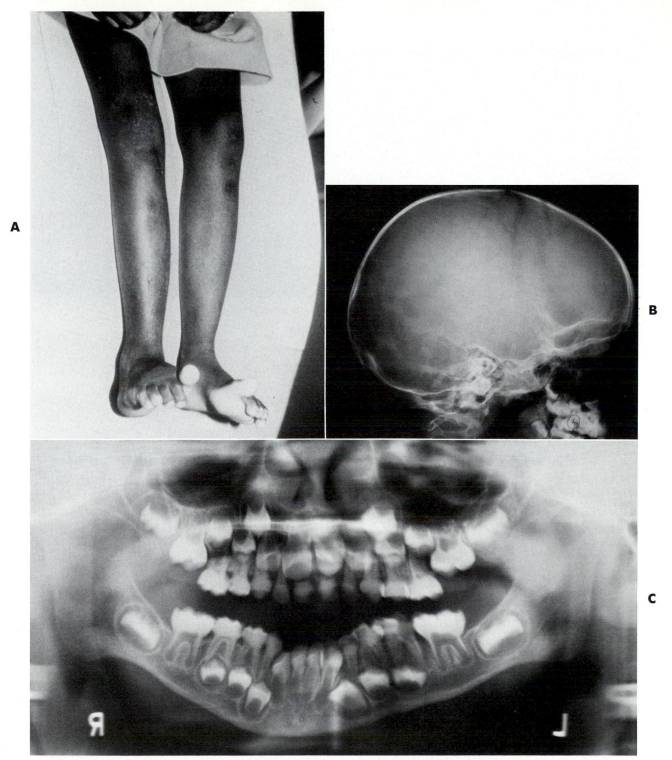

Fig. 4-19 **A,** Deformed legs following multiple fracture episodes in osteogenesis imperfecta. **B,** Same patient as in **A.** Lateral radiograph shows thin calvarium and relative radiolucency of skull. **C,** Same patient as in **A.** Panoramic radiograph shows a relatively thin mandibular cortex and teeth with short, bulbous crowns. The remaining primary teeth show pulp calcification. The first permanent molars have widened pulp canals. *Continued.*

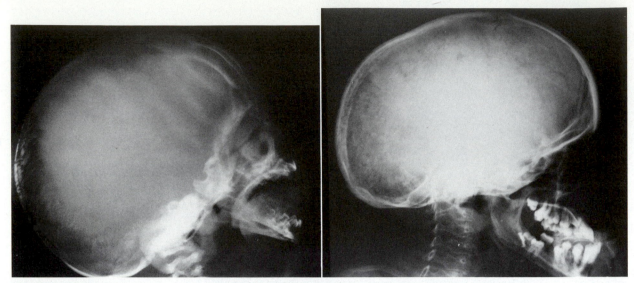

Fig. 4-19, cont'd.   D, Lateral skull radiograph of newborn child with extremely thin calvarium and general radiolucency of skull from osteogenesis imperfecta. Wormian bones are apparent. **E,** Lateral skull radiograph showing generalized porosity.

OSTEOPETROSIS (ALBERS-SCHÖNBERG DISEASE, MARBLE BONES)

Overview

Definition: In osteopetrosis, a cellular fault in osteoclasis causes a net excess deposition of bone.

Pathogenesis: There are two major forms of osteopetrosis, a clinically benign form that is inherited as a dominant trait and a clinically malignant form that is inherited as a recessive trait. The two forms occur with equal frequency.

Clinical Features

Symptoms and signs: Most of the bones of the body are involved in a diffuse sclerosis. In the malignant, recessive form of osteopetrosis, the disease is detected at or soon after birth; 75% of these patients develop optic atrophy. Other features of the malignant form of osteopetrosis are hepatosplenomegaly resulting from compensatory extramedullary hematopoiesis; susceptibility to infection as a result of granulocytopenia; poor growth; frontal bossing; pathologic fractures; and (as a result of narrowing of the cranial foramina) facial palsy, hearing loss, and genu valgum. Thrombocytopenia and pancytopenia have also been reported. Patients commonly die before 20 years of age from anemia or secondary infection.

Involvement is less severe in the benign, dominant form of osteopetrosis. This type is generally diagnosed later in life, sometimes not until middle age. Nearly half of patients with the benign form are asymptomatic.

Laboratory tests: Serum calcium, phosphorus, and alkaline phosphatase levels are within normal range. Reduced red blood cell count and granulocytopenia may be noted in the malignant form. A carbonic anhydrase II enzyme defect related to an autosomal recessive gene has also been reported.

RADIOLOGIC FEATURES

Cardinal Signs

Homogeneous diffuse sclerosis of bones
Reduced medullary spaces
Thickened cortices

Ancillary Signs

Clubbing and transverse striation of ends of long bones
Fractures
Osteomyelitis secondary to dental infection
Enamel hypoplasia
Thickened lamina dura
Unerupted teeth
Obscured dental roots because of opacity of bone
Wormian bones
Thickened base of skull

Differential Diagnosis

Pyknodysostosis
Oculodentoosseous dysplasia
Metaphyseal dysplasia
Paget disease of bone
van Buchem syndrome
Florid osseous dysplasia

Text continued on page 145.

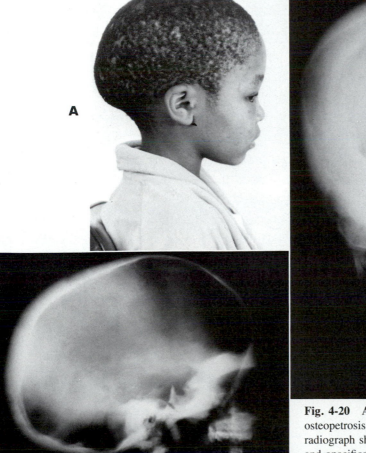

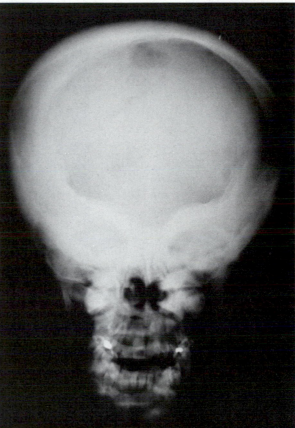

Fig. 4-20   A, Clinical appearance of child with osteopetrosis. **B,** Same patient as in **A.** Lateral skull radiograph showing thickening of skull and cranial base and opacification of maxilla. **C,** Same patient as in **A.** Posteroanterior projection showing thickened and sclerotic skull vault and cranial base.   *Continued.*

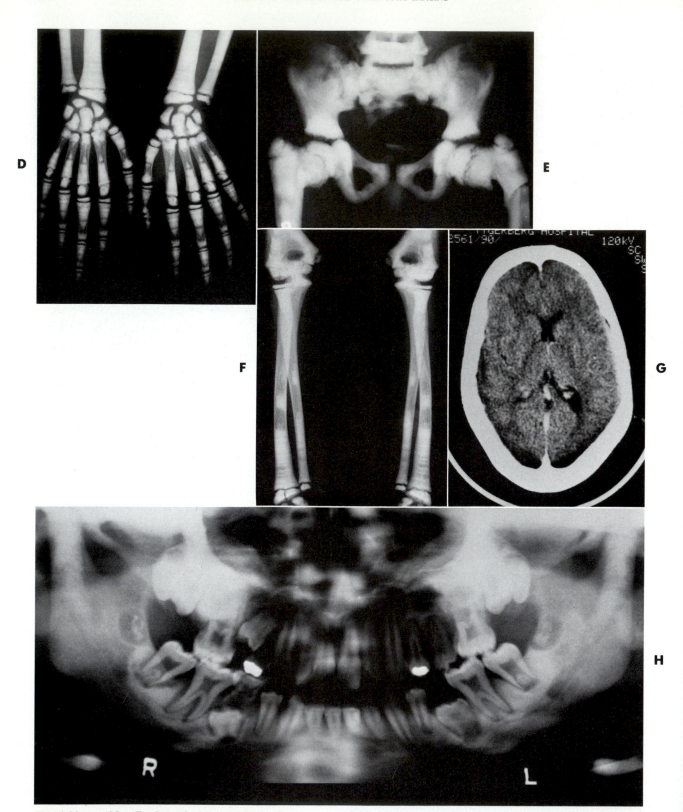

Fig. 4-20, cont'd. For legends see opposite page.

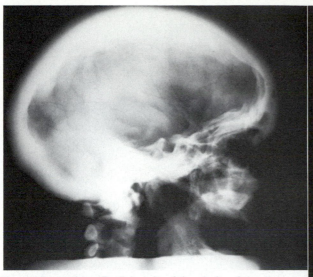
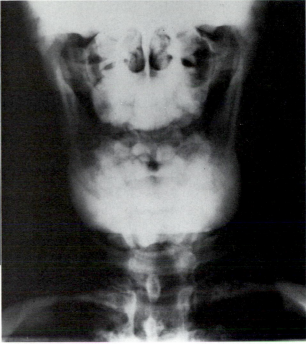

Fig. 4-20, cont'd.   D, Sclerosis of the shafts of the digits and long bones in patient with osteopetrosis. **E,** Osteosclerosis of sacrum and both femurs in patient with osteopetrosis. Note multiple pathologic fractures. **F,** Patchy sclerosis in long bones of patient with osteopetrosis. **G,** Axial CT scan showing gross thickening of skull in patient with osteopetrosis. **H,** Panoramic radiograph of teenager with osteopetrosis. Note sclerosis in both jaws, especially prominent in the mandibular alveolar bone surrounding the erupted teeth. **I,** Lateral skull radiograph showing gross thickening of skull and cranial base. **J,** Posteroanterior projection showing sclerosis and thickening of both jaws.

PYKNODYSOSTOSIS

Overview

Definition: Pyknodysostosis is a rare, inherited form of dwarfism that is associated with dense, fragile bones.

Clinical Features

Symptoms and signs: Affected patients are short with short phalanges and possible history of fracture. They are predisposed to osteomyelitis.

RADIOLOGIC FEATURES

Cardinal Signs
   Dwarfism
   Dense bones

Partial agenesis of terminal phalanges of hands and
   feet
Open fontanelles

Ancillary Signs
   Short-rooted teeth
   Fractured bones
   Obtuse mandibular angles
   Hypoplastic maxilla and mandible
   Small paranasal sinuses
   Thin calvarium
   Thickening of base of skull
   Premature or delayed dental eruption
   Malocclusion of teeth

Differential Diagnosis
   Osteopetrosis (Albers-Schönberg disease)

Text continued on page 147.

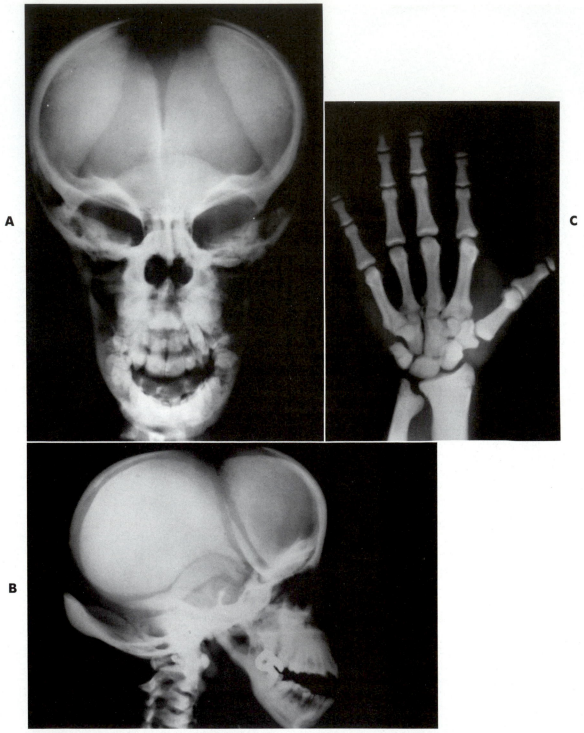

Fig. 4-21 **A,** Posteroanterior radiograph showing open anterior fontanelle, dense bones, and small maxillary sinuses in patient with pyknodysostosis. **B,** Same patient as in **A.** Note open fontanelles and sutures, dense bones, and obtuse mandibular angles. **C,** Hand-wrist film demonstrating incomplete terminal phalanges.

SICKLE CELL ANEMIA

Overview

Definition: Sickle cell anemia is an inherited condition affecting the red blood cells. It confers some resistance to malaria. Affected individuals have an altered form of the oxygen-carrying compound hemoglobin.

Clinical Features

Demographics: Sickle cell anemia is most serious when affected genes are inherited from both parents; this occurs in about 10% of cases. Sickle cell trait is found in more than 40% of the population in certain regions of Africa. Approximately 10% of African Americans carry the sickle cell trait, but only 0.5% actually have the disease. It also occurs in the oasis

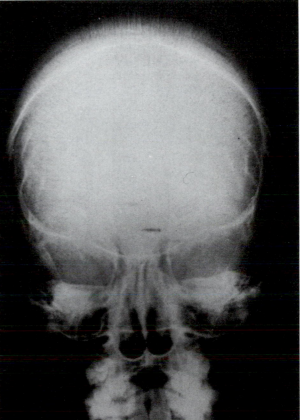
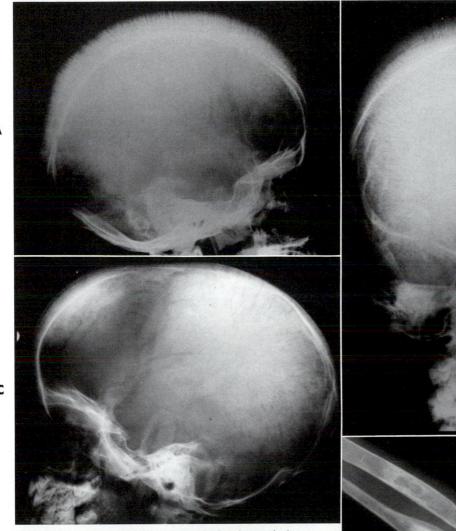
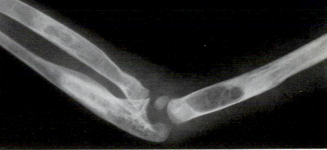

Fig. 4-22   A, Lateral skull radiograph showing typical "hair-on-end" calvarium of sickle cell anemia. **B,** Posteroanterior projection of patient in **A.** Note "hair-on-end" calvarium and granular trabeculation of bone in skull. **C,** Lateral skull radiograph showing coarse trabeculations and "hair-on-end" calvarium with thinned cortices. **D,** Same patient as in **C.** Widened marrow spaces with sparse trabeculation in long bones of arm represent an attempt at increased red blood cell manufacture. Patchy sclerosis can also be seen.

population of Saudi Arabia, the Veddoid tribes of southern India, and in some individuals in Greece. Through migration it is also found in other parts of the world.

Symptoms and signs: Patients with the homozygous form of sickle cell anemia usually manifest symptoms before 30 years of age. Commonly the patient is weak, breathless, and fatigued. There may be nausea and vomiting and pain in the joints, limbs, and abdomen. Peripheral infarcts may result from erythrostasis within the microvasculature; such infarcts have been reported in the mandible. A sickle cell crisis may develop through hypoxia, and this is a particular risk during general anesthesia.

Laboratory tests: The erythrocyte count can be as low as 1 million or less per mm^3 of blood. Sickle-shaped cells are characteristically seen on blood smears. Nuclear enlargement, binucleation, and atypical chromatin distribution can be seen in epithelial cells in scrapings from the buccal mucosa in 90% of homozygotes.

RADIOLOGIC FEATURES

Cardinal Signs
"Hair-on-end" calvarium
Thickened diploë
Enlarged medullary spaces in all bones

Ancillary Signs
Thinned cortices in all bones
Increased radiolucency of jaws
Diminished trabeculation and enlarged marrow spaces
Coarse, well-defined trabeculation of jaws
Occasional localized increase in bone density

Differential Diagnosis
Thalassemia (Cooley anemia)

STAFNE DEFECT (LINGUAL SALIVARY GLAND DEPRESSION)

Overview
Definition: In Stafne defects, aberrantly positioned salivary gland tissue causes a deep depression, or inclusion, at the angle of the mandible during development.

Clinical Features
Demographics: Stafne defect is an asymptomatic radiographic finding in 0.1% to 1.3% of sample populations. Although it is rarely seen in children it is generally considered to be a congenital defect. However, it has been shown to occur over a 5-year period in a middle-aged man and to have arisen in an 11-year-old boy. It is apparently more frequent in males than in females.

RADIOLOGIC FEATURES

Cardinal Signs
Ovoid radiolucency situated between mandibular canal and lower border, just anterior to angle of mandible.

Ancillary Signs
Occasionally bilateral
Occasionally double unilaterally
Salivary gland tissue demonstrated by sialography in 40% of cases.

Differential Diagnosis
Hemorrhagic bone cyst
Early ossifying fibroma
Benign nonodontogenic tumor, such as neurofibroma
Myeloma
Idiopathic histiocytoses, including eosinophilic granuloma
Central giant cell granuloma
Ectopic benign odontogenic tumor or keratocyst; unusual below mandibular canal

Text continued on page 150.

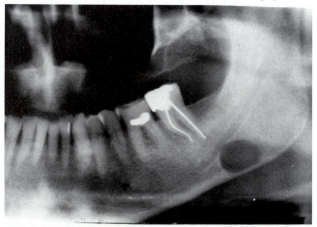

A

Fig. 4-23. For legend see opposite page.

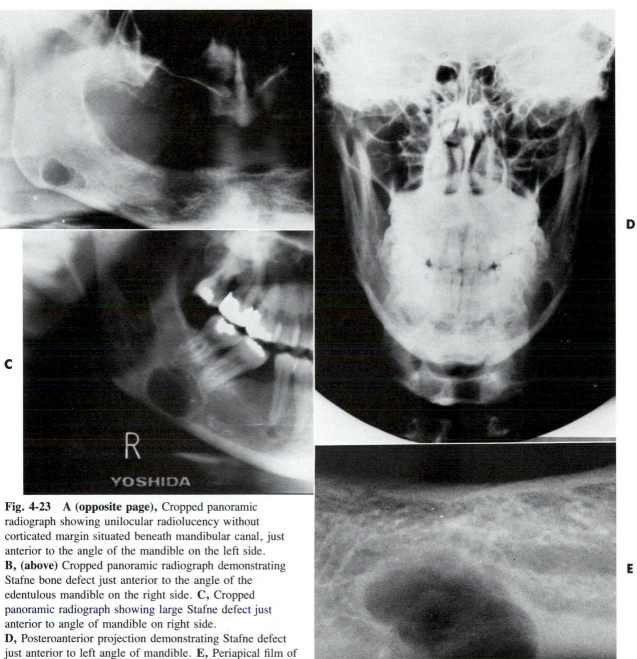

Fig. 4-23   A (opposite page), Cropped panoramic radiograph showing unilocular radiolucency without corticated margin situated beneath mandibular canal, just anterior to the angle of the mandible on the left side. **B, (above)** Cropped panoramic radiograph demonstrating Stafne bone defect just anterior to the angle of the edentulous mandible on the right side. **C,** Cropped panoramic radiograph showing large Stafne defect just anterior to angle of mandible on right side.
D, Posteroanterior projection demonstrating Stafne defect just anterior to left angle of mandible. **E,** Periapical film of edentulous mandible demonstrating Stafne defect with adjacent thinning of lower cortex of mandible.

STURGE-WEBER SYNDROME (ENCEPHALOTRIGEMINAL ANGIOMATOSIS)

Overview

Definition: Sturge-Weber syndrome is one of the phakomatoses, a group of congenital and hereditary developmental anomalies. These conditions are characterized by the presence of tumorlike malformations with blastomatous tendencies and pigmented patches, or angiomata, in tissues of ectodermal origin, particularly the skin, eye, and central and peripheral nervous systems. Neurofibromatosis (von Recklinghausen disease) is another of the phakomatoses.

Clinical Features

Symptoms and signs: Seizures, facial port-wine stain (nevus flammeus) in the trigeminal distribution, and ipsilateral curvilinear cortical calcifications are the classic features of Sturge-Weber syndrome. Other typical manifestations include glaucoma, mental retardation, hemiparesis, and hemiatrophy. Although one third of all patients with Sturge-Weber syndrome exhibit bilateral port-wine stains, only 15% have involvement of both cerebral hemispheres. Seizures usually commence between 3 and 9 months after birth, but cortical calcifications are rarely seen on plain radiographs within the first year. Computed tomography has been used to advantage for early detection of minimal intracranial calcifications. Carotid angiography of the leptomeningeal angiomatosis may aid diagnosis in the very young patient. Nuclear scintigraphy of the brain using technetium 99m pertechnetate shows uptake in major regions of hemisphere involvement but does not detect small lesions.

RADIOLOGIC FEATURES

Cardinal Signs

"Railroad track" calcifications in brain cortex
Unilateral curvilinear calcifications of brain cortex

Ancillary Signs

Bilateral calcification of brain cortex
Technetium 99m pertechnetate uptake in established brain lesions
Prominent medullary veins and sparse superficial cortical veins on contrast angiography
Intraoral soft tissue (angiomatous mass)
Localized hyperplasia or hypoplasia of alveolar bone
Delayed or accelerated dental eruption
Macrodontia

Differential Diagnosis

Klippel-Trenaunay-Weber syndrome
Childhood leukemia

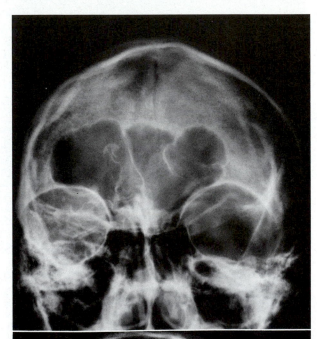

A

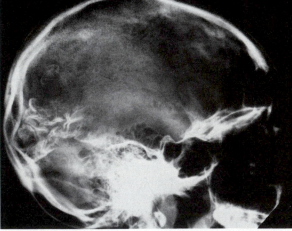

B

Fig. 4-24 A, Posteroanterior projection of patient with Sturge-Weber syndrome, demonstrating "railroad track" calcification of brain superimposed over right side of frontal sinus. **B,** Multiple curved "railroad track" calcifications of brain in occipital region and patchy calcifications more anteriorly.

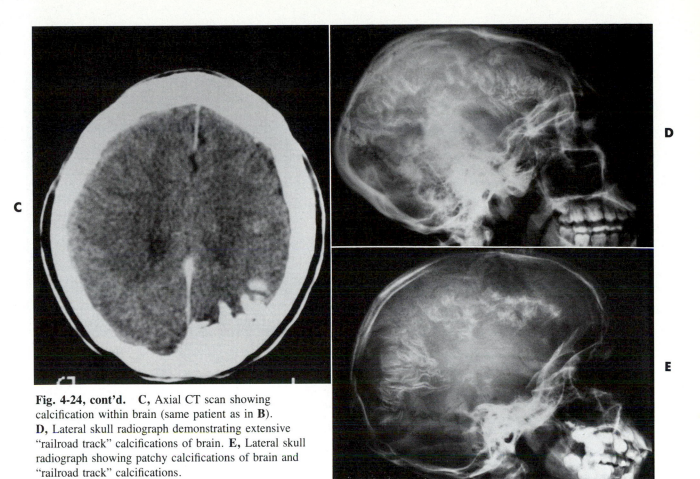

Fig. 4-24, cont'd. **C,** Axial CT scan showing calcification within brain (same patient as in **B**). **D,** Lateral skull radiograph demonstrating extensive "railroad track" calcifications of brain. **E,** Lateral skull radiograph showing patchy calcifications of brain and "railroad track" calcifications.

THALASSEMIA (COOLEY ANEMIA)

Overview

Definition and pathogenesis: *Thalassemia* refers to a group of autosomal dominant anemias caused by diminished synthesis of either the α- or β-globulin chain of hemoglobin A. The condition most commonly affects individuals of Mediterranean or Armenian origin and their descendants. In heterozygotes the disease is mild and termed *thalassemia minor;* homozygotes have the full disease, which is termed *thalassemia major.*

Clinical Features

Symptoms and signs: Thalassemia major is generally detected in the first 2 years of life. The child typically has yellowish, pallid skin and exhibits slight pyrexia, malaise, hepatosplenomegaly, and lethargy. The face may have mongoloid features with slanting eyes, prominent zygomatic arches, prominent maxilla with protrusion of the maxillary anterior teeth, and depressed nasal bridge. This is the so-called rodent facies. The oral mucosa may exhibit anemic pallor. Patients with thalassemia minor generally lack clinical signs.

Laboratory findings: Patients with thalassemia have hypochromic microcytic anemia with poikilocytosis and anisocytosis of erythrocytes. Nucleated red blood cells (normoblasts) and "safety pin" cells are characteristically present. Leukocytosis may exceed 25,000 white blood cells per mm^3 of blood. Serum bilirubin may be raised as a result of hemosiderosis.

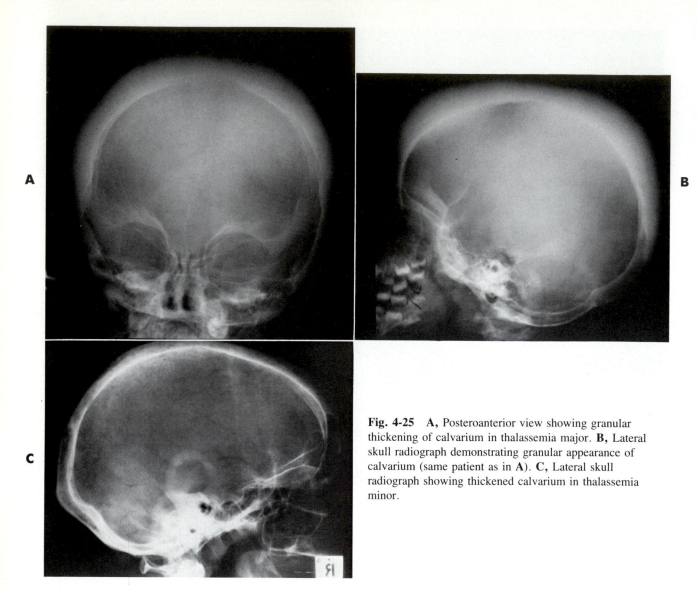

Fig. 4-25 **A,** Posteroanterior view showing granular thickening of calvarium in thalassemia major. **B,** Lateral skull radiograph demonstrating granular appearance of calvarium (same patient as in **A**). **C,** Lateral skull radiograph showing thickened calvarium in thalassemia minor.

RADIOLOGIC FEATURES

Cardinal Signs

Granular thickening of calvarium
Widened medullary spaces in skull and long bones
Thinned cortices in skull and long bones

Ancillary Signs

Thinned inferior cortex of mandible
Extreme thickening of diploë
Enlargement of jaws, especially in a vertical dimension
Spacing of teeth
Increased overbite and overjet of teeth
Maxillary hyperplasia with associated alveolar enlargement
Reduced size of maxillary sinuses
Relative osteoporosis of skull and long bones
Coarse trabeculae in both jaws
Thinning of lamina dura
Circular radiolucencies in alveolar bone

Differential Diagnosis

Down syndrome
Sickle cell anemia

TORUS MANDIBULARIS AND PALATINUS

Overview

Definition: Torus mandibularis and palatinus are slowly growing, flat-based bony protuberances found either in the midline of the hard palate or on the lingual aspect of the mandible, generally adjacent to the premolar teeth.

Pathogenesis: The lesions appear to be inherited as separate mendelian dominant traits.

Clinical Features

Demographics: Torus palatinus is found more commonly in women than men, with a prevalence of 20% to 25% in the U.S. general population. It can be found in any age group, but often becomes noticeable during the third decade of life.

When one or both parents are affected with mandibular torus, children have a 40% to 60% chance of occurrence, compared with 5% to 8% for children of unaffected parents.

There is no known correlation between the incidence of mandibular and maxillary tori, but both are reported to be most frequent in mongoloid groups such as the Alaskan Eskimo and Aleuts. The incidence is higher in Eskimo women than in Eskimo men.

Symptoms and signs: Torus palatinus is a bony, hard swelling in the midline of the hard palate. It can be flat, spindle-shaped, nodular, or lobular. The overlying mucosa is intact.

Torus mandibularis is an exostosis found on the lingual surface of the mandible and is bilateral in 80% of cases. The lesion is bony, hard and covered by intact oral mucosa.

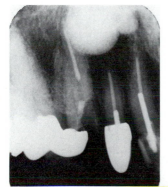

A

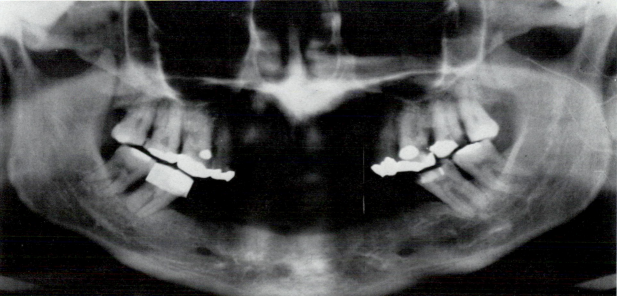

B

Fig. 4-26 **A,** Periapical radiograph demonstrating maxillary torus above roots of endodontically treated anterior teeth. **B,** Maxillary torus seen in midline of panoramic radiograph. Only relatively large tori are seen on panoramic radiographs because they are not usually in the image layer.

Continued.

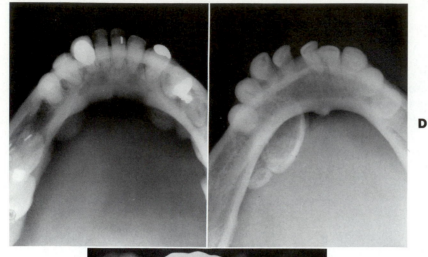

C

D

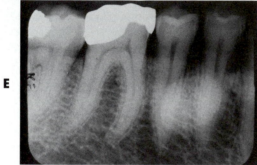

E

Fig. 4-26, cont'd. **C,** Mandibular occlusal radiograph showing bilateral mandibular tori on lingual surface of the mandible in the premolar regions. **D,** Unilateral mandibular torus as demonstrated by occlusal radiography. **E,** Mandibular torus seen on periapical radiograph as a well-defined radiopacity superimposed over premolar roots.

RADIOLOGIC FEATURES

Cardinal Signs

Smooth-surfaced radiopacity in maxillary midline

Radiopacities superimposed on midroot region of mandibular premolars

Differential Diagnosis

Focal osteosclerosis

Condensing osteitis

Mucocele of maxillary sinus

Antrolith

Gardner syndrome

Buccal exostoses

Osteochondroma

BIBLIOGRAPHY

Achondroplasia

Shafer WG, Hine MK, Levy BN: *Textbook of oral pathology,* ed 4, Philadelphia, 1983, W.B. Saunders p 696.

Apert Syndrome

Bu B, Kaban LB, Vargervik K: Effect of LeFortIII osteotomy on mandibular growth in patients with Crouzon and Apert syndromes, *J Oral Maxillofac Surg* 47:666, 1989.

Costas-Volarich M, Pruzansky S: Is the mandible intrinsically different in Apert and Crouzon syndromes? *Am J Orthod* 86:475, 1984.

Singh M, Hadi F, Aram GN: Craniosynostosis—Crouzon's disease and Apert syndrome, *Indian Pediatr* 20:608, 1983.

Caffey Disease

Burbank PM, Lovestedt SA, Kennedy RL: The dental aspects of infantile cortical hyperostosis, *Oral Surg Oral Med Oral Pathol* 11:1126, 1958.

Edeiken J, Nodes PJ: Roentgen diagnosis of diseases of the bone, ed 2, Baltimore, 1973, Williams & Wilkins.

Saul RA, Lee WH, Stevenson RE: Caffey's disease revisited, *Am J Dis Child* 136:56, 1982.

Cherubism

Coope JW, Ireland SL, Burke PH: Cherubism with serial stereophotogrametric assessment, *Br Dent J* 155:127, 1983.

McClendon JL, Anderson DE, Cornelius EA: Cherubism: hereditary fibrous dysplasia of the jaws, II. Pathologic considerations, *Oral Surg Oral Med Oral Pathol* 15(suppl 2):17, 1962.

Peters WJ: Cherubism: a study of twenty cases from one family, *Oral Surg Oral Med Oral Pathol* 47:307, 1979.

Von Wowern N: Cherubism, *Int J Oral Surg* 1:240, 1972.

Cleft Palate

Morrison G, et al: The incidence of cleft lip and palate in the Western Cape, *S Afr Med J,* 68:576, 1985.

Natsume N, Suzuki T, Kawai T: The prevalence of cleft lip and palate in the Japanese: their birth prevalence in 40,304 infants born during 1982, *Oral Surg Oral Med Oral Pathol* 63:421, 1987.

Sandham A: Classification of clefting deformity, *Early Hum Dev* 12:81, 1985.

Cleidocranial Dysplasia

Kalliala E, Taskinen PJ: Cleidocranial dysostosis, *Oral Surg Oral Med Oral Pathol* 15:808, 1962.

McKusick VA, Scott CL: A nomenclature for constitutional disorders of bone, *J Bone Joint Surg* 53A:978, 1971.

Shafer WG, Hine MK, Levy BM: *Textbook of oral pathology,* ed 4, Philadelphia, 1983, W.B. Saunders, p 678.

Craniofacial Dysostosis

Shafer WG, et al: *Textbook of oral pathology,* ed 4, Philadelphia, 1983, WB Saunders, p 680.

Ectodermal Dysplasias

Freire-Maia N: Ectodermal dysplasia, *Hum Hered* 21:309, 1971.

Nortje CJ, et al: X-linked hypohidrotic ectodermal dysplasia—an unusual prosthetic problem. *J Prosthet Dent* 40:137, 1978.

Witkop CJ Jr, Brearley LJ, Gentry WC Jr: Hypoplastic enamel, onycholysis and hypohidrosis inherited as an autosomal dominant trait, *Oral Surg Oral Med Oral Pathol* 39:71, 1975.

Frontonasal Malformation

Cohen MM: Craniofrontonasal dysplasia, *Birth Defects* 15:85, 1979.

Day O: Unique subpopulations in the diagnostic category of frontonasal dysplasia, *Birth Defects* 19:12, 1983.

DeMeyer W: Median facial malformations and their implications for brain malformations, *Birth Defects* 11:155, 1975.

Gollop TR, Fontes LF: The Greig cephalopolysyndactyly syndrome: report of a family and review of the literature, *Am J Med Genet* 22:59, 1985.

Grutzner E, Gorlin RJ: Craniofrontonasal dysplasia: phenotypic expression in females and males and genetic considerations, *Oral Surg Oral Med Oral Pathol* 65:436, 1988.

Sedano NO, Gorlin RJ: Frontonasal malformation as a field defect and its syndromic associations, *Oral Surg Oral Med Oral Pathol* 65:704, 1988.

Gardner Syndrome

Watne AL, Core SK, Carrier JM: Gardner's syndrome, *Surg Gynecol Obstet* 141:53, 1975.

Goldenhar Syndrome

Cavom JW Jr, Pratt LL, Alonso WA: First brachial cleft syndrome and associated hearing loss, *Laryngoscope* 86:739, 1976.

Converse JM, et al: On hemifacial microsomia: the 1st and 2nd branchial arch syndrome, *Plast Reconstr Surg* 51:268, 1973.

Gorlin RJ, et al: Oculoauriculovertebral dysplasia, *J Pediatr* 63:991, 1963.

Hemifacial Hypertrophy

Fraumeni JF Jr, Geises CF, Marmay ND: Wilms' tumor and congenital hemihypertrophy: report of 5 new cases and review of the literature, *Pediatrics* 40:886, 1967.

Rowe NH: Hemifacial hypertrophy: review of the literature and addition of four cases, *Oral Surg Oral Med Oral Pathol* 15:572, 1962.

Mandibulofacial Dysostosis

Fernandez AO, Ronis ML: The Treacher-Collins syndrome, *Arch Otolaryngol* 80:505, 1964.

Rogers BO: Berry-Treacher-Collins syndrome: a review of 200 cases, *Br J Plast Surg* 17:109, 1964.

Rovin S, et al: Mandibulofacial dysostosis: a family study of five generations, *J Pediatr* 64:215, 1964.

Stovin JJ, Lyons JA Jr, Clemmens RA: Mandibulofacial dysostosis, *Radiology* 74:225, 1960.

Marfan Syndrome

Baden E, Spirgi M: Oral manifestations of Marfan's syndrome, *Oral Surg Oral Med Oral Pathol* 19:757, 1965.

Boucek RJ, et al: The Marfan syndrome: a deficiency in chemically stable collagen cross-links, *N Engl J Med* 305:988, 1981.

Oatis GW Jr, Burch MS, Samuels HS: Marfan's syndrome with multiple maxillary and mandibular cysts: report of case, *J Oral Surg* 29:515, 1971.

Shafer WG, et al: *Textbook of oral pathology,* ed 4, Philadelphia, 1983, W.B. Saunders, p 683.

Mucopolysaccharoidoses

Gorlin RJ: Genetic disorders affecting mucous membranes, *Oral Surg Oral Med Oral Pathol* 28:512, 1962.

Hofer PA, Bergenholtz A: Oral manifestations in Urbach-Wiethe disease, *Odont Rev* 26:39, 1975.

McKusick VA, et al: The genetic mucopolysaccharidoses, *Medicine* 44:445, 1965.

Neufeld EF, Fratatoni JC: Inborn errors of mucopolysaccharide metabolism: faulty degradative mechanisms are implicated in this group of human diseases, *Science* 169:141, 1970.

Weidner WA, Wenzi JE, Swischuk LE: Roentgenographic findings in lipoid proteinosis: a case report, *AJR* 110:457, 1970.

Neurofibromatosis

Cherrick HM, Eversole LR: Benign neural sheath neoplasia of the oral cavity: report of thirty-seven cases, *Oral Surg Oral Med Oral Pathol* 32:900, 1971.

Hosoi K: Multiple neurofibromatosis with special transformation, *Arch Surg* 22:258, 1931.

Prescott GH, White RE: Solitary central neurofibroma of the mandible: report of a case and review of the literature, *J Oral Surg* 28:305, 1971.

Oculodentoosseous Dysplasia

Farman AG, Smith SN, Nortje CJ: Oculodentodigital dysplasia, *Br Dent J* 142:405, 1977.

Odontogenic Keratocyst – Basal Cell Nevus Syndrome

Gorlin RJ, Goltz RW: Multiple nevoid basal-cell epithelioma, jaw cysts and bifid rib, *N Engl J Med* 262:908, 1960.

Gorlin RJ: Nevoid basal cell carcinoma syndrome, *Medicine* 66:98, 1987.

Gundlach KK, Kiehn M: Multiple basal cell carcinomas and keratocysts—the Gorlin and Goltz syndrome, *J Maxillofac Surg* 7:229, 1979.

Woolgar JA, Rippin JW, Browne RM: The odontogenic keratocyst and its occurrence in the nevoid basal cell carcinoma syndrome, *Oral Surg Oral Med Oral Pathol* 64:727, 1987.

Osteogenesis Imperfecta

Bauze RJ, Smith R, Francis MJ: A new look at osteogenesis imperfecta, *J Bone Joint Surg* 53B:72, 1971.

Falvo HA, Root L, Bullough PC: Osteogenesis imperfecta: clinical evaluation and management, *J Bone Joint Surg* 56A:783, 1974.

King JO, Bobeckko WP: Osteogenesis imperfecta: an orthopaedic description and surgical review, *J Bone Joint Surg* 53B:72, 1971.

Osteopetrosis

Albers-Schönberg N: Rontgenbilder einer Selt enen Knochen emkrankung. Demonstration vor dem Artzlichen verein in Hamburg. Sitzung vom 10.2. *Munich Med Wochenschr* 41:365, 1904.

Bjorvtan K, Gilhuus-Noe O, Asrskog D: Oral aspects of osteopetrosis, *Scand J Dent Res* 87:245, 1979.

Dick NM, Simpson WJ: Dental changes in osteopetrosis, *Oral Surg Oral Med Oral Pathol* 34:408, 1972.

Dyson DP: Osteomyelitis of the jaws in Albers-Schönberg disease, *Br J Oral Surg* 17:178, 1980.

Sly WS, Emmett DH: Carbonic anhydrase II deficiency identified as the primary defect in autosomal recessive syndrome of osteopetrosis with renal tubular acidosis and cerebral calcification, *Proc Natl Acad Sci USA* 80:2752, 1983.

Steiner M, Gould AR, Mears WR: Osteomyelitis of the mandible associated with osteopetrosis, *J Oral Maxillofac Surg* 41:395, 1983.

Wong ML, Balkany TJ: Head and neck manifestations of malignant osteopetrosis, *Otolaryngology* 86:585, 1978.

Younai F, Eisenbud L, Scuibba JJ: Osteopetrosis: a case report including gross and microscopic findings in the mandible at autopsy, *Oral Surg Oral Med Oral Pathol* 65:214, 1988.

Pyknodysostosis

Elmore SM: Pyknodysostosis: a review, *J Bone Joint Surg* 49A:153, 1967.

Sickle Cell Anemia

Calabrese EJ: Ecogenetics: historical foundation and current status, *J Occup Med* 28:1096, 1986.

Canter EF: Employment discrimination implications of genetic screening in workplace under Title VII and the Rehabilitation Act, *Am J Law Med* 10:323, 1984.

Goldsby JW, Staats OJ: Characteristic cellular changes in oral epithelial cells in sickle cell diseases, *Cent Afr J Med* 10:336, 1964.

Mourshed F, Tuckson CR: A study of the radiographic features of the jaws in sickle cell anemia, *Oral Surg Oral Med Oral Pathol* 37:812, 1974.

Roberts JA, Pembrey ME: *An introduction to medical genetics,* ed 8, New York, 1985, Oxford University Press.

Walker RD, Schenck KL Jr: Infarct of the mandible in sickle cell anemia, *J Am Dent Assoc* 87:661, 1973.

Stafne Defect

Gorab GN, Brahney C, Aria AA: Unusual presentation of a Stafne bone cyst, *Oral Surg Oral Med Oral Pathol* 61:213, 1986.

Hansson L-G: Development of a lingual mandibular bone cavity in an 11-year-old boy, *Oral Surg Oral Med Oral Pathol* 49:376, 1980.

Langlais RP, Cottone J, Kasle MJ: Anterior and posterior lingual depressions of the mandible, *J Oral Surg* 34:502, 1976.

Karmiol M, Walsh RF: Incidence of static bone defect of the mandible, *Oral Surg Oral Med Oral Pathol* 26:225, 1968.

Oikarinen VJ, Julku M: An orthopantomographic study of developmental mandibular bone defects, *Int J Oral Surg* 3:71, 1974.

Wolf J, Mattila K, Ankkuriniemi O: Development of a Stafne mandibular bone cavity, *Oral Surg Oral Med Oral Pathol* 61:519, 1986.

Sturge-Weber Syndrome

Borns PF, Rancier LR: Cerebral calcification in childhood leukemia mimicking Sturge-Weber syndrome, *Am J Roentgenol Radiat Ther Nucl Med* 122:52, 1974.

Farman AG, Wilson S: Diagnostic imaging in Sturge-Weber syndrome, *Dentomaxillofac Radiol* 14:97, 1985.

Garcia JC, Roach ES, McLean WT: Recurrent thrombotic deterioration in Sturge-Weber syndrome, *Child Brain* 8:427, 1981.

Garwicz S, Mortensson W: Intracranial calcification mimicking Sturge-Weber syndrome, *Pediatr Radiol* 5:5, 1976.

Gordeur D, Palmieri A, Mashaly R: Cranial computed tomography in the phakomatoses, *Neuroradiology* 25:293, 1983.

Maki Y, Semba A: Computed tomography of Sturge-Weber disease, *Child Brain* 5:51, 1979.

Rothman L, Tenner M, Quencher R: Non-filling of the subependymal veins of the lateral ventricles, *Acta Radiol Suppl (Stockh)* 347:223, 1975.

Thalassemia

Logothesis J, et al: Cephalofacial deformities of thalassemia major, *Am J Dis Child* 121:300, 1971.

Novak AJ: The oral manifestations of erythroblastic (Cooley's) anemia, *Am J Orthod Oral Surg* 30:539, 1944.

Poyton HG, Davey KW: Thalassemia: changes visible in radiographs used in dentistry, *Oral Surg Oral Med Oral Pathol* 25:564, 1968.

Torus Mandibularis and Palatinus

Kolas S, et al: The occurrence of torus palatinus and torus mandibularis in 2,478 dental patients, *Oral Surg Oral Med Oral Pathol* 6:1134, 1953.

Moorrees CF: The dentition as a criterion of race with special reference to the Aleut, *J Dent Res* 30:815, 1951.

Suzuki JA, Sukai T: A familial study of torus palatinus and torus mandibularis, *Am J Phys Anthropol* 18:263, 1960.

5

TRAUMATIC INJURIES

TRAUMATIC DENTAL INJURY

Overview

We arbitrarily define recent trauma as injury occurring within 48 hours of the patient's presentation. The term *nonrecent trauma* is therefore reserved for patients who present after 48 hours from the time of injury. We realize that every patient is different and that a great deal of overlap in radiologic features exists between these two groups.

Traumatic injury to the dentition is not uncommon, and many of these injuries may go untreated. It is therefore important to know both the immediate and long-term radiographic appearances of dental injury. Radiographic assistance is particularly valuable in patients in whom the radicular portions of the teeth may be involved.

Except in determining pulpal involvement, which is better achieved clinically, the use of radiographic techniques may be helpful in ascertaining the degree of root apex closure, the presence of intrusion and luxation, and the existence of previous or concomitant periapical disease. Many classifications of trauma to the dentition exist, but none are universally accepted.

Clinical Features

Demographics: The most common cause of dental fracture is a direct blow to the incisor teeth. Maxillary teeth are more commonly affected than mandibular teeth, and the maxillary central incisors are most likely to be fractured. Males are more likely to suffer dental trauma than females, and most incidents occur in children between the ages of 10 and 15 years.

RADIOLOGIC FEATURES

Recent Traumatic Injury

Cardinal Signs

Thin radiolucent line or lines extending through any portion of the tooth (Such radiolucent fracture lines continue only for the length or breadth of a tooth and not beyond the confines of the radiographic shadow of the tooth. If the central ray of the x-ray beam passes directly through the fracture line, a single line will be evident. If it does not pass directly through a fracture line, then two thin radiolucent lines may be evident.)

"Step defect," in which an edge of the radiographic shadow of a structure exhibits a sudden change in direction

Well-defined yet soft radiolucent band confined to the radiographic shadow of the tooth (This is present when the central ray of the x-ray beam cuts the fracture line obliquely.)

Ancillary Signs

Radiopaque zone, usually visible in association with a step defect, caused by telescoping of the

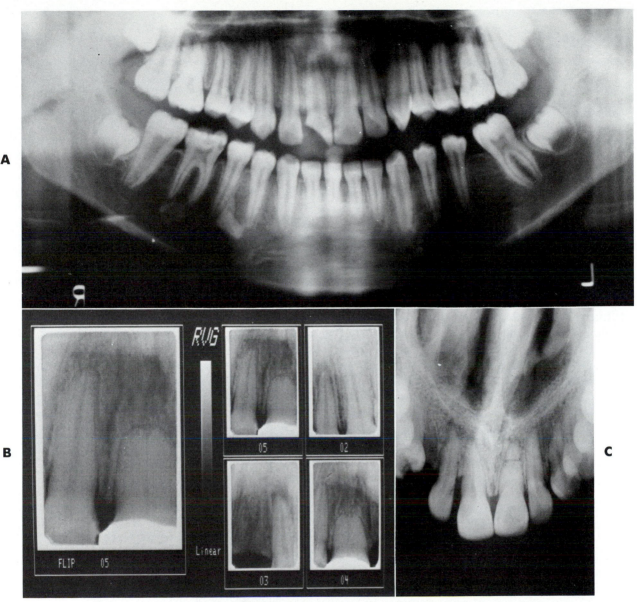

Fig. 5-1 A, Fractured central incisor (panoramic radiograph). **B,** External root resorption of apex of central incisor subsequent to fracture. Pulpal sclerosis is also present. Contralateral lateral incisor has periapical lesion. **C,** Topographic occlusal radiograph showing root fracture of left central incisor. There is also associated fracture of the alveolar bone.

tooth root when severe direct apical pressure to a tooth results in crushing the root

Splaying of the mesial and distal alveolar bone away from the tooth consequent to forceful intrusive apical pressure on tooth

Apparent elevation of the tooth in the socket, presumably caused by a combination of luxation and accumulation of inflammatory products at the apex of the tooth

Localized widening of the periodontal ligament space, the degree of which is determined by the amount of luxation

Dental fractures sometimes undetected if the fracture is incomplete, the beam does not transect the fracture, or there is no displacement of fracture segments

Nonrecent Traumatic Injury

Cardinal Signs

Fracture line discernible as thin radiolucent line or lines, as in recent fracture

Interposition of a radiolucent connective tissue zone between two radicular fracture segments, the edges of which have become rounded

Interposition of granulation tissue between two radicular fracture segments with widening of the fracture line and adjacent region of radiolucency

External root resorption confined to the neck of a tooth root and extending around its circumference

Widening of periodontal ligament shadow space adjacent to fracture (If this occurs at apex of tooth, periapical radiolucency results.)

Ancillary Signs

Dilaceration of tooth root caused by traumatic injury to a developing tooth

Partial or complete pulpal calcification best demonstrated when comparing the pulpal outlines of adjacent teeth

Paradoxically, the pulp of the traumatized tooth is possibly enlarged compared with adjacent normal teeth (This happens when pulpal necrosis occurs and secondary dentin is not laid down inside the traumatized tooth.)

Enostosis (external root resorption with bone ingrowth) resulting in radiolucency overlying the root of the tooth with apparent cancellous bone structure extending into the tooth root

Interposition of bone and connective tissue between two radicular segments with radiopaque bony trabecula between two root fragments

Gross localized periodontal bone loss associated with a vertical fracture

Localized enlargement of the pulp chamber or canals with resultant internal resorption

Gross external root resorption

Differential diagnosis

Vascular canal

Periodontal ligament shadow of an accessory or adjacent root

Overlying soft tissue shadow such as a lip shadow, nasolabial fold, alar shadow, or cheek shadow

Crimp in the radiographic film before exposure or processing

Fractured alveolus

DISPLACEMENT OF TEETH

Overview

In addition to causing coronal or radicular fractures, traumatic forces can cause changes in tooth position. A significant number of accidents result in displacement of a tooth to other areas of the body, including the lips, tongue, and even the lungs. This has prompted some to suggest soft tissue radiographs in cases in which teeth remain unaccounted for.

Classification: Andreasen and Andreasen have divided displaced or traumatized teeth into three broad categories: concussion, subluxation, and luxation. Concussion is said to occur when the tooth-supporting structures are injured without resultant tooth loosening or displacement. Clinically, the teeth are sensitive to percussion. Subluxation occurs when trauma results in abnormal tooth loosening without radiographically demonstrable loosening of the tooth. Luxated teeth are classified as extrusive, intrusive, or lateral, depending on the direction of the blow and the movement of the tooth.

Radiographic Assessment: Regardless of the nature of the injury, it is imperative that several exposures (at various vertical and horizontal angulations) of the traumatized tooth be made to detect luxations. Furthermore, bodily movement of the teeth does not exclude the possibility of a fracture. For this reason luxated teeth must be examined for the radiographic signs of radicular and coronal fractures. Finally, radiographs should be obtained serially to detect changes that can occur after the dental injury.

RADIOLOGIC FEATURES

Concussion

Often no radiologic signs

Localized widening of the radiographic shadow of the periodontal ligament space, most frequently at apical region of root

Subluxation

Often no radiologic changes

Marked tooth mobility usually accompanied by localized or generalized widening of the periodontal ligament space shadow

Luxation

Straight extrusive luxation results in widening of the periodontal ligament space.

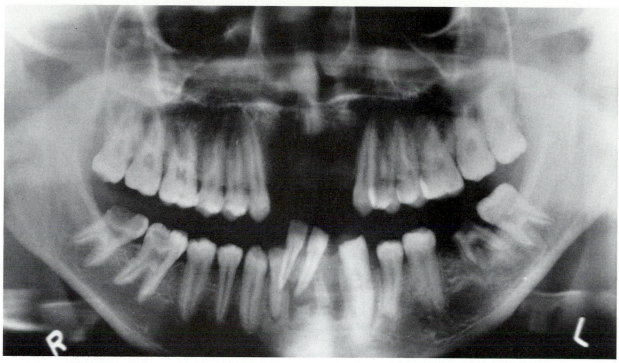

Fig. 5-2 Subluxation of mandibular anterior teeth following trauma. The maxillary central incisors have been lost completely.

Widening is uniform or restricted to the apical portion of the tooth.

Severe blow that moves the tooth bodily results in uniform increase in the width of the periodontal ligament on the side of tooth struck by the blow. If, however, the blow causes a levering of the tooth in the socket bone, periodontal ligament widening will occur on the side of the blow above the axis of rotation and on the opposite side below the axis of rotation.

Minor alveolar fractures will occur in lateral and extrusive luxation of the teeth and can be radiographically demonstrable when occurring on the mesial or distal aspects of the involved tooth.

Minor alveolar fractures on the buccal or lingual aspects of a tooth can be masked by the radiographic shadow of the tooth itself.

Luxated tooth will often be located either inferiorly or superiorly in relation to the normal occlusal plane.

Intrusive Luxation

Diminution of the periodontal ligament space shadow present, being marked in the apical regions

Splaying of alveolar bone adjacent to intruded tooth

Improper relationship between the crest of the alveolar bone and the cementoenamel junction (With intrusion the alveolar crest will be located coronal to the cementoenamel junction.)

Direct contact between root of the intruded tooth and the adjacent cancellous bone

Long-term changes associated with luxated teeth

About half of traumatized teeth develop pulp necrosis. Radiographically, pulp necrosis should be suspected in a tooth that has an enlarged pulp compared with its neighbors (absence of continued secondary dentin production).

Periapical inflammation, often a sequela of pulpal necrosis, is not uncommon after luxation injuries. Radiographically, an area of periapical rarefaction with or without an adjacent region of osseous sclerosis is visible.

External root resorption is usually visible in a few weeks and is typified radiographically by an irregular moth-eaten appearance of the root. It usually occurs within 3 to 4 months of the injury.

Pulpal obliteration (calcification of the dental pulp) occurs in about one in five cases.

Loss of crestal or marginal alveolar bone occurs in a small number of cases and is indistinguishable from simple periodontitis.

Ankylosis of teeth occurs more commonly with intrusion and reimplantation of avulsed teeth but can occur in association with luxated teeth. Radiographically, there is close approximation of root and cancellous bone and merging of the two tissues.

Damage to permanent tooth buds after trauma to primary teeth has been reported. This consists of arrest in root formation, gross deformity of resultant tooth structures, dilaceration, obliteration of the pulp chamber, and transposition of teeth.

In many cases no long-term radiographic signs are present.

Gross displacement of teeth

If a tooth is present in bone, it should cast a periodontal ligament space shadow.

If the tooth is outside bone, it can be in soft tissue, beneath the periosteum, in a body cavity such as the sinus, in one of the fascial planes, in the gastrointestinal tract, or in a lung. Teeth usually go into the right lung, because the right bronchus has a relatively straight course compared with the left.

ALVEOLAR FRACTURE

Overview

Definition: Alveolar fractures are restricted to those contained in the alveolar processes of the maxilla or mandible.

Pathogenesis: The most common cause of alveolar fractures is probably tooth extraction accompanied by removal of a portion of the maxilla (commonly) or mandible. Alveolar fractures can also be caused by direct blunt trauma to the teeth and indirect trauma resulting from a severe blow to the chin point with resultant force transfer to mandibular and maxillary teeth. Direct and indirect trauma can occur in motor vehicle accidents, work accidents, or sports or as a result of violence.

Clinical Features

Demographics: Alveolar fractures unassociated with more profound jawbone features reportedly constitute about 3% of maxillofacial fractures. Alveolar fractures are likely to be more common than this because of underreporting of iatrogenic (extraction) incidents and alveolar fractures associated with minor dentofacial trauma.

Symptoms and Signs: Fractures of the alveolar processes are often accompanied by fractures of teeth. It is prudent to evaluate teeth for dental fractures, intrusion or extrusion, and extent of root development. There is usually displacement of a single tooth or segment of teeth so that finger pressure exerted on one corner of the segment is accompanied by movement of the whole segment. Malocclusion can result from such fractures. There is usually tenderness and occasionally crepitation with digital movement of the segment. Ecchymosis of the adjacent sulci is also not uncommon. Edema, gingival laceration, contusions, and abrasions can also be present.

Radiographic assessment: For radiographic evaluation of an alveolar fracture, intraoral periapical or occlusal radiographs offer adequate definition to best determine and outline the fracture line. For a fracture to be evident, the beam must transect the fracture line directly. For this reason multiple views are beneficial, with two views in different planes being the minimum requirement.

RADIOLOGIC FEATURES

Cardinal Signs

Sharply defined, uncorticated, and occasionally jagged radiolucent line at any level of the alveolus

Fracture lines most often horizontal

Step defects between the fracture segment and the normal adjacent bone (Border of the fracture will show a sharp jag relative to the normal bony contour.)

Segment of teeth in region of displaced bone

Splintering of bone at the margin of the segment

Widening of periodontal ligament if the fracture line runs through tooth periodontal space

Text continued on page 164.

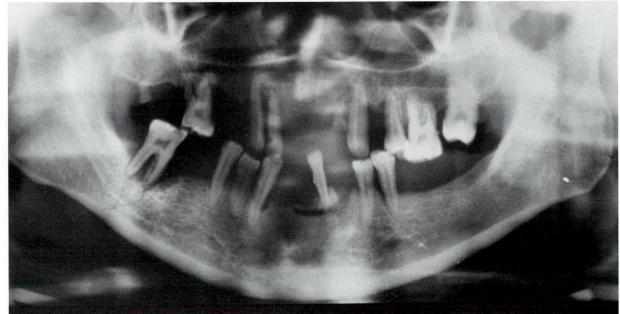

Fig. 5-3 **A,** Alveolar fracture in anterior mandible (panoramic radiograph). There is also a mandibular fracture in the right molar region, extending apical to the anterior root. **B,** Topographic occlusal radiograph of mandible showing alveolar fracture associated with the right canine and incisors and the left central incisor. There is also a fracture through the mandibular symphysis region. **C,** Panoramic radiograph showing alveolar fracture in anterior mandible.

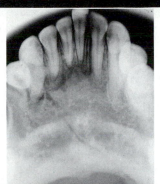

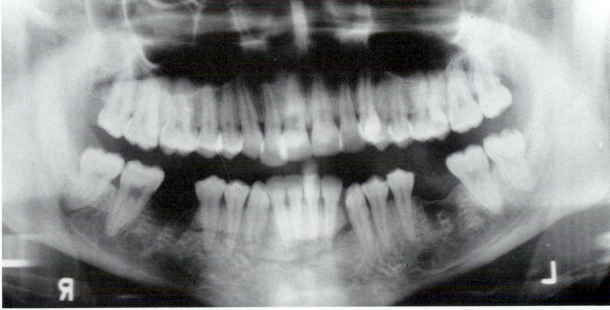

Continued.

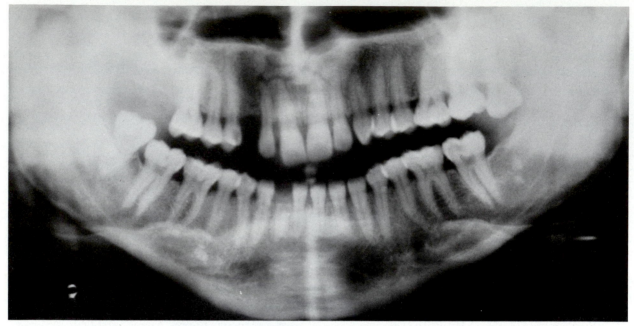

D

Fig. 5-3, cont'd.   D, Panoramic radiograph demonstrating alveolar fracture in anterior maxilla.

Ancillary Signs

Root fractures affecting teeth in the fractured segment

Little or no radiographic evidence in single-surface fracture (in which one side is bent and the other fractured)

Vertical intrusion of teeth sometimes accompanied by outward splaying of adjacent support bone so that fracture is evidenced by submergence of tooth with bordering spurs of alveolar bone projecting from either side

Increased uptake of technetium 99mdp at site of fracture

Differential Diagnosis

Nutrient canals

Overlapping normal periodontal ligament space shadows

Overlapping lip lines or nasolabial soft tissue margins

Fracture of teeth uncomplicated by alveolar fracture

MANDIBULAR CONDYLAR FRACTURE

Overview

The mandible may be likened to an archer's bow. The body and rami constitute the arch of the bow, with the condylar necks and heads as the supporting ends. Therefore any force directed to the arch is transferred to the condyles.

Pathogenesis: Condylar fractures can occur in motor vehicle accidents, work accidents, or sports or as a result of violence. Motor vehicle accidents and personal violence are the most common causes.

Text continued on page 166.

Fig. 5-4   A, (opposite page) Panoramic radiograph showing fracture of right mandibular condyle and left mandibular angle. **B,** Reverse Towne projection of left condylar head fracture showing lateral displacement. **C,** Reverse Towne projection of left condylar head fracture showing medial displacement. **D,** Panoramic radiograph showing fracture of left mandibular condyle and mandibular symphyseal region.

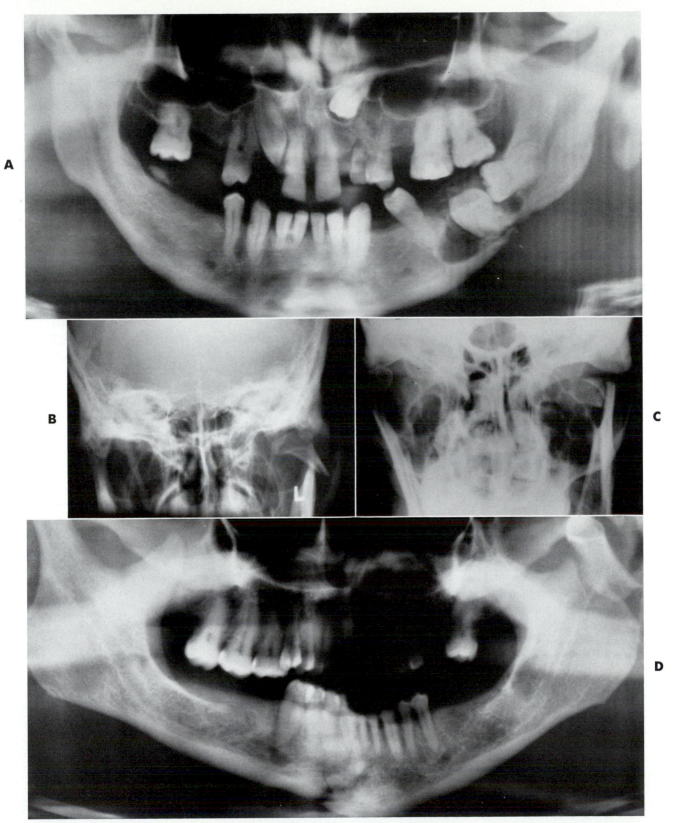

Fig. 5-4, cont'd. For legend see opposite page.

Clinical Features

Demographics: The mandible is the most commonly fractured facial bone. Condylar fractures are also common. They constitute up to 30% of all mandibular fractures and affect all age groups.

Symptoms and Signs: Patients with condylar fractures may have evidence of trauma to the symphysis region of the jaw, with localized pain and swelling over the joint region and limited opening. In addition, occlusal disharmony of recent onset, open bite on the contralateral side, and deviation to the affected side on maximal opening are also often present. If the fracture is of sufficient severity, a soft tissue defect or evidence of hemorrhage can be present in the external acoustic meatus. On palpation there may be no evidence of translational condylar movement, and when maximal opening of the jaw is attempted, a step defect may be palpable over the joint region.

Condylar fractures may be classified as simple, compound, comminuted, or greenstick. They may be horizontally favorable or unfavorable, depending on the relationship between the fracture ends and the lateral pterygoid muscle pull. Condylar fractures can also be differentiated on the basis of their location. They are either confined to the joint capsule (intracapsular) or located outside of it (extracapsular).

RADIOLOGIC FEATURES

Cardinal Signs

Intracapsular fractures seen as crush injuries in which the condylar head is telescoped inward on itself (Step defects are often visible at the anterior edge of the summit of the condylar head.)

Overlap of trabecular pattern visualized as band of increased opacity at the fracture site

Condylar head split in two when viewed on a posteroanterior projection, such as the reverse Towne or transorbital views.

Ancillary Signs

Condyle is "sheared off" and displaced to one side (usually the medial) with displacement on the posteroanterior view and increased radiopacity on lateral projections.

Articular portion of the condylar head can be crushed by heavy force, resulting in marked radiopacity of the condylar head region, appearing not as a normal condyle but as "a bag of fragmented bone."

Bilateral condylar neck fractures are not uncommonly associated with symphyseal or parasymphyseal fractures.

Step defect can be present at the distal border of the mandible with the condylar neck portion extending medially and anteriorly.

Medial displacement of the condylar head is common in horizontally unfavorable condylar neck fractures. Lateral displacement of the condylar fracture segment is said to be rare.

On computed tomography (axial and coronal views) displaced condylar heads are readily visualized as radiopacities immediately medial to the residual condylar necks.

Deviation of the mandible to the affected side is evidenced on posteroanterior views of the mandible.

Anterior open bite is visible on lateral projections in bilateral fractures of the condylar necks.

In rare instances the condylar head maintains its integrity, but the force of the blow drives the entire head superiorly, breeching the articular fossa so that the condyles come to rest in the middle cranial fossa.

Differential Diagnosis

Charcot joint, also known as neuropathic joint (This is the result of fracture, but the mechanism is different in that chronic overloading of the joint creates the so-called bag of bones.)

Severe degenerative joint disease mimicking the sclerosis of telescoped fracture segments—can be differentiated on the basis of lack of a trauma history

Pathologic fracture (malignancy or infection)

Bifid condylar head (normal variant)

MANDIBULAR BODY FRACTURES

Overview

Definition: Mandibular body fractures are fractures involving portions of the bone, excluding the condylar heads or necks and alveolar processes.

Pathogenesis: Fractures of the mandible have a variety of causes, including motor vehicle accidents, personal violence, and sports injuries.

Clinical Features

Demographics: Fractures of the mandible are more common than fractures of the maxilla. The most common site of mandibular body fracture is the junc-

Text continued on page 171.

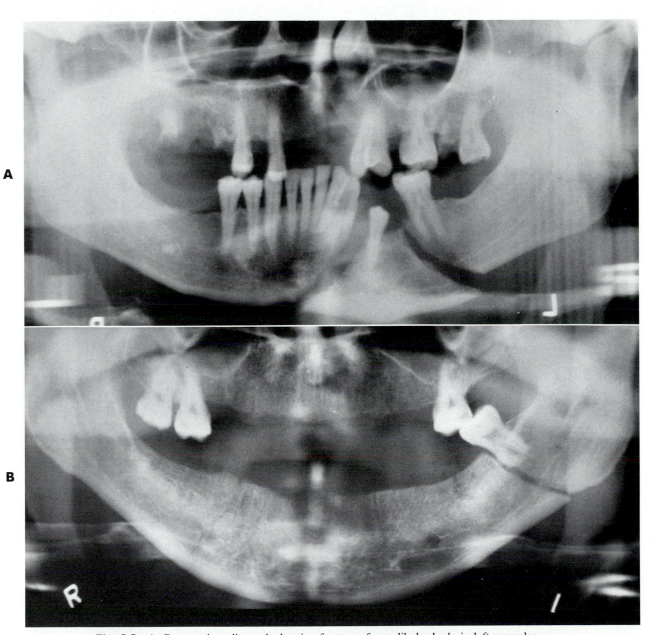

Fig. 5-5 A, Panoramic radiograph showing fracture of mandibular body in left premolar region. The affected segment is relatively depressed, taking the left mandibular premolar below the occlusal level. **B,** Fracture of left mandibular angle. The panoramic radiograph shows a single line as the x-ray beam is parallel to the fracture.   *Continued.*

C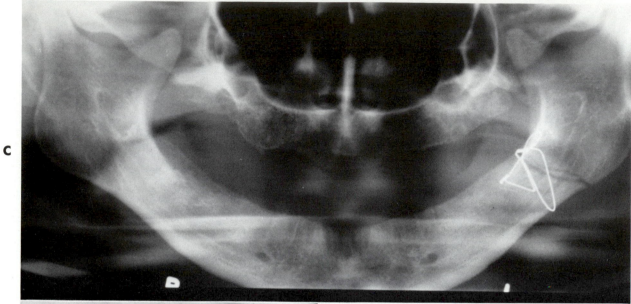

D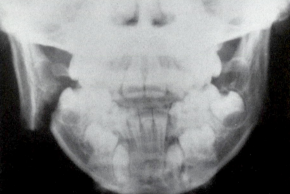

Fig. 5-5, cont'd.   **C,** Same patient as in **B.** After surgical fixation of the separated segments, another panoramic radiograph was taken. The x-ray beam was no longer parallel to the fracture line, hence the fracture lines through the buccal and lingual plates are not superimposed. This leads to an apparent "double fracture." **D,** Posteroanterior projection showing fracture of right mandibular angle. **E,** Panoramic radiograph of same patient as in **D** shows the importance of having at least two views at right angles when a fracture is suspected. The fracture is not as obvious with this projection.

E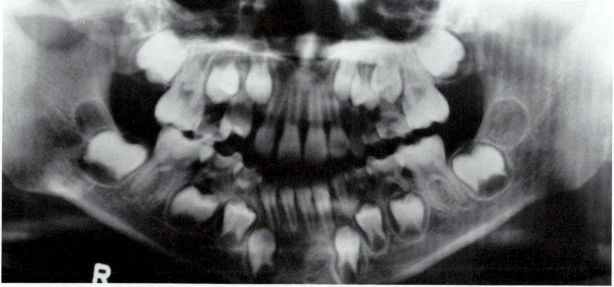

Continued.

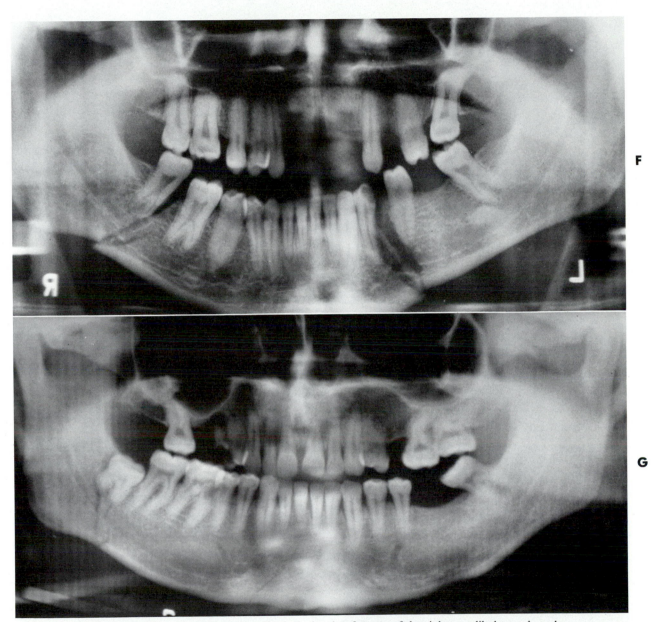

Fig. 5-5, cont'd.   F, Panoramic radiograph showing fracture of the right mandibular angle and left premolar region. **G,** Fracture of right side of mandible extending through distal periodontal membrane space of unerupted third molar (panoramic radiograph).   *Continued.*

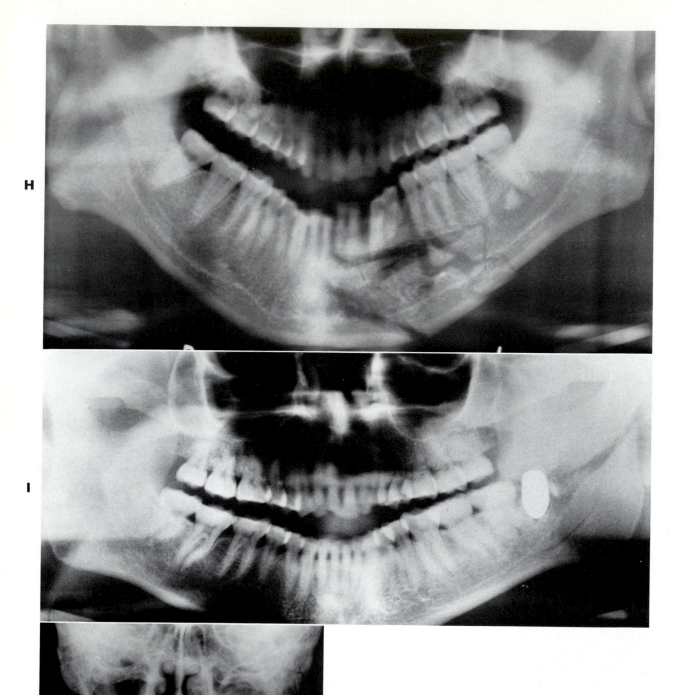

Fig. 5-5, cont'd.   H, Comminuted fracture of left mandibular body (panoramic radiograph). **I,** Panoramic radiograph of comminuted fracture caused by bullet. **J,** Posteroanterior projection of patient in **I.**

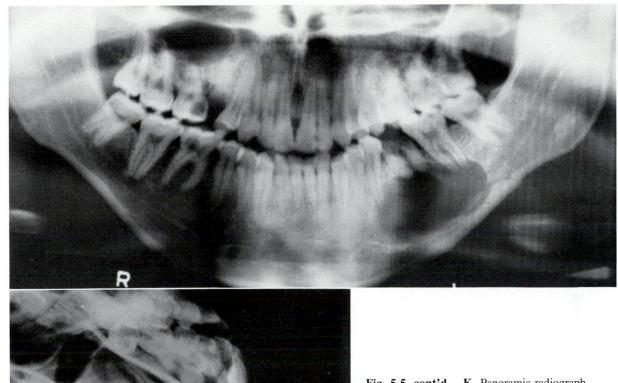

K

R

L

Fig. 5-5, cont'd. **K,** Panoramic radiograph showing pathologic fracture associated with large apical radicular cyst. **L,** Lateral-oblique projection of patient in **K.**

tion of the body and ramus, followed by the molar region, the mental portion, the symphyseal and parasymphyseal region, and the mid ramus.

Symptoms and Signs: Mandibular fractures are characterized by depressed or raised fragments, alterations in the occlusal plane, mucosal lacerations, crepitus on palpation, inability to perform the normal range of mandibular motion, movement of segments of the jaw, pain, and ecchymosis of the adjacent sulci.

There are three ways to classify mandibular body fractures, based on the nature of the fracture, the favorability of the fracture, and the fracture site.

Favorability of a fracture refers to the relationship of the fracture line to the direction of muscle pull.

Generally, fractures are either vertically favorable or unfavorable or horizontally favorable or unfavorable. In favorable fractures normal muscle action causes approximation of the fracture segments. In the unfavorably fractured jaw the segments are distracted by the paramandibular musculature. The nature of a fracture is simple, compound, comminuted, or greenstick. Greenstick fractures are those in which one plate of the bone fractures and the other is bent. This type is more commonly seen in younger patients because of the malleability of juvenile bone. The term *simple fracture* refers to a single complete fracture that has not breeched the integument, so that the fracture segments are not connected to the outside air. In compound fractures, a fracture segment contacts the outside surface, either mucosal or skin. Comminuted fractures are those in which more than one fracture is present in the same bone. These often appear as if the bone has been crushed into many parts.

Radiologic assessment: Radiologic investigation of mandibular body fractures is best performed using high-quality conventional radiographic views. These should include panoramic dental views, lateral oblique projections of the mandible, posteroanterior mandibular projections, reverse Towne views, and basal or occlusal views.

RADIOLOGIC FEATURES

Cardinal signs

Mandibular fractures are characterized by a radiographically visible line of cleavage.

If the x-ray beam passes directly through and parallel to the fracture line, then a single, ragged edged, uncorticated fracture line results.

If the x-ray beam passes oblique to the fracture, then the line of cleavage might not be seen.

Double fracture lines may be present in simple fractures, depending on the relationship between the fracture lines in the buccal and lingual plates.

Fracture line can involve a tooth socket (or tooth), in which case the fracture line may disappear into a widened periodontal ligament space.

Ancillary signs

Jaw fractures that involve tooth-bearing areas may be accompanied by radiographic signs consistent with fractures of teeth.

Mandibular body fractures are frequently accompanied by fractures of the contralateral condylar head or neck.

Impaction of the fracture segments results in a band of slightly increased opacity at the fracture site. If intraoral views with sufficient resolution are obtained, an overlapping of individual trabeculae may be visible.

Step defects are visible in lateral or occlusal projections.

Greenstick fractures can result in a sharp angulation. Small spicules of bone away from the surface are visible at the fracture site.

Comminuted fractures show a multitude of radiolucent fracture lines.

Differential diagnosis

Normal soft tissue superimpositions (A common misinterpretation of mandibular fracture is the shadow of the pharynx superimposed over the mandibular angle in lateral projections and panoramic views.)

LE FORT TYPE MAXILLOFACIAL FRACTURE

Overview

Definition: Le Fort facial fractures involve the middle third of the facial skeleton and its relationship to the cranial base. The three basic categories of Le Fort fractures are conveniently called Le Fort I, Le Fort II, and Le Fort III. They may occur unilaterally or bilaterally.

Pathogenesis: Motor vehicle accidents are the most common cause of Le Fort fractures.

Clinical Features

Demographics: Mid-third facial fractures are about one fourth as common as fractures of the mandible. The peak age incidence is in the third decade of life. Men constitute more than 80% of patients with these fractures. Le Fort type injuries in children are comparatively rare.

Symptoms and signs: Le Fort fractures are accompanied by specific signs. Le Fort I fractures are defined as those occurring above the level of the maxillary teeth apices and include fractures of the alveolar processes, the palate, and the pterygoid processes of the sphenoid. In one study Le Fort I comprised about a quarter of Le Fort fractures. Clinically the fracture block can be manipulated as if it were a maxillary denture. If there is displacement, there may be an open bite or alteration in the occlusal relationship. Swelling of the facial region, periorbital ecchymosis, and epistaxis can also be present. The mid-facial contour may be flattened, and the patient may report diplopia, paresthesia, or pain.

Le Fort II fractures constitute about 60% of Le Fort fractures and are accompanied by more serious clinical signs. A typical Le Fort II fracture, termed a *pyramidal fracture,* is a fracture across the nasal bones and frontal processes of the maxilla. It then characteristically extends laterally through the lacrimal bone and inferior rim of the orbit, transversing the orbital rim near the zygomaticomaxillary suture. Finally, the fracture extends laterally and backward along the lateral wall of the maxilla and through the pterygoid plates.

Text continued on page 174.

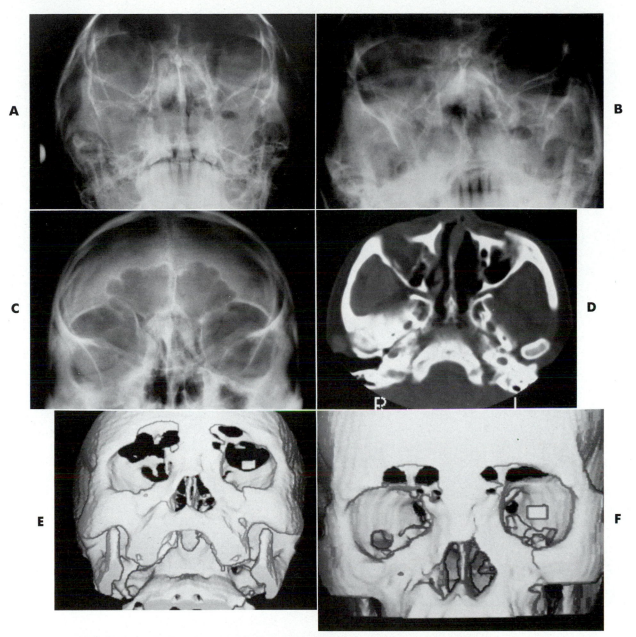

Fig. 5-6 A, Posteroanterior radiograph. Le Fort I midfacial fracture with bilateral fractures of the lateral walls of the left and right maxillary sinuses. Both sinuses show opacification. **B,** Posteroanterior radiograph. Le Fort II midfacial fracture. Note bilateral fracture lines extending obliquely through the nasofrontal sutures, through the medial and inferior aspects of both orbits and lateral walls of both maxillary sinuses. **C,** Posteroanterior view of Le Fort II fractures. **D,** Axial CT scan of patient in **C. E,** Three-dimensional CT reconstruction of Le Fort II fractures (same patient as in **C**). **F,** Three-dimensional CT reconstruction of patient in **C.**

Continued.

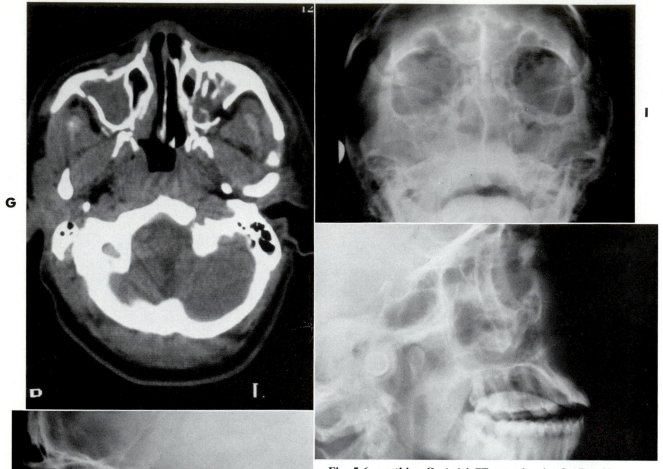

Fig. 5-6, cont'd. **G,** Axial CT scan showing Le Fort II fractures. Note discontinuities of walls of maxillary sinuses. **H,** Lateral radiograph demonstrating fracture lines in the nasoethmoidal and anterior maxillary regions (both Le Fort I and Le Fort III). **I,** Posteroanterior projection of Le Fort III midfacial fractures involving the lateral walls of the maxillary sinuses and concomitant opacification of both maxillary sinuses. Also note the fracture lines involving the glabella and left and right zygomaticofrontal sutures. **J,** Lateral view demonstrating a Le Fort III fracture involving the nasoethmoidal region.

Clinically, Le Fort II facial fractures are accompanied by swelling of the involved area, orbital edema, and ecchymosis and subconjunctival hemorrhage. The contour of the nose is displaced laterally or anteroposteriorly and is accompanied by epistaxis. The mid-third facial height is often increased. The occlusal re-lationship of the teeth is altered by displacement of the maxilla.

Le Fort III fractures are also termed *craniofacial dysjunction,* which describes the shearing of the facial complex from the cranial base that typically occurs with this severe injury. This fracture involves the na-sofrontal, maxillofrontal, and zygomaticofrontal su-tures, as well as the orbital, ethmoid, and sphenoid sinus floors. They are the least common of the Le Fort fractures. Clinically there is often massive edema, increased length of the mid face, subconjunctival bleeding, paresthesia, displacement of the mid face in one or more directions, and alteration in the occlusal relationships of the teeth. Finally, this fracture is often associated with cerebrospinal fluid rhinorrhea, resulting from the disruption of the integrity of the cranial base.

Radiographic assessment: The radiographic assessment of these patients should be based on a thorough clinical examination after the patient is stabilized. Technetium bone scans can also assist in outlining the areas to be studied radiographically. Facial fractures can be associated with craniocerebral or spinal injuries and are best assessed with high-resolution computed tomography.

RADIOLOGIC FEATURES

Le Fort I

Clouding of the maxillary sinus shadows on one or both sides

Sharp horizontal line or lines of cleavage through the maxilla or pterygoid plates of the sphenoid

Canted maxilla relative to the cranial base and mandibular teeth

Discontinuity of the lateral maxillary sinus walls visible on plane films or computed tomography

Le Fort II

Increased width of frontonasal suture with or without concomitant fracture of one or both nasal bones

Radiolucent line of cleavage extending across one or both frontal processes of the maxilla

Step defect with or without line of cleavage visible in one or both infraorbital rims

Separation of zygomaticomaxillary suture unilaterally or bilaterally

Obscuring of radiolucent maxillary sinus shadows as a consequence of bleeding into the air spaces

Radiolucent line of cleavage extending through one or both pterygoid plates of the sphenoid bone

Disruption of the maxillomandibular occlusal relationship

Le Fort III

Widening of the normal nasofrontal suture with or without fracture of the nasal bones themselves

Widening of the maxillofrontal suture

Enlargement of the zygomaticofrontal suture

Enlargement of the zygomaticotemporal suture

Radiolucent line of cleavage extending through the frontal processes of the maxilla

Radiolucent line of cleavage extending through one or both pterygoid plates

Radiolucent line of cleavage or step defects associated with one or both orbital floors

Disruption of the normal radiolucent appearance of all the paranasal sinuses as a consequence of hemorrhage into them after injury

Differential Diagnosis

Shadows of the cranial base or intervertebral shadows

ZYGOMATICOMAXILLARY FRACTURES

Overview

Pathogenesis: Zygomaticomaxillary fractures are most often caused by a direct blow to the height of zygomatic arch, which can occur during sports, in motor vehicle accidents, or as a result of personal violence.

Clinical Features

Demographics: Zygomaticomaxillary fractures are less common than mandibular fractures but more common than Le Fort type facial fractures. Le Fort III account for about 10% of facial fractures in children.

Radiographic assessment: Radiographs are obtained when the patient is clinically stable. Radiographically the projections best suited to demonstrate zygomaticomaxillary arch fractures include posteroanterior skull views, lateral projections, and Waters views, which are especially good for evaluating the presence of coronoid impingement. A basal skull projection allows for examination of the contour of the zygomaticomaxillary prominence.

Symptoms and signs: The affected side is flattened. It is best examined by viewing the face superoinferiorly from the top of the patient's head. Because of the medial displacement of most of these fractures, the skin overlying the fracture dimples, and the lower part of the cheek feels full. When the region is palpated, the patient experiences pain. Subconjunctival hemorrhage is also associated with malar fractures, as is swelling of the involved tissue and epistaxis. If the fracture is severe, paresthesia of the cheek may be present.

Text continued on page 177.

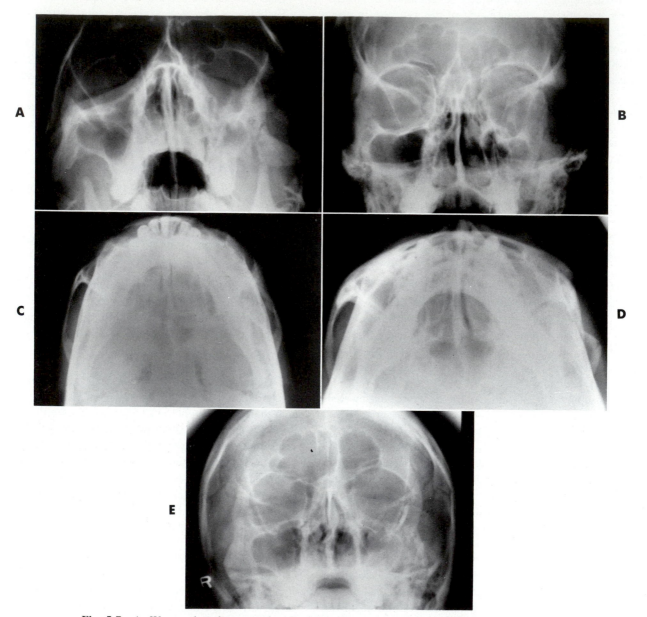

Fig. 5-7 A, Waters view demonstrating displaced tripod fracture on the left side.
B, Posteroanterior view demonstrating displaced tripod fracture of left zygomatic arch. Note separation of zygomaticofrontal suture. **C,** Submentovertex projection showing depressed fracture of left zygomatic arch. **D,** Submentovertex projection showing depressed fracture of left zygomatic arch. **E,** Waters projection showing fracture of left zygomatic arch and blow-out fracture of left orbital floor.

RADIOLOGIC FEATURES

Cardinal signs

Depression of zygomatic arch as viewed on the basal, Waters, and posteroanterior skull views

Widening of zygomaticofrontal, zygomaticomaxillary, or zygomaticotemporal suture lines

Step defects at junction of frontal and zygomatic bones, zygomatic and maxillary bones, or temporal and zygomatic bones

Ancillary signs

Close proximity of the coronoid process to the medial aspect of the zygomatic arch on the affected side as viewed on the basal, Waters, and posteroanterior skull views

V-shaped depression fracture of the zygomatic prominence with the apex of the V directed medially (best demonstrated on basal view)

Fracture line obscured by soft tissue swelling, visible as an increased soft tissue shadow overlying the prominence of the zygomatic bone on the affected side

Maxillary sinus shadow obscured by hemorrhage into the sinus as a consequence of breeching of its lateral wall

Zygomatic bone possibly rotated upward and inward on the Waters projection, so that a greater portion of the lateral aspect of this bone is visible on the affected side

Multiple lines of cleavage in cases of comminuted fractures of the zygomatic arch (rare)

Step defect possibly at junction of zygomatic bone and orbital floor on the posteroanterior projection

Differential Diagnosis

Infraorbital canal

Zygomaticomaxillary suture

Zygomaticotemporal suture

BLOW-OUT FRACTURE

Overview

Definition and pathogenesis: Blow-out fractures result from a blow to the orbit by an object too large to enter the orbit (e.g., a fist or tennis ball). The force is transmitted to the thin orbital floor, which generally fractures near the infraorbital canal.

Clinical Features

Demographics: Blow-out fractures represent 3% to 5% of all mid-facial fractures.

Symptoms and Signs: A history of trauma is usually elicited. Diplopia results from periorbital edema and hemorrhage or occasionally muscle entrapment in the fracture line. Ecchymosis is apparent. Enophthalmos can be noticeable. Less frequently, communication with the anterior cranial fossa can lead to cerebrospinal fluid leakage into the orbit or herniation of the meninges or brain through the fracture lines.

RADIOLOGIC FEATURES

Cardinal Signs

Soft tissue swelling over the orbital rim

Opacification of affected maxillary sinus

Displaced orbital floor (occasionally hidden by soft tissue swelling); "trap door" appearance

Polypoid density in roof of maxillary sinus (teardrop herniation of orbital content)

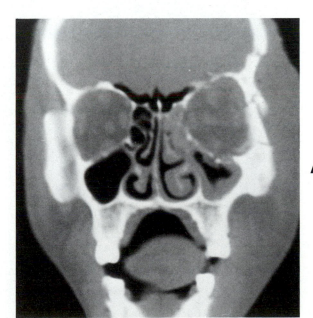

A

Fig. 5-8 **A,** Coronal CT showing fracture of lateral margin of left orbit and blow-out fracture into left maxillary sinus. Note lack of continuity of orbital margin and floor and thickening of the left maxillary sinus mucosa on the left side. *Continued.*

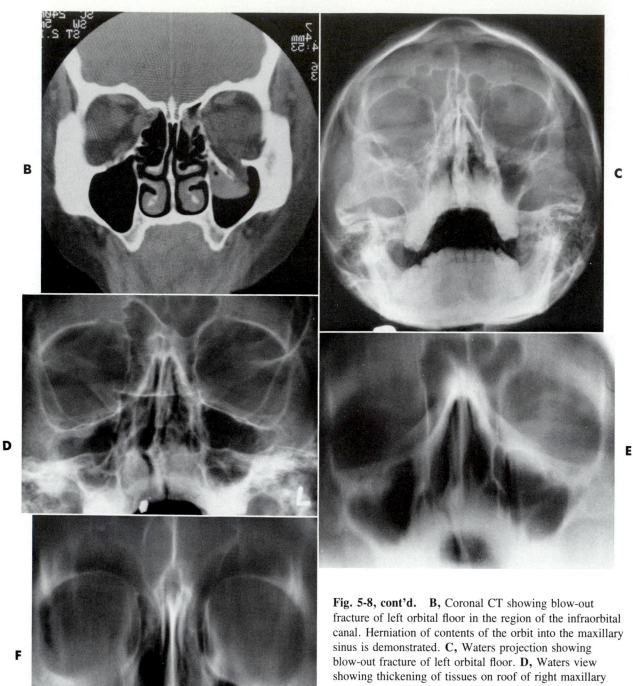

Fig. 5-8, cont'd. **B,** Coronal CT showing blow-out fracture of left orbital floor in the region of the infraorbital canal. Herniation of contents of the orbit into the maxillary sinus is demonstrated. **C,** Waters projection showing blow-out fracture of left orbital floor. **D,** Waters view showing thickening of tissues on roof of right maxillary sinus, representing a blow-out fracture of the right orbital floor. **E,** Tomograph of same patient as in **D.** The discontinuity of the orbital floor is apparent on this view. **F,** Tomograph showing classical "trap door" sign of right-side blow-out fracture. There is a general haziness from associated maxillary sinusitis.

Ancillary Signs

Orbital fat higher than normal attenuation on computed tomography from hemorrhage

Orbital emphysema

Differential Diagnosis

Maxillary sinus polyp

Mucous extravasation phenomenon

REFERENCES

Tooth Fractures

Andreasen FM, et al: Occurrence of pulp canal obliteration (PCO) after luxation injuries in the permanent dentition, *Endod Dent Traumatol* 3:103, 1987.

Andreasen JO, Hjorting-Hansen E: Intra-alveolar root fractures: radiographic and histologic study of 50 cases, *J Oral Maxillofac Surg* 25:414, 1967.

Artun J, Aamdal HMA: Severe root resorption of fractured maxillary lateral incisor following endodontic treatment and orthodontic extrusion, *Endod Dent Traumatol* 3:263, 1987.

Beeching BW: *Interpreting dental radiographs,* London, 1981, Update Books, pp 45-49.

Bennett DJ: Traumatized anterior teeth, *Br Dent J* 115:309, 1963.

Birch R, Rock DP: The incidence of complications following root fracture in permanent anterior teeth, *Br Dent J* 160:119, 1986.

Chow MH: Radiographic appearance of root fracture caused by a bend on the radiograph, *Oral Surg Oral Med Oral Pathol* 55:220, 1983.

Galea H: An investigation of dental injuries treated in an acute care general hospital, *J Am Dent Assoc* 109:434, 1984.

Goaz PW, White SC: *Oral radiology: principles and interpretation,* ed 2, St. Louis, 1987, Mosby–Year Book, pp 719-727.

Goldstein AR: Periodontal defects associated with root fracture, *J Am Dent Assoc* 102:863, 1981.

Kreutz RW, Kinni ME: Pseudo-fracture of mandibular first molar, *Oral Surg Oral Med Oral Pathol* 64:774, 1987.

Macko DJ, et al: A study of fractured anterior teeth in a school population, *J Am Soc Dent Child* 46:130, 1979.

Moule AJ, Thomas RP: Cervical external root resorption following trauma: a case report, *Int Endod J* 18:277, 1985.

Oikarnen K, Kassila O: Causes and types of traumatic tooth injuries treated in a public dental health clinic, *Endod Dent Traumatol* 3:172, 1978.

Oluwole TO, Leverett DH: Clinical and epidemiological survey of adolescents with crown fractures of permanent anterior teeth, *Pediatr Dent* 8:221, 1986.

Orkin DA, Naidoo C: Radiolucent artifacts simulating root or tooth fractures, *J Dent Assoc S Afr* 34:179, 1979.

Poyton HG: *Oral radiology,* Baltimore, 1982, Williams & Wilkins, pp 260-279.

Ravn JJ: Follow-up study of permanent incisors with enamel fractures as a result of an acute trauma, *Scand J Dent Res* 89:213, 1981.

Worth HM: *Principles and practice of oral radiologic interpretation,* Chicago, 1963, Year Book Medical, pp 373-383.

Displacement of Teeth

Allen FJ: Dental fragments in the lips, *Int J Oral Maxillofac Surg* 10(suppl 1):260, 1981.

Andreasen FM, et al: Occurrence of pulp canal obliteration after luxation injuries in the permanent dentition, *Endod Dent Traumatol* 3:103, 1987.

Andreasen FM, Andreasen JO: Diagnosis of luxation injuries: the importance of standardized clinical, radiographic, and photographic techniques in clinical investigations, *Endod Dent Traumatol* 1:160, 1985.

Andreasen FM, Yu Z, Thomsen BL: Relationship between pulpal dimensions and the development of pulp necrosis after luxation injuries in the permanent dentition, *Endod Dent Traumatol* 2:90, 1986.

Andreasen JO: Luxation of permanent teeth due to trauma: a clinical and radiographic follow-up study of 184 injured teeth, *Scand J Dent Res* 78:273, 1970.

Andreasen JO: Replantation of teeth. I. Radiographic and clinical study of 110 human teeth replanted after accidental loss, *Acta Odontol Scand* 24:263, 1966.

Belostoky L: Undiagnosed intrusion of a maxillary primary incisor tooth: 15-year follow-up, *Pediatr Dent* 8:294, 1986.

Gibilsco JA: *Stafne's oral radiographic diagnosis,* ed 5, Philadelphia, 1985, W.B. Saunders, pp 341-345.

Goaz PW, White S: *Oral radiology principles and interpretation,* St Louis, 1987, Mosby–Year Book, pp 719-722.

McIntosh GC, Steadman RK, Gross B: Aspiration of an erupted permanent tooth during maxillofacial trauma, *J Oral Maxillofac Surg* 40:448, 1982.

Oikarinen K, Gunlach K, Pfeifer G: Late complications of luxation injuries to the teeth, *Endod Dent Traumatol* 3:296, 1987.

Poyton HG: *Oral radiology,* Baltimore, 1982, Williams & Wilkins p 279.

Symons AL: Root resorption: a complication following traumatic avulsion, *ASDC J Dent Child* 53:271, 1986.

Worth HM: *Principles and practice of oral radiologic interpretation,* Chicago, 1963, Year Book Medical, pp 373-383.

Zilberman Y, et al: Effect of trauma to primary incisors on root development of their permanent successors, *Pediatr Dent* 8:289, 1986.

Maxillofacial Fracture

Afzelius L, Rosen C: Facial fractures: a review of 368 cases, *Int J Oral Maxillofac Surg* 9:25, 1980.

Daffner RH, et al: Computed tomography in the evaluation of severe facial trauma, *Comput Radiol* 7:91, 1983.

DelBalso AM, Hall RE, Margarone JE: Radiographic evaluation of maxillofacial trauma. In DelBalso AM, editor: *Maxillofacial imaging,* Philadelphia, 1990, W.B. Saunders, pp 35-128.

Dolan KD, Jacoby CG: Facial fractures, *Semin Roentgenol* 13:37, 1978.

Duval AJ, Banovetz JD: Maxillary fractures, *Otolaryngol Clin North Am* 9:489, 1976.

Ellis E, El-Attar A, Moos KF: An analysis of 2,067 cases of zygomatico-orbital fracture, *J Oral Maxillofac Surg* 43:417, 1985.

Ellis E, Moos KF, El-Attar A: Ten years of mandibular fractures: an analysis of 2,137 cases, *Oral Surg Oral Med Oral Pathol* 59:120, 1985.

Finkle DR, et al: Comparison of the diagnostic methods used in maxillofacial trauma, *Plast Reconstr Surg* 75:32, 1985.

Hagan EG, Huelke DF: An analysis of 319 reports of mandibular fracture, *J Oral Maxillofac Surg* 19:93, 1961.

Jacoby JG, Dolan KD: Fragment analysis in maxillofacial injuries: the tripod fracture, *J Trauma* 20:292, 1980.

Johnson DH: CT of maxillofacial trauma, *Radiol Clin North Am* 22:131, 1984.

Jurkiewicz MJ, Nickell WB: Fractures of the skeleton of the face, *J Trauma* 11:947, 1971.

Le Fort R: Étude experimentale sur les fractures de la machoire superieure, *Rev Chir* 23:208, 360, 479, 1901.

Lindahl L: Condylar fractures of the mandible. I. Classification and relation to age, occlusion, and concomitant injuries of teeth and teeth supporting structures and fractures of the mandibular body, *Int J Oral Maxillofac Surg* 2:12, 1977.

Moilanen, A: Skull radiography in patients with facial trauma, *Int J Oral Maxillofac Surg* 11:89, 1982.

Noyek AM, et al: Contemporary radiologic evaluation in maxillofacial trauma, *Otolaryngol Clin North Am* 16:473, 1983.

Olsen RA, et al: Fractures of the mandible: review of 580 cases, *J Oral Maxillofac Surg* 40:23, 1982.

Rowe NL, Miller E, Brandt-Zawadzki M: Computed tomography in maxillofacial trauma, *Laryngoscope* 91:745, 1981.

Smiler DG, Linz AM, Wenngole CF: Signs and symptoms of zygomaticomaxillary fractures involving the orbit, *Oral Surg Oral Med Oral Pathol* 29:103, 1971.

Som PM, Bergeron RT: *Head and neck imaging,* ed 2, St. Louis, 1991, Mosby–Year Book, pp 227-249.

Zilkha A: Computed tomography of facial trauma, *Radiology* 144:545, 1982.

Zizmore J, Noyek AM: Fractures of the paranasal sinuses, *Otolaryngol Clin North Am* 6:473, 1973.

Blow–Out Fracture

Berkowitz RA, Putterman AN, Patel DB: Prolapse of the globe into the maxillary sinus after orbital fracture, *Am J Ophthalmol* 91:253, 1981.

Gozum G: Blow-out fractures of the orbit, *Otolaryngol Clin North Am* 9:477, 1976.

Grove AS: Computed tomography in the management of orbital trauma, *Ophthalmology* 89:433, 1982.

Hammerschlag SB, et al: Blow-out fractures of the orbit: a comparison of computed tomography and conventional radiography with anatomic correlation, *Radiology* 143:487, 1982.

6

INFECTIONS OF THE TEETH AND JAWS

DENTAL CARIES

Overview

Definition: Dental caries may be defined as the progressive destruction of tooth substance, initiated by microbial activity at the tooth surface and leading to cavity formation. Dental caries is therefore characterized by dental enamel decalcification followed by disintegration.

Clinical Features

The prevalence of dental caries in many areas of the developed world has shifted, becoming less prevalent in children; still, dental caries occurs in all ages, both sexes, and all populations of the world. The value of radiographs in detecting caries is well documented; however, it must be borne in mind that no investigation of caries is complete without a thorough clinical examination.

RADIOLOGIC FEATURES

Because there is a loss of tooth material, the density of the affected part of the tooth will be decreased, appearing radiolucent on radiographs.

Clinically the early lesion is usually larger than depicted radiographically, because early decalcification does not produce sufficient changes in density to be detected radiographically.

PROXIMAL DENTAL CARIES

Proximal caries occurs on the proximal surface of teeth, between the contact point and the free gingiva.

Signs and symptoms: The first presentation of proximal caries is a chalky white spot without any apparent loss of continuity of the enamel surface. Later, because of decalcification of the superficial enamel, the white spot becomes slightly roughened. As the caries progresses, the lesion appears bluish white in appearance; this is especially evident when it reaches the dentinoenamel junction (DEJ).

RADIOLOGIC FEATURES

Cardinal Signs

Extremely small radiolucent notching of the enamel surface just below the contact point

Triangular radiolucency (in enamel) of varying size, with the base of the triangle being the orig-

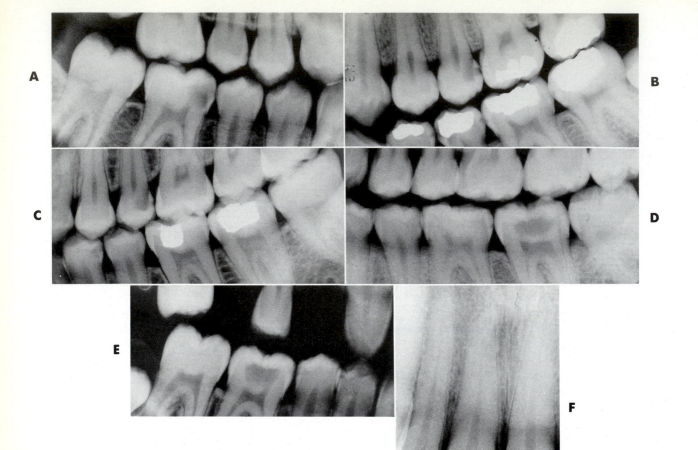

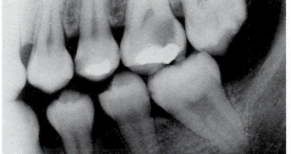

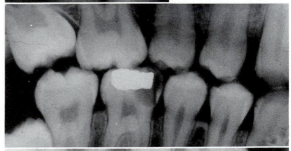

Fig. 6-1 **A,** Bitewing radiograph demonstrating proximal dental caries. Incipient lesions (radiolucent notching) are seen between the maxillary premolar teeth. **B,** Bitewing radiograph showing moderate proximal dental caries in the mandibular premolars and maxillary first premolar (classic triangular proximal lesions). Extensive dentinal caries is present on the distal-proximal surface of the maxillary second premolar tooth. **C,** Bitewing radiograph showing proximal dental caries with dentinal involvement of the maxillary second premolar and mandibular first premolar. Note spread of caries along dentin-enamel junction.
D, Occlusal dental caries of mandibular second permanent molar and distal proximal lesion of mandibular first molar.
E, Early occlusal (radiolucent shadow under dentin-enamel junction) and mesial proximal caries of mandibular second molar, with more advanced lesions in mandibular first molar. **F,** Advanced labial dental caries seen as well-defined radiolucency. **G,** Recurrent dental caries around restoration in maxillary first permanent molar.
H, Recurrent dental caries beneath occlusal restoration in maxillary first permanent molar.

Continued.

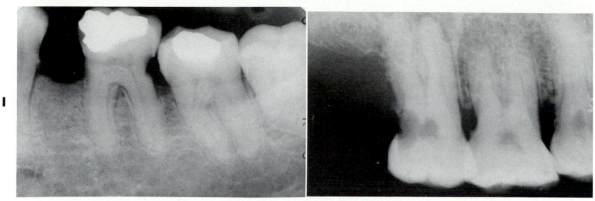

Fig. 6-1, cont'd.   I, Cervical dental caries seen as ill-defined saucer-shaped radiolucency on distal root surface of mandibular first molar. **J,** Cervical dental caries on distal aspect of maxillary second permanent molar (third molar is missing).

inal contour of the tooth surface and the apex pointing towards the DEJ
Second triangular radiolucency (in dentin) with apex towards pulp
Thin radiolucent line in enamel
Diffuse radiolucency in dental crown

OCCLUSAL CARIES

Occlusal caries occurs on the occlusal surfaces of posterior teeth, starting in pits and fissures.

Signs and symptoms: Occlusal caries presents with brown or black pits and fissures, into which an explorer probe may stick. The adjacent enamel may appear opaque bluish white.

RADIOLOGIC FEATURES

Cardinal Signs
Dark radiolucent shadow or line just under the DEJ
Diffuse radiolucencies of varying size

Ancillary Signs
Band of increased opacity between the carious lesion and pulp chamber

BUCCAL AND LINGUAL/PALATAL CARIES

Buccal and lingual or palatal caries usually occurs in the pits and grooves or in the region of the free margin of the gingiva.

RADIOLOGIC FEATURES

Cardinal Signs
Well-defined radiolucency with clear demarcation between carious and noncarious enamel

CERVICAL CARIES

Cervical caries (cemental caries, radicular caries, senile caries) develops in the area between the enamel border and the free margin of the gingiva and involves both cementum and dentin.

Clinical Features

Demographics: Studies of cervical caries in the United States and Scandinavia have shown that the prevalence of root caries increases with age, approximately doubling between the ages of 30 and 60 years.

Signs and symptoms: Classically, the active lesion of cervical caries presents either as a yellow-orange tan or light brown lesion. Lesions in remission are darker, sometimes almost black. The anterior and premolar teeth are most commonly involved.

RADIOLOGIC FEATURES

Cardinal Signs
Poorly defined, saucer-shaped, cupped-out radiolucency on the surface of the root

RECURRENT DENTAL CARIES

Recurrent or secondary dental caries occurs in the immediate vicinity of a restoration. Recurrent caries may result from either poor cavity preparation, inadequate adaptation of restorations, or incomplete removal of caries.

Demographics: Common in association with poor oral hygiene.

RADIOLOGIC FEATURES

Cardinal Signs

Similar to primary caries

Areas of increased radiolucency adjacent to the margins of restoration

PERIODONTITIS

Overview

Definition: Periodontitis can be defined as an inflammation of the supporting tissues of the teeth, involving the gingiva and alveolar mucosa and extending to the periodontal ligament, cementum, and alveolar bone.

Pathogenesis: Various hypothesis have been suggested for the progression from gingivitis to periodontitis:

1. Direct tissue destruction caused by bacterial plaque and its metabolic products
2. Immune hyperresponsiveness precipitated by immune complexes, lymphocyte blastogenesis, or activation of complement pathways
3. Immune deficiencies involving neutrophil function (chemotaxis, phagocytosis), neutropenia, or the autologous mixed lymphocyte response

The classification of periodontitis is based on such features as age of onset, sexual predilection, familial background, abnormalities of host defense, and local etiologic factors. Other distinguishing features included the rate of distribution and severity of periodontal breakdown. The classification included the following:

1. Adult periodontitis
2. Early-onset periodontitis
   a. Prepubertal periodontitis (localized and generalized forms)
   b. Juvenile periodontitis (localized and generalized forms)
   c. Rapidly progressive periodontitis
3. Periodontitis associated with systemic disease
4. Necrotizing ulcerative periodontitis
5. Refractory periodontitis

ADULT PERIODONTITIS

Adult periodontitis usually occurs after the age of 35 years. There seems to be no sex predilection. The quantity of plaque and calculus is closely related to the presence and severity of adult periodontitis. It has been suggested that the rate of progression of periodontal breakdown may not be slow and continuous, but rather characterized by bursts of periodontal breakdown followed by periods of quiescence. The caries rate is variable but usually high. The host response is apparently normal. The associated microbial flora is variable but typically includes spirochetes, gram-negative rods, *Actinomyces* species, and *Bacteroides* species. Periodontal breakdown may be localized in one area of the dental arch or generalized throughout the mouth. Destruction may be mild, moderate, or severe.

RADIOLOGIC FEATURES

Cardinal Signs

Loss of density and break in the continuity of the crest of the alveolar bone

Blunting of the crest at the alveolar bone in the anterior region

Loss of sharp angle between lamina dura and crest of alveolar bone in posterior region

Horizontal bone loss

Interproximal crater

Vertical bone loss

Furcation involvement

Ancillary Signs

Presence of dental calculus

Overhanging restorations

Poorly contoured restorations

Open interproximal dental contacts

Differential Diagnosis

Other types of periodontitis

Idiopathic histiocytosis

Malignancy

Text continued on page 188.

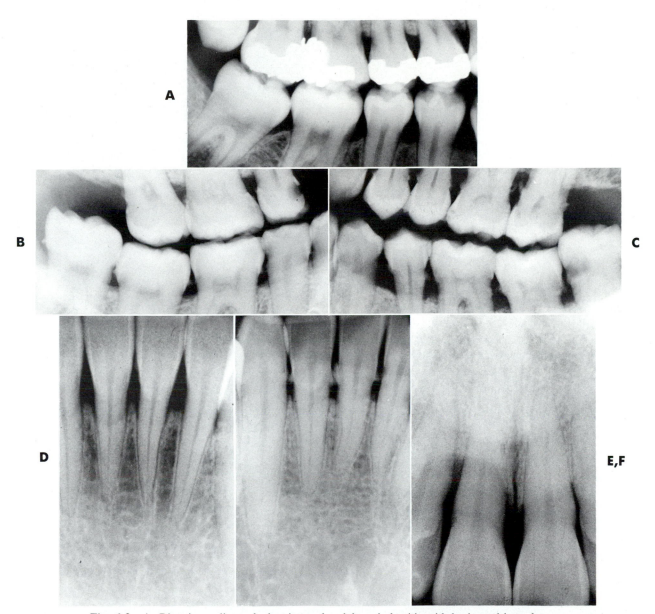

Fig. 6-2 A, Bitewing radiograph showing early adult periodontitis with horizontal bone loss. Note loss of density of alveolar crest and break in continuity of crest between lower first molar and second premolar. **B,** Bitewing radiograph showing early adult periodontitis in patient with marked interproximal dental calculus deposition. **C,** Bitewing radiograph demonstrating moderate horizontal bone loss with adult periodontitis. The mandibular first molar shows furcation involvement. **D,** Periapical radiograph showing early horizontal bone loss in adult periodontitis. There is blunting of alveolar bone crests interproximally. **E,** Moderate horizontal bone loss in adult periodontitis in patient with noticeable deposits of dental calculus. **F,** Vertical bone loss in adult periodontitis is evident around the right maxillary central incisor.

Continued.

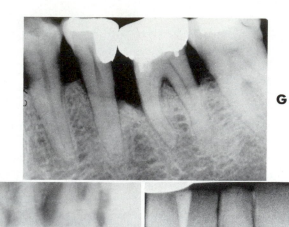

G

H

I

Fig. 6-2, cont'd.   **G,** Periapical radiograph demonstrating vertical bone loss and furcal involvement in region of left mandibular first molar. **H,** Detail from panoramic radiograph showing furcation involvement in adult periodontitis. **I,** Severe horizontal bone loss in adult periodontitis. **J,** Juvenile periodontitis showing bilateral angular defects in incisor and molar regions.

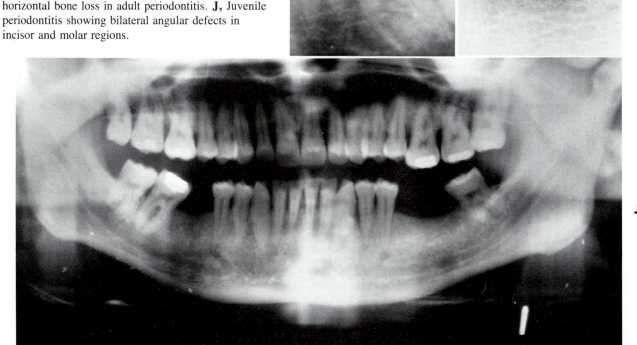

J

Continued.

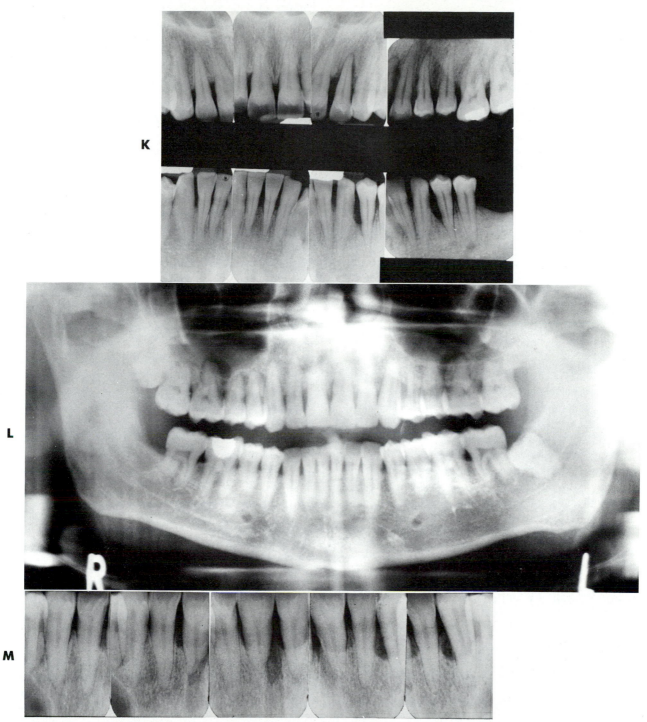

Fig. 6-2, cont'd. **K,** Periapical radiographs showing juvenile periodontitis. **L,** Panoramic radiograph of patient with rapidly progressing periodontitis. There is generalized horizontal bone loss, particularly severe in maxilla. **M,** Periapical radiographs showing rapidly progressive periodontitis.

PREPUBERTAL PERIODONTITIS

Prepubertal periodontitis is defined as periodontitis affecting the primary dentition or mixed dentition in young children. The prevalence is unknown but the condition is probably rare; it appears to be more common in females than males. The onset of disease is during or immediately after eruption of the primary teeth. The possibility of a genetic basis has been suggested in some instances. The organisms associated with prepubertal periodontitis appear to be *Bacteroides intermedius* and *Capnocytophaga sputigena*. The disease may occur in a localized or generalized form.

Localized Form

In the localized form, only a few teeth are affected. This form usually occurs around the age of 4 years or younger, with minimal gingival inflammation and plaque. The rate of destruction is more rapid than in adult periodontitis but slower than in the generalized form of prepubertal periodontitis. Functional defects of neutrophils and monocytes are seen.

Generalized Form

In the generalized form, all the primary teeth are affected with or without involvement of the permanent teeth. Onset is at the time of tooth eruption. There is a fiery-red acute inflammation of the gingiva around all the teeth, with gingival proliferation, cleft formation, and recession. The rate of destruction of alveolar bone and gingiva is very rapid. Functional defects of either neutrophils and monocytes, but not both, may be seen. The peripheral white blood cell count is markedly elevated. Otitis media and upper respiratory infections are common findings.

RADIOLOGIC FEATURES

Cardinal Signs
Extensive bone loss associated with primary teeth
Furcation involvement

JUVENILE PERIODONTITIS

The rate of destruction in juvenile periodontitis is three to five times faster than in adult periodontitis. The lack of clinical inflammation and the presence of minimal plaque and calculus deposits are striking features of the disease. It appears to be more common in females than in males by a ratio of 3:1, and blacks tend to be affected more than whites. Patients often present with mobility and migration of teeth. Other complaints may include radiating pain on chewing and root sensitivity to thermal change. A large proportion of patients show a depressed neutrophil chemotaxis effect. The autologous mixed lymphocyte response is frequently elevated. A familial distribution has been suggested.

Localized Form

In the localized form, only the first molars and incisors are involved. The onset of this form is generally around puberty (11 to 13 years). *Actinobacillus actinomycetemcomitans* appears to be the most common associated organism.

Generalized Form

The generalized form involves the first molars and incisors as well as other teeth. The onset of disease is generally between 12 and 26 years of age.

RADIOLOGIC FEATURES

Cardinal Signs
Bilateral, arc-shaped, angular defects especially of the molars and incisors (often symmetrical—so-called mirror images)
Generalized bone loss around teeth

RAPIDLY PROGRESSIVE PERIODONTITIS

In rapidly progressive periodontitis, there is relatively rapid loss of attachment and alveolar bone. It is clinically very similar to the generalized form of juvenile periodontitis; however, differences do exist. The age of onset is between puberty and about 35 years of age. Involvement is generalized with no predilection for specific areas. The initial destructive process may cease spontaneously or greatly slow down. The gingiva is acutely inflamed, with marginal proliferation during the active phase of the disease. Approximately 83% of patients have defects of the neutrophils and/or monocytes. Patients may have systemic manifestations such as weight loss, mental depression, and general malaise.

RADIOLOGIC FEATURES

Cardinal Signs

Extensive generalized horizontal bone loss
Furcation involvement

INFLAMMATORY PERIAPICAL DISEASE

Overview

Inflammatory changes in the periapical region usually result from pulpal degeneration. Other less common causes are infections from extraction wounds, the periodontal ligament, or fracture sites. It rarely results from hematogenous spread. When the infection reaches the periapical tissue, a number of different tissue reactions may occur, depending on the nature of the infection and the resistance of the host. These reactions may be acute or chronic.

APICAL PERIODONTITIS

Apical periodontitis results largely from edema of the apical periodontal ligament.

Clinical Features

The pulp is nonvital. The tooth is elevated in its socket and very sensitive to pressure and percussion. There may be spontaneous pain, ranging from a slight tenderness to a constant, throbbing pain. In the chronic phase the only symptom is some intermittent discomfort.

RADIOLOGIC FEATURES

Cardinal Signs

No radiographic features initially
Widening of periodontal ligament space at the apex of the tooth
Radiopaque sclerotic band outside the widened periodontal ligament space (seen in chronic phase) called *focal sclerosing osteomyelitis* or *condensing osteitis*

Ancillary Signs

Tooth with large carious cavity or large restorations or evidence of previous trama

APICAL ABSCESS

Apical abscesses may be acute or chronic. The acute type result from necrosis of the periodontal tissue with pus formation. The chronic type may develop from an acute apical abscess or, more commonly, from an apical granuloma.

Clinical Features

The tooth is nonvital. There is intense, constant, throbbing pain. The tooth is extremely sensitive to percussion. There may be swelling and redness of the soft tissues in the region of the involved tooth, and cellulitis may be present. Pus may drain with eventual fistula formation; acute symptoms may ease as the abscess goes into the chronic phase.

RADIOLOGIC FEATURES

Cardinal Signs

No radiologic features during acute phase other than possible raising of tooth in socket
Widening of periodontal ligament space
Diffuse radiolucency at the apex of the tooth blending into the surrounding bone (chronic phase)
Radiolucent canal (fistulous tracts) extending toward the surface of the bone—only in chronic phase

PERIAPICAL GRANULOMA

Periapical granuloma is the most common chronic reaction of the periapical tissues to pulpal degeneration. It is basically a localized mass of granulation tissue, fending off a source of irritation. The apical foramen of a tooth is too narrow to allow granulation tissue to grow back into the tooth more than about 2 mm; hence, untreated teeth with necrotic pulps constitute a chronic source of irritation.

Clinical Features

The involved tooth is nonvital and asymptomatic. It may appear darker in color or have a large carious cavity or restoration.

RADIOLOGIC FEATURES

Cardinal Signs

Loss of lamina dura
Round or oval radiolucency at apex of the involved tooth, with or without well-circumscribed borders
Small radiolucency—usually less than 1.5 cm in diameter

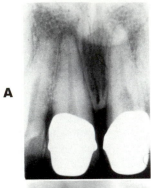

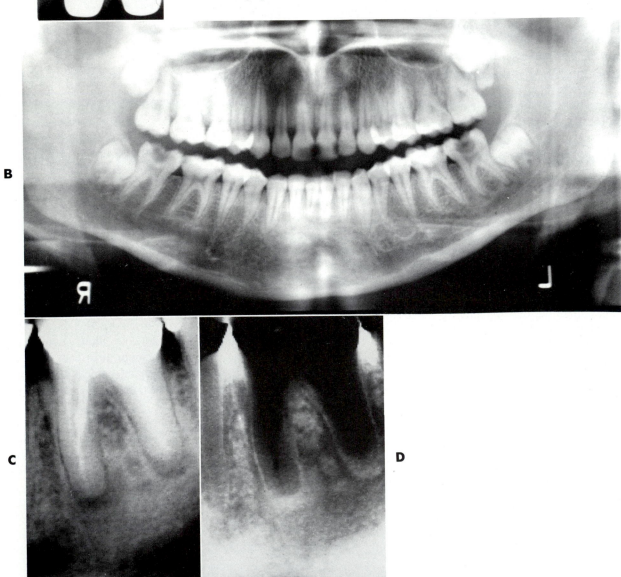

Fig. 6-3   A, Early periapical radiolucency with widening of periodontal ligament space at apex of right maxillary central incisor. The left central incisor shows the normal apical periodontal ligament space. **B,** Periapical periodontitis of carious right mandibular second molar and periapical granuloma of carious left mandibular first molar. **C,** Direct digital radiograph of healing periapical lesions on endodontically treated tooth. **D,** Same patient as in **C.** Inverse radiographic contrast.

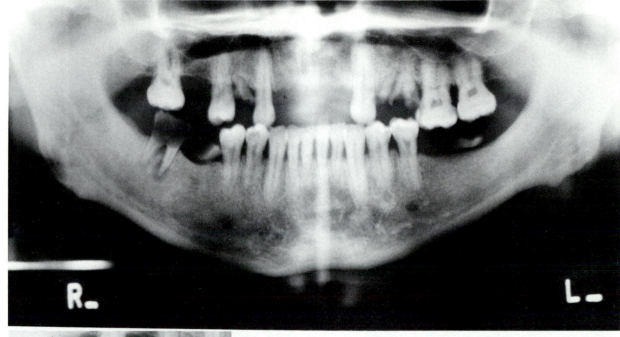

E

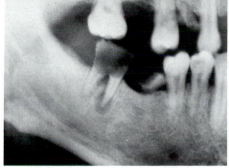

F

Fig. 6-3, cont'd. **E,** Panoramic radiograph showing chronic periapical abscess. This lesion is indistinguishable from apical granuloma or radicular cyst using radiologic features alone. **F,** Same patient as in **E.** Detail from panoramic radiograph.

Indistinguishable radiographically from periapical cyst (see Chapter 7).

Differential diagnosis
Periapical abscess
Periapical granuloma
Periapical cyst
Periapical scar/surgical defect
Periapical cemental dysplasia (early stages)
Traumatic bone cyst

OSTEOMYELITIS

Overview

Definition: *Osteomyelitis* literally means inflammation of the bone marrow.

Pathogenesis: Most cases of osteomyelitis of the jaws result from odontogenic infections; infections from a fracture site; or, rarely, hematogenous spread from a distant site. Factors that lower host resistance or reduce the local blood supply of the bone may predispose to osteomyelitis. Other causes of osteomyelitis of the jaws include syphilis, tuberculosis, and actinomycosis. It starts in the medullary cavity and haversian system and extends to involve the periosteum. The calcified portion of the bone becomes necrotic when the accumulation of pus in the medullary spaces or beneath the periosteum compromises the blood supply of the bone.

Text continued on page 194.

A

B

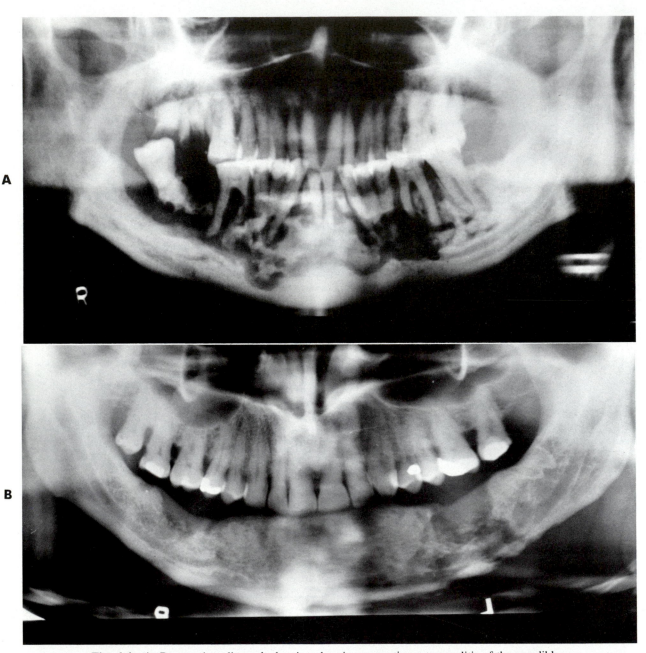

Fig. 6-4 A, Panoramic radiograph showing chronic suppurative osteomyelitis of the mandible. Note irregular radiolucency with sequestration of dead bone including the right mandibular molars. **B,** Panoramic radiograph showing chronic suppurative osteomyelitis of mandible bilaterally in premolar and molar regions.   *Continued.*

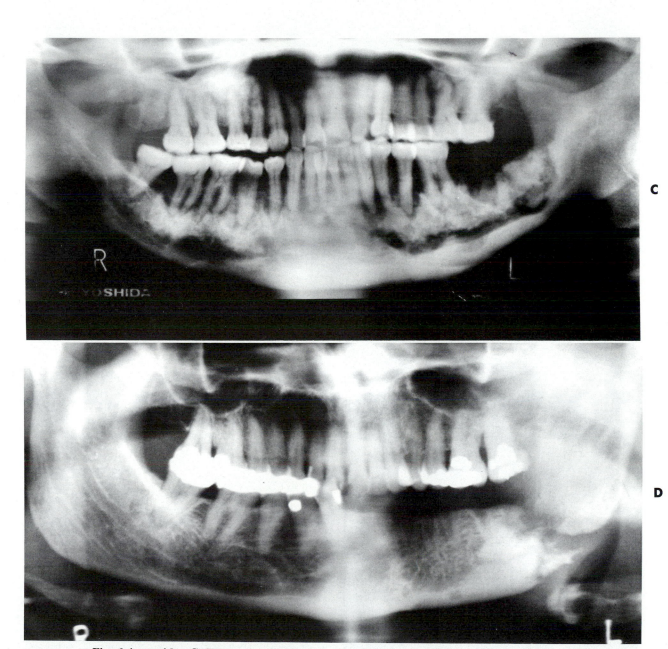

Fig. 6-4, cont'd. **C,** Panoramic radiograph showing chronic suppurative osteomyelitis of both jaws. **D,** Panoramic radiograph showing pathologic fracture through chronic supurative osteomyelitis in left mandibular third molar and angle regions.

Continued.

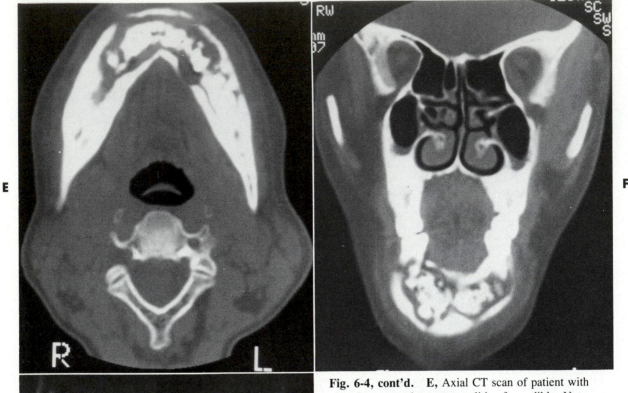

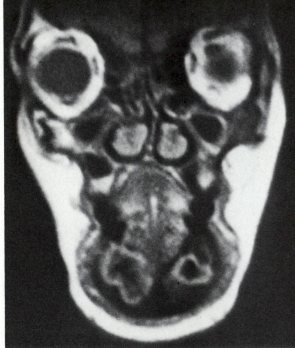

Fig. 6-4, cont'd. E, Axial CT scan of patient with chronic suppurative osteomyelitis of mandible. Note sequestration of bone in anterior mandible. **F,** Same patient as in **E.** Coronally reformatted CT scan. **G,** Same patient as in **E.** Coronal T2-weighted MR scan. The sequestrated bone (no signal) is surrounded by zones of high signal intensity representing the regions of active inflammation.

Clinical Features

Demographics: Osteomyelitis of the jaws is rare in Europe and North America but remains common in some developing countries. It is more common in the mandible than the maxilla.

Signs and symptoms: Osteomyelitis may be acute or chronic and may present with one of the following reactions predominating:

1. Bone destruction and pus formation—"suppurative osteomyelitis"
2. Bone sclerosis—"sclerosing osteomyelitis"
3. Periosteal reaction—"periostitis ossificans"

SUPPURATIVE OSTEOMYELITIS

Signs and symptoms: The acute phase of suppurative osteomyelitis is sudden in onset and rapid in course. The patient experiences severe pain, fever, regional lymphadenopathy, and leukocytosis. An indurated swelling may develop with multiple sinuses draining pus. Teeth in the region become loose and tender to percussion. When the mandible is involved there may be paresthesia or anesthesia of the lower lip on the affected side. As soon as drainage is established, the pain eases, the temperature drops, and the patient becomes much more comfortable. Without treatment the infection may progress into a protracted chronic phase, with bone destruction and pus formation continuing to predominate. Sinuses develop, drain pus, and close again, and the cycle repeats itself.

RADIOLOGIC FEATURES

Cardinal Signs

No detectable radiographic features in first 8 to 10 days

Blurred or "fuzzy" appearance of trabeculae in affected area as result of loss of density of trabeculae

Single or multiple irregular radiolucencies with poorly defined margins

Classic moth-eaten appearance resulting from sequestrum formation

Ancillary Signs

Pathologic fractures of the jaw

Differential Diagnosis

Infections
Malignancies
Osteoradionecrosis

CHRONIC SCLEROSING OSTEOMYELITIS

Overview

Definition: Sclerosing osteomyelitis can be described as a predominantly proliferative reaction of bone to infection occurring in patients with high host resistance or a low-grade infection.

Pathogenesis: In patients with chronic sclerosing osteomyelitis, infection acts as a stimulus rather than an irritant; this results in proliferation instead of destruction. Bone is deposited along existing trabeculae, resulting in thickening of the trabeculae and reduction or obliteration of the marrow spaces.

Two types of sclerosing osteomyelitis have been described:

1. Localized type—focal sclerosing osteomyelitis
2. Generalized type—diffuse sclerosing osteomyelitis

FOCAL SCLEROSING OSTEOMYELITIS (CONDENSING OSTEITIS)

Focal sclerosing osteomyelitis is a localized proliferative reaction occurring in the periapical region as a result of pulpal necrosis.

Clinical Features

Demographics: Focal sclerosing osteomyelitis is a rather common condition. It is usually found in young individuals, especially before the age of 20 years. The mandibular first molar seems to be the most commonly involved tooth.

Signs and symptoms: Focal sclerosing osteomyelitis is usually asymptomatic, but some patients have mild symptoms. The only classical sign may be a large carious tooth or a large restoration with marginal deficiencies.

RADIOLOGIC FEATURES

Cardinal Signs

Widening of apical periodontal ligament space

Well-circumscribed to diffuse radiopaque mass of sclerotic bone of varying size and shape surrounding the apex

Area of rarefying osteitis adjacent to sclerotic bone

Differential Diagnosis

Osteosclerosis
Periapical cemental dysplasia
Hypercementosis
Cementoblastoma
Soft tissue calcification (lymph node, salivary gland)

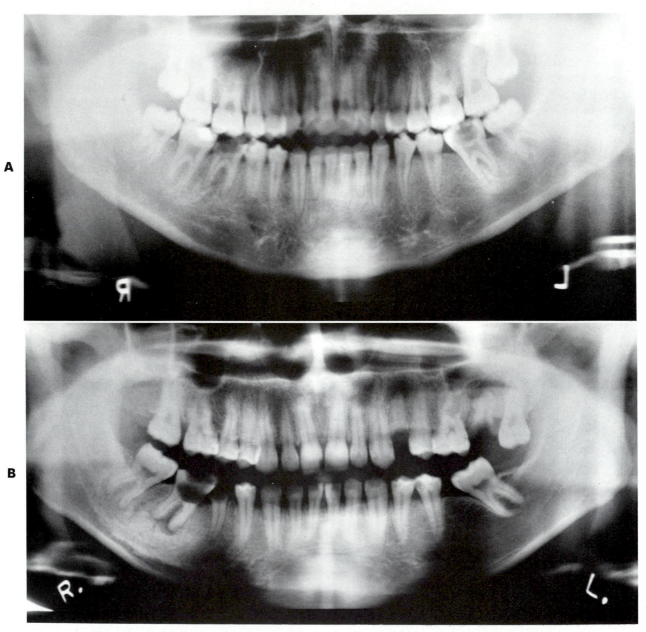

Fig. 6-5 **A,** Focal sclerosing osteomyelitis (condensing osteitis) is seen beyond the apical rarefactions around the carious mandibular first permanent molars. **B,** Extensive focal sclerosing osteomyelitis is evident subjacent to the carious right mandibular first molar tooth.

Continued.

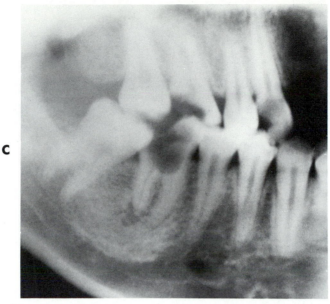

Fig. 6-5, cont'd.   C, Detail from panoramic radiograph demonstrating focal sclerosing osteomyelitis (condensing osteitis) subjacent to carious right mandibular first permanent molar.

DIFFUSE SCLEROSING OSTEOMYELITIS

Diffuse sclerosing osteomyelitis is similar to the focal form except that the proliferative reaction is more generalized and commonly results from generalized periodontal disease instead of pulpal degeneration.

Clinical Features

Demographics: Diffuse sclerosing osteomyelitis is not a very common condition. It can occur at any age but, in contrast to focal sclerosing osteomyelitis, is more common in older individuals. It tends to be more common in females, especially black females. It is more common in the mandible, especially in edentulous regions.

Signs and symptoms: Diffuse sclerosing osteomyelitis is usually symptomatic. The patient complains of tenderness and pain in the affected part of the jaw. These exacerbations are usually accompanied by suppuration and elevated temperature and erythrocyte sedimentation rate. In young patients facial asymmetry is a common feature, resulting from swelling along the lower border of the mandible.

RADIOLOGIC FEATURES

Cardinal Signs

Diffuse areas of sclerosis of bone without a sharp demarcation from the neighboring unaffected bone

Enlargement of bone

Subperiosteal bone deposition, especially in children

Poorly defined osteolytic and osteosclerotic areas during acute exacerbations

Ancillary Signs

Cortical bone deficit, especially at the angle of the mandible

Shortening of tooth roots in affected area

Differential Diagnosis

Florid osseous dysplasia

Fibrous dysplasia

Paget disease of bone

Osteopetrosis

Osteoblastic malignancies

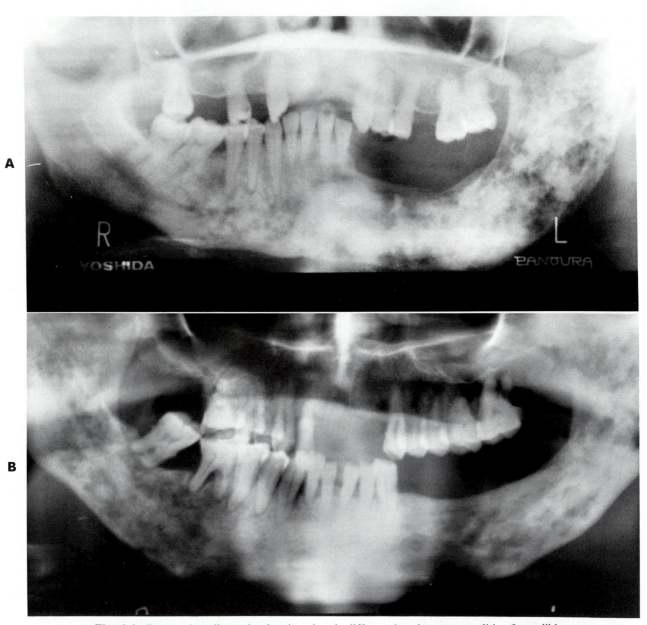

Fig. 6-6 Panoramic radiographs showing chronic diffuse sclerosing osteomyelitis of mandible. In **C (opposite page),** osteomyelitis may be superimposed over preexisting florid osseous dysplasia. *Continued.*

C

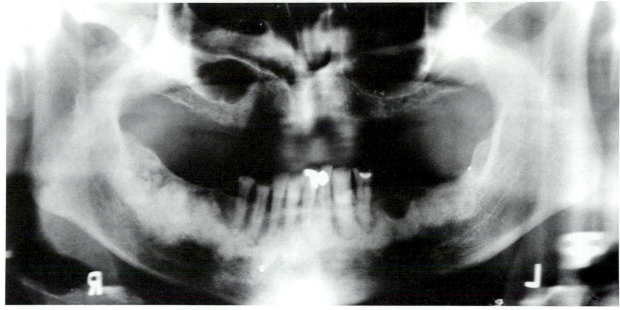

Fig. 6-6 C.

OSTEOMYELITIS WITH PERIOSTITIS (PERIOSTITIS OSSIFICANS)

Overview

Definition: Osteomyelitis with periostitis has been erroneously described in the past as Garré osteomyelitis. It is simply a variant of osteomyelitis in which a periosteal reaction predominates, leading to subperiosteal deposition of new bone.

Pathogenesis: Infective periapical lesions resulting from caries are the most common cause of osteomyelitis with periostitis.

Clinical Features

Demographics: Osteomyelitis with periostitis occurs mainly in young people, with a mean age at detection of 13 years. There appears to be a slight predilection for males. The most common site is the lower border of the mandible, adjacent to the first molar.

Signs and symptoms: Patients have facial asymmetry resulting from a bony, hard swelling of the mandible. The overlying skin and mucosa usually appear normal. Patients may have a low-grade fever, but pain is not usually a feature.

RADIOLOGIC FEATURES

Cardinal Signs

Laminar periosteal new bone (so-called onion skin pattern), most evident on the inferior, buccal, or lingual aspect of the mandible

Thickening of entire mandible and endosseous structure; their appearance is mottled, with fuzzy radiopaque and radiolucent areas

Maintenance of the radiographic shadow of the former mandibular cortex.

Ancillary Signs

Presence of grossly carious tooth, usually a first mandibular molar

Intense uptake of technetium 99m methylene diphosphonate on bone scintigraphy

Effacement of follicular cortices of adjacent unerupted teeth

Bony sequestra if associated with suppurative osteomyelitis

Differential Diagnosis

Caffey syndrome (infantile cortical hyperostosis)

Syphilitic osteomyelitis

Healing fracture callus

Osteogenic sarcoma

Text continued on page 202.

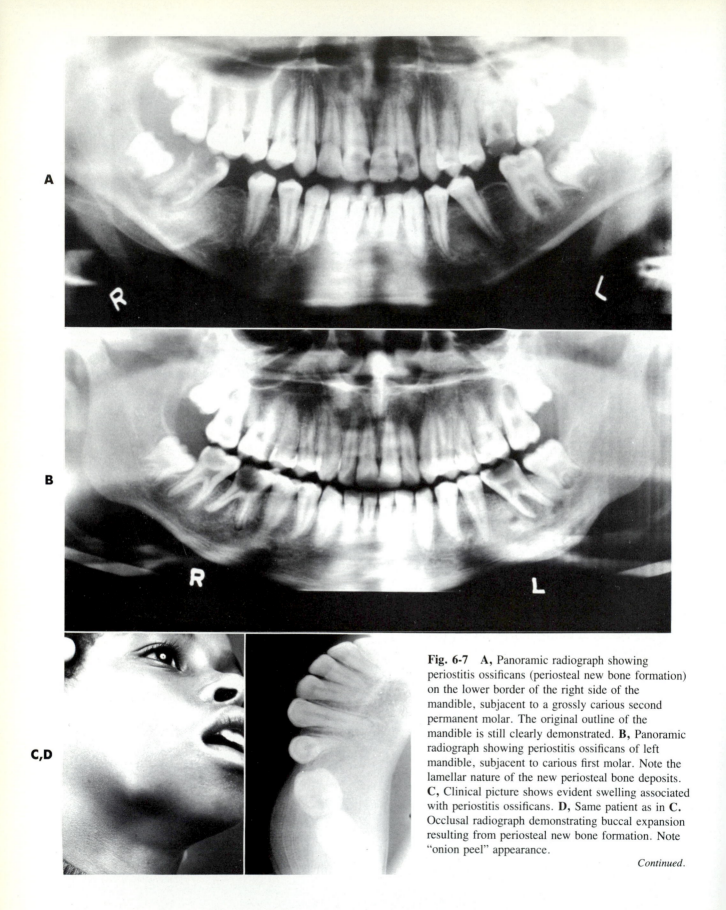

Fig. 6-7 **A,** Panoramic radiograph showing periostitis ossificans (periosteal new bone formation) on the lower border of the right side of the mandible, subjacent to a grossly carious second permanent molar. The original outline of the mandible is still clearly demonstrated. **B,** Panoramic radiograph showing periostitis ossificans of left mandible, subjacent to carious first molar. Note the lamellar nature of the new periosteal bone deposits. **C,** Clinical picture shows evident swelling associated with periostitis ossificans. **D,** Same patient as in **C.** Occlusal radiograph demonstrating buccal expansion resulting from periosteal new bone formation. Note "onion peel" appearance.

Continued.

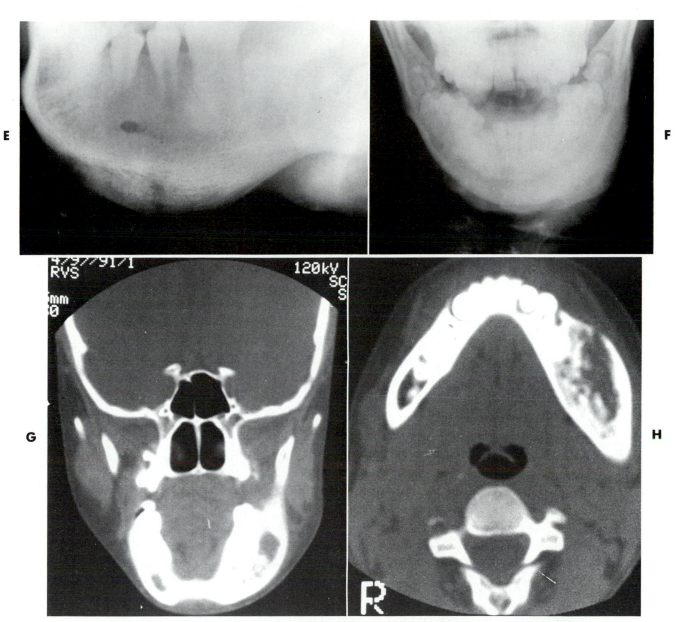

Fig. 6-7, cont'd.   E, Lateral-oblique view showing periostitis ossificans of no obvious cause. Note persistence of original mandibular outline and lamellar structure of new bone deposition. **F,** Posteroanterior projection showing periostitis ossificans of left mandible with marked bony swelling of affected region. **G,** Same patient as in **F.** Coronally reconstructed CT scan showing expansion of left side of mandible. Note sclerosis of medullary bone, which is hidden by the periosteal reaction on the posteroanterior projection. **H,** Same patient as in **F.** Axial CT scan showing mandibular expansion and the presence of bony sequestra.

TUBERCULOUS OSTEOMYELITIS

Overview

Definition: Tuberculous osteomyelitis is a specific infection caused by the acid-fast bacillus *Mycobacterium tuberculosis.*

Pathogenesis: Almost all cases arise from known pulmonary disease. The oral tissue is involved via three routes: direct inoculation, extension from other infection sites, or hematogenous seeding.

Clinical Features

Demographics: Involvement of the oral region is rare, occurring in less than 2% of all persons with tuberculosis. Tuberculous osteomyelitis of the jaws is more common in the mandible than the maxilla, but even mandibular involvement accounts for less than 2% of osseous lesions in tuberculosis.

Signs and symptoms: Patients complain of repeated attacks of pain, described as toothache, and swelling of the affected area. The swelling is firm initially and softens later. Sinus tracts develop as the swellings rupture spontaneously and drain intraorally and/or extraorally. Trismus may be present.

RADIOLOGIC FEATURES

Cardinal Signs
None

Ancillary Signs
Rarefaction with ill-defined borders and formation of sequestra
Periosteal new bone formation

Differential Diagnosis
Nonspecific osteomyelitis
Malignancies
Eosinophilic granuloma

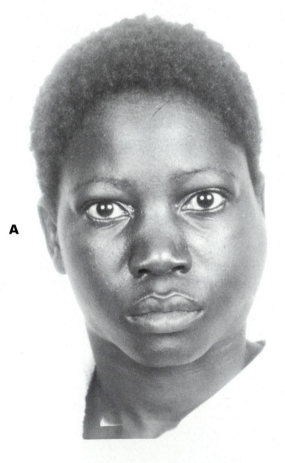

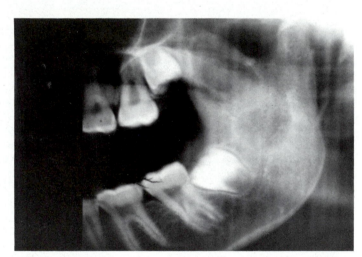

Fig. 6-8   **A,** Swelling of left cheek in patient with tuberculous osteomyelitis of mandibular ramus. **A** to **F** are all of the same patient. **B,** Detail from panoramic radiograph. Irregular radiolucency below mandibular notch was tuberculous osteomyelitis.   *Continued.*

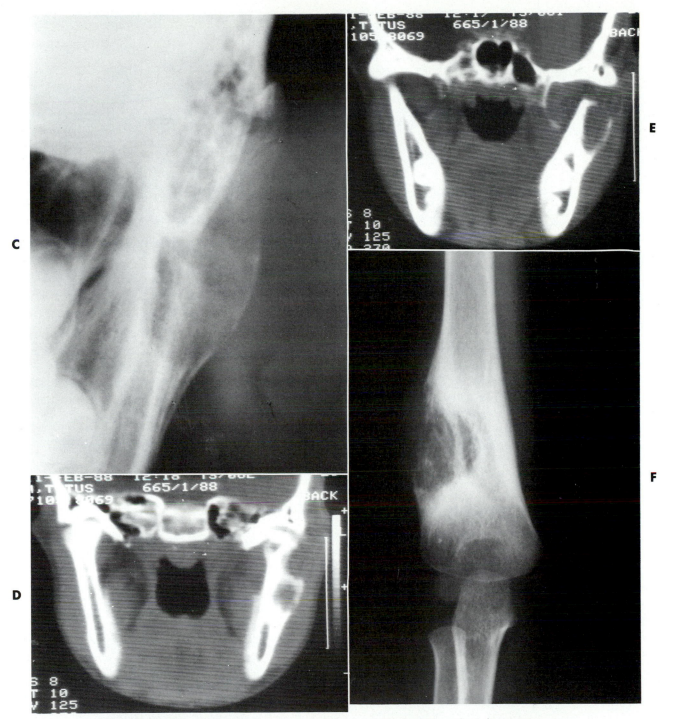

Fig. 6-8, cont'd. **C,** Posteroanterior view. Buccal expansion of the cortical plate of the mandible is evident. **D,** Coronally reconstructed CT scan showing irregular radiolucency of left mandibular ramus and buccal expansion of cortex. **E,** Coronally reconstructed CT scan with more anteriorly positioned cut showing loss of cortical continuity. **F (right),** Tuberculous osteomyelitis was also present in this long bone. Note the similarity to the radiographic features of the mandible.   *Continued.*

G 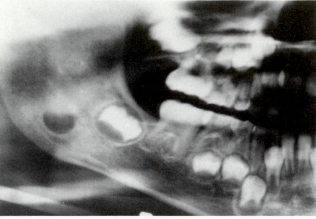 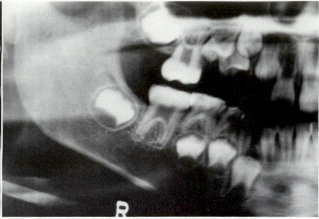 H

Fig. 6-8, cont'd.   G, Tuberculous osteomyelitis of right mandible subjacent to mandibular canal. This patient had a fairly well-delineated radiolucency. **H,** Same patient as in **G** after treatment for tuberculosis. Note complete resolution of the mandibular lesion.

SYPHILIS

Overview

Definition: Syphilis is caused by the infection with the spirochete *Treponema pallidum.*

Pathogenesis: Syphilis may be congenital or acquired. The acquired form is usually further subclassified into three distinctive stages: primary, secondary, and tertiary. The bone may be affected in congenital syphilis and in both the secondary and tertiary stages of acquired syphilis.

Clinical Features

Demographics: The jaws are rarely affected in syphilis. When they are the palate is more frequently involved than the mandible.

Signs and symptoms: The characteristic lesion of primary syphilis is the chancre, which clinically presents as an ulcerated, indurated, painless lesion. Oral lesions of secondary syphilis include mucous patches and maculopapular eruptions. Two types of lesions occur in tertiary syphilis: the gumma and atrophic syphilitic glossitis.

_____

RADIOLOGIC FEATURES

Cardinal Signs

Deposition of subperiosteal new bone along inferior border of mandible (syphilitic periostitis)

Destruction of bone, especially the palate, causing perforation of palate and appearing as large radiolucent areas (gumma)

Well-demarcated destruction along cortical margin, especially the mandible (cortical gumma)

Multiple radiolucencies with poorly defined margins and sequestrum formation (syphilitic osteomyelitis)

Differential Diagnosis

Periostitis ossificans
Caffey syndrome (infantile cortical hyperostosis)
Healing fracture
Osteogenic sarcoma

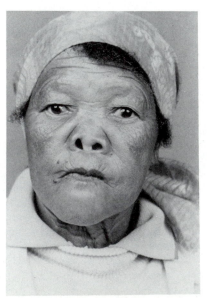

A

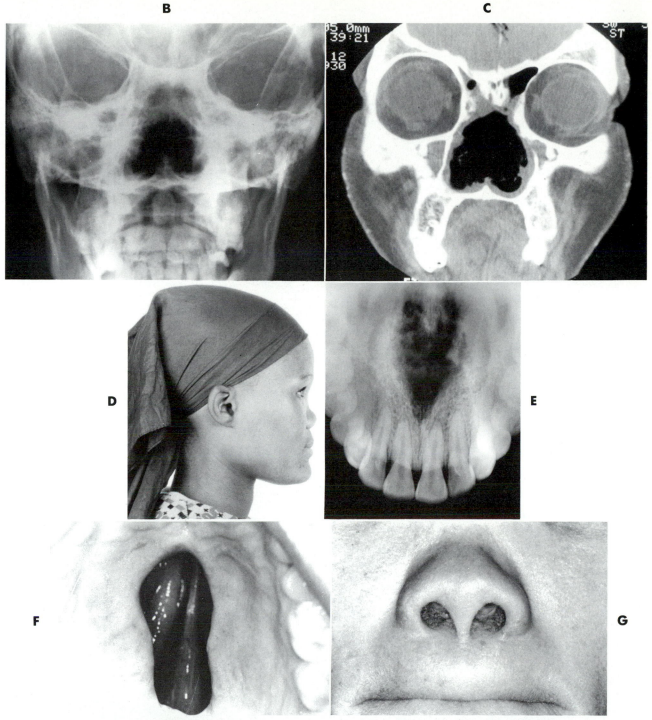

Fig. 6-9 A (left), Gummatous destruction of bridge of nose. **B (above),** Same patient as in **A.** Posteroanterior view showing gummatous destruction of nasal septum and conchae. **C,** Same patient as in **A.** Coronal CT reconstruction showing gummatous destruction of nasal septum and conchae. **D,** Deficient bridge of nose in patient with congenital syphilis. **E,** Same patient as in **D.** Topographic occlusal radiograph demonstrating gummatous destruction of palate/floor of nasal passage. **F,** Same patient as in **D.** Gummatous destruction of palate. **G,** Same patient as in **D.** Careful examination of the nose reveals gummatous destruction of the floor of the nose.

OSTEORADIONECROSIS COMPLICATED BY OSTEOMYELITIS

Overview

Definition: Osteoradionecrosis is defined as bone necrosis secondary to radiation damage. Osteomyelitis does not occur until infection is introduced into the devitalized bone.

Pathogenesis: The classic sequence is radiation, trauma, and infection. Osteoradionecrosis is not a primary infection but a complex metabolic and tissue homeostatic deficiency caused by radiation-induced cellular damage. Microorganisms only play a contaminant role, leading to superimposed osteomyelitis.

Clinical Features

Demographics: Osteoradionecrosis with osteomyelitis is more common in the mandible than the maxilla and more common in males than females. Patients usually have severe pain and swelling, with or without draining sinuses. There may be sloughing of the oral mucosa with subsequent exposure of large areas of bone.

RADIOLOGIC FEATURES

Cardinal Signs
No change in early stages
Areas of bone rarefaction
Radiolucent areas with poorly defined borders and enlarged and irregular trabecular spaces (typical moth-eaten appearance)
Evidence of bone sequestration

Ancillary Signs
Pathologic fractures
Rampant dental caries

Differential Diagnosis
Osteomyelitis
Malignancies

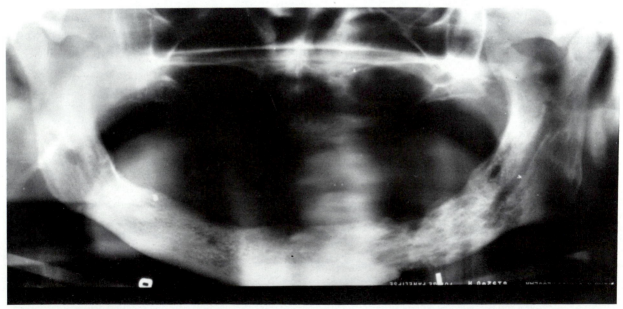

Fig. 6-10   A, Panoramic radiograph showing osteoradionecrosis of left side of mandible. Note "moth eaten" appearance.   *Continued.*

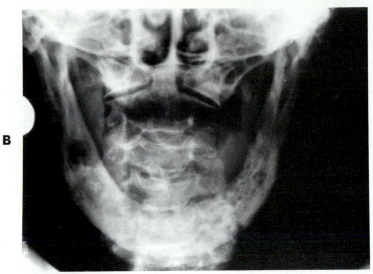

Fig. 6-10, cont'd.   B, Same patient as in **A.** Posteroanterior view.

CANCRUM ORIS (NOMA)

Overview

Definition: Cancrum oris, or noma, is a gangrenous infection of the mouth. It starts off as an ulcer of the mucous membrane and progresses rapidly, leading to destruction of bone and soft tissue. It is almost always quickly fatal.

Clinical Features

Demographics: Cancrum oris is predominantly seen in 2- to 5-year-old children in underdeveloped countries with widespread malnutrition, dehydration, and epidemic infections. In the Western world, it is sometimes found in immunosuppressed adults with predisposing conditions such as leukemia and malnutrition-associated infections. It appears to have a predilection for females.

Signs and symptoms: Cancrum oris usually starts as a painful red or purplish area or an indurated papule on the alveolar margin. The lesion progresses rapidly to involve the surrounding tissues of the jaws, lips,

and cheeks by gangrenous necrosis. The overlying skin becomes inflamed, edematous, and finally necrotic. Masses of necrotic tissue may slough off, denuding the underlying bone. The commencement of gangrene is denoted by blackening of the skin and a foul odor. Patients have high temperatures during the course of the disease; they may develop secondary infections and die from toxemia or pneumonia.

RADIOLOGIC FEATURES

Cardinal Signs

Occasionally none if destruction is rapid
Moth-eaten radiolucencies similar to those of acute osteomyelitis
Gross loss of soft tissues visible on CT or MRI

Differential Diagnosis

Acute necrotizing ulcerative gingivitis
Osteomyelitis
Malignant neoplasia

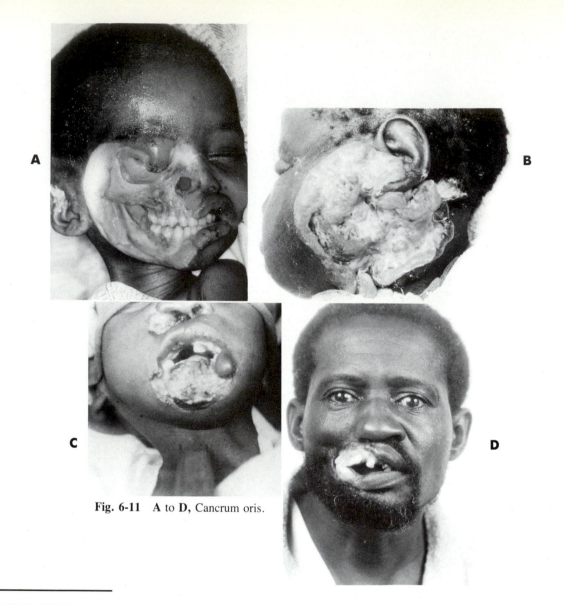

Fig. 6-11   **A** to **D,** Cancrum oris.

BIBLIOGRAPHY

Dental Caries

Banting D, Ellen RP, Fullery E: Prevalence of root surface caries among institutionalized elderly people, *Community Dent Oral Epidemiol* 8:84, 1980.

Buchholz R: Histological-radiographic relation of proximal carious lesions, *J Prev Dent* 4:23, 1977.

Edward S, et al: A comparative study of clinical and roentgenological recording of proximal caries in primary molars of preschool children, *Odont Rev* 24:317, 1973.

Elderton RJ: The causes of failure of restorations: a literature review, *J Dent* 4:257, 1976.

Gwinnet A: A comparison of proximal carious lesions as seen by a clinical radiograph, contact microradiography and light microscopy, *J Am Dent Assoc* 83:1078, 1971.

Hellyer PH, et al: Root caries in older people attending a general dental practice in East Sussex, *Br Dent J* 169:201, 1990.

Kidd EA, Pitts NB: A reappraisal of the value of bitewing radiographs in the diagnosis of posterior approximal caries, *Br Dent J* 169:195, 1990.

Locker D, Shade GD, Leake JL: Prevalence of and factors associated with root decay in older adults in Canada, *J Dent Res* 68:768, 1989.

Silverstone LM, et al: *Dental caries—aetiology, pathology and prevention,* ed 4, London, 1981, Macmillan.

Zamir T, et al: A longitudinal radiographic study of the rate of spread of human approximal dental caries, *Arch Oral Biol* 21:523, 1976.

Periodontitis

Baer PN: The case for periodontosis as a clinical entity, *J Periodontol* 42:516, 1971.

Clemons GP, et al: Current concepts in the diagnosis and classification of periodontitis, *Can Dent J* 18:33, 1990.

Page RC, et al: Prepubertal periodontitis. Definition of a clinical disease entity, *J Periodontol* 54:257, 1983.

Pruthi VK, Angier JE, Gelskey SC: Localized juvenile periodontitis: a case analysis and rational approach to treatment, *Can Dent J* 56;427, 1990.

Suzuki JB: Diagnosis and classification of the periodontal diseases, *Dent Clin North Am* 32:195, 1988.

Suzuki JB, Park S, Falker WA: Immunological profile of localized and generalized juvenile periodontitis. Lymphocyte blastogenesis and autologous mixed lymphocyte response, *J Periodontol* 55:453, 1984.

Inflammatory Periapical Disease.

Shafer WG, Hine MK, Levy BM: *Textbook of oral pathology,* ed 4, Philadelphia, 1983, W.B. Saunders.

Wood NK, Goaz PW: *Differential diagnosis of oral lesions,* ed 4, St Louis, 1991, Mosby–Year Book.

Suppurative Osteomyelitis

Adekeye EO, Cornah J: Osteomyelitis of the jaws: a review of 141 cases, *Br J Oral Maxillofac Surg* 23:24, 1985.

Gibilisco JA: *Stafne's oral radiographic diagnosis,* ed 5, Philadelphia, 1985, W.B. Saunders.

Killy HC, Kay TW: *Inflammatory diseases of the jaw bones.* In Gorlin RJ, Goldman HM, editors: *Thoma's Oral Pathology,* ed 6, St Louis, 1970, Mosby–Year Book.

Shafer WG, Hine MK, Levy BM: *Textbook of oral pathology,* ed 4, Philadelphia, 1983, W.B. Saunders.

Worth HM: *Principles and practice of oral radiographic interpretation,* Chicago, 1963, Year Book Medical.

Chronic Sclerosing Osteomyelitis

Jacobson S: Diffuse sclerosing osteomyelitis of the mandible, *Int J Oral Surg* 13:363, 1984.

Shafer WG: Chronic sclerosing osteomyelitis, *Oral Surg Oral Med Oral Pathol* 15:138, 1957.

Shafer WG, Hine MK, Levy BM: *A textbook of oral pathology,* ed 4, Philadelphia, 1983, W.B. Saunders.

Worth HM: *Principles and practice of radiologic interpretation,* Chicago, 1963, Year Book Medical.

Osteomyelitis With Periostitis

Jacobson S, et al: Chronic sclerosing osteomyelitis of the mandible, *Oral Surg Oral Med Oral Pathol* 45:167, 1978.

Nortje CJ, Wood RE, Grotepass F: Periostitis ossificans versus Garre's osteomyelitis. Part II. Radiologic analysis of 93 cases in the jaws, *Oral Surg Oral Med Oral Pathol* 66:249, 1988.

Smith S, Farman AG: Osteomyelitis with proliferative periostitis (Garre's osteomyelitis), *Oral Surg Oral Med Oral Pathol* 43:315, 1977.

Wood RE, et al: Periostitis ossificans versus Garre's osteomyelitis. Part I. What did Garre really say? *Oral Surg Oral Med Oral Pathol* 65:773, 1982.

Worth HM: *The periosteum in disease of the jaw: a radiologic study.* In Walker RV, editor: *Transactions of the Third International Conference on Oral Surgery,* Edinburgh, 1970, E&S Livingstone.

Tuberculous Osteomyelitis

Jones WC, Miller WE: Skeletal tuberculosis, *South Med J* 57:964, 1963.

Sephariadou-Mavropoulo T, Yannoulopolous A: Tuberculosis of the jaws, *Oral Maxillofac Surg* 44:158, 1986.

Wood RE, Housego T, Nortje CJ: Tuberculous osteomyelitis in the mandible of a child, *Pediatr Dent* 9:317, 1987.

Syphilis

Killey HC, Kay TW: *Inflammatory disease of the jaw bones.* In Gorlin RJ, Goldman HM, editors: *Thoma's Oral Pathology,* ed 6, St Louis, 1970, Mosby–Year Book.

Meyer I, Shklar G: Oral manifestation of acquired syphilis, *Oral Surg Oral Med Oral Pathol* 23:45, 1967.

Shafer WG, Hine MK, Levy BM: *Textbook of oral pathology,* ed 4, Philadelphia, 1983, WB Saunders.

Worth HM: *Principles and practice of oral radiologic interpretation,* Chicago, 1963, Year Book Medical.

Osteoradionecrosis Complicated by Osteomyelitis

Bedwinck JM, et al: Osteoradionecrosis in patients treated with definitive radiotherapy for squamous cell carcinoma of the oral cavity and naso and oropharynx, *Radiology* 119:665, 1976.

Marx RE: Osteoradionecrosis, a new concept in its pathology, *J Oral Maxillofac Surg* 1:283, 1983.

Marx RE, Johnson RD: Studies in the radiobiology of osteoradionecrosis and their clinical significance, *Oral Surg Oral Med Oral Pathol* 64:379, 1987.

Meyer I: Infectious diseases of the jaws, *J Oral Surg* 28:17, 1970.

Cancrum Oris

Shafer WG, Hine MM, Levy BM: *Textbook of oral pathology,* ed 4, Philadelphia, 1983, WB Saunders.

7

Cysts of the Jaws

CALCIFYING ODONTOGENIC CYST

Overview

Definition: Calcifying odontogenic cysts are developmental odontogenic lesions that occasionally behave aggressively. When they suggest a neoplasm, they are called *odontogenic ghost cell tumors*.

Pathogenesis: Calcifying odontogenic cysts are believed to arise from odontogenic epithelial remnants in the gingivae or in the mandible or maxilla.

Clinical Features

Demographics: An incidence of 3 calcifying odontogenic cysts per 10,000 oral biopsies has been reported. Patients range widely in age (1 to 87 years), with a peak incidence for detection in the second decade of life. These cysts usually appear in patients less than 40 years of age. Some reports suggest that the cysts have a predilection for females, whereas other studies show no gender bias. More than 70% of calcifying odontogenic cysts are associated with the maxilla; one fourth of these occur extraosseously as localized masses involving the gingivae. The anterior segments of the jaws are most commonly affected.

Signs and symptoms: A calcifying odontogenic cyst may initially appear as a localized slow-growing mass. Occasionally pain is a symptom. Displacement of teeth is also seen. The lesion is sometimes associated with unerupted teeth.

RADIOLOGIC FEATURES

Cardinal Signs

The central calcifying odontogenic cyst may appear initially as a unilocular or multilocular radiolucency with discrete, well-demarcated margins.

Irregularly sized calcifications may be scattered in the radiolucency, producing variable degrees of opacity. This may produce a "salt and pepper" appearance.

The lesion may be a homogeneous radiolucency.

Ancillary Signs

If seen along with a complex odontoma, the opaque components may be blending.

Root resorption is occasionally seen.

Differential Diagnosis

Before calcification
    Dentigerous cyst
    Keratocyst
    Ameloblastoma
After calcification
    Adenomatoid odontogenic tumor
    Cystic odontoma
    Calcifying epithelial odontogenic tumor
    Extraosseous variant
    Peripheral giant cell granuloma
    Peripheral ossifying fibrous hyperplasia
    Pyogenic granuloma

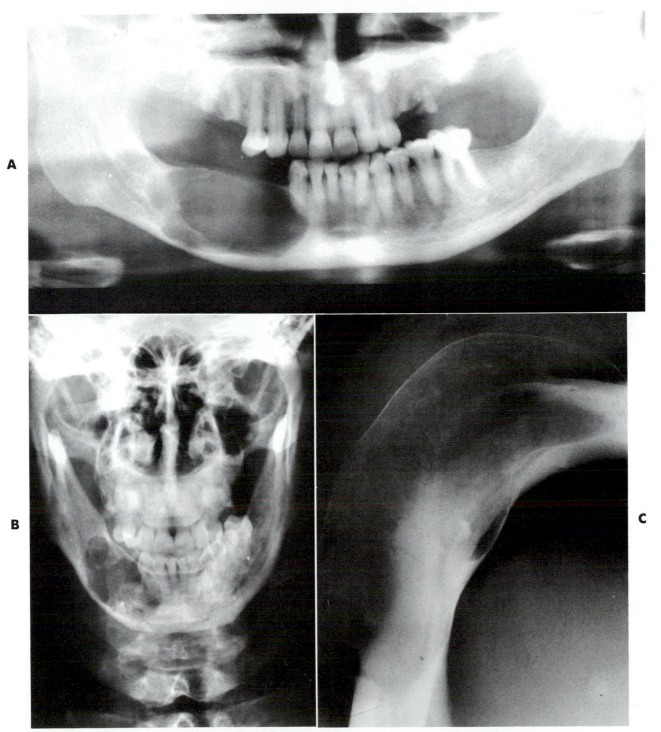

Fig. 7-1 A, Panoramic radiograph. The homogeneous, well-circumscribed radiolucency in the right mandibular premolar and molar regions was a calcifying odontogenic cyst.
B, Posteroanterior radiograph of the patient in **A. C,** True occlusal radiograph of calcifying odontogenic cyst in anterior mandible, extending to the premolar region. Fine ("salt-and-pepper") calcifications are evident in the lumen of the cystic cavity. Note buccal expansion of the mandibular cortex.   *Continued.*

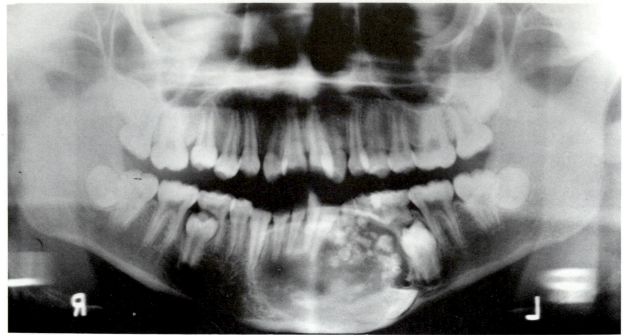

D

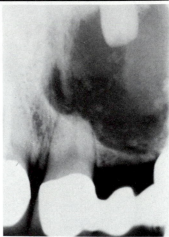

E

Fig. 7-1, cont'd.   D, Panoramic radiograph. Calcifying odontogenic cyst in mandibular midline. Note the extensive calcification seen in this case and the apparent dentigerous relationship to an impacted and displaced mandibular canine. **E,** Calcifying odontogenic cyst in anterior maxilla. This patient also demonstrates a dentigerous relationship to an unerupted tooth. Note the external resorption of the root of the overlying tooth.

DENTIGEROUS CYST

Overview

Definition: Dentigerous cysts arise in the follicular region of an unerupted tooth and are attached to the tooth at the cementoenamel junction in the cervical region.

Pathogenesis: A dentigerous cyst develops after fluid accumulates between the remnants of the enamel organ and the subjacent tooth crown. The enamel organ remnant, or reduced enamel epithelium, forms one of the delimiting surfaces of the cyst, and the mature tooth crown forms the other. Fluid accumulates between the reduced enamel epithelium and the crown and occasionally in the enamel organ itself. The expansion of the dentigerous cyst is related to a secondary increase in cyst fluid osmolality, resulting from passage of inflammatory cells and desquamative epithelial cells into the cyst lumen. The increased intracystic osmotic pressure results in net ingress of fluid and secondary centrifugal growth of the cyst.

Clinical Features

Demographics: Dentigerous cysts are the most common odontogenic cysts, next to radicular cysts. The most common sites are the third molar regions of

Text continued on page 216.

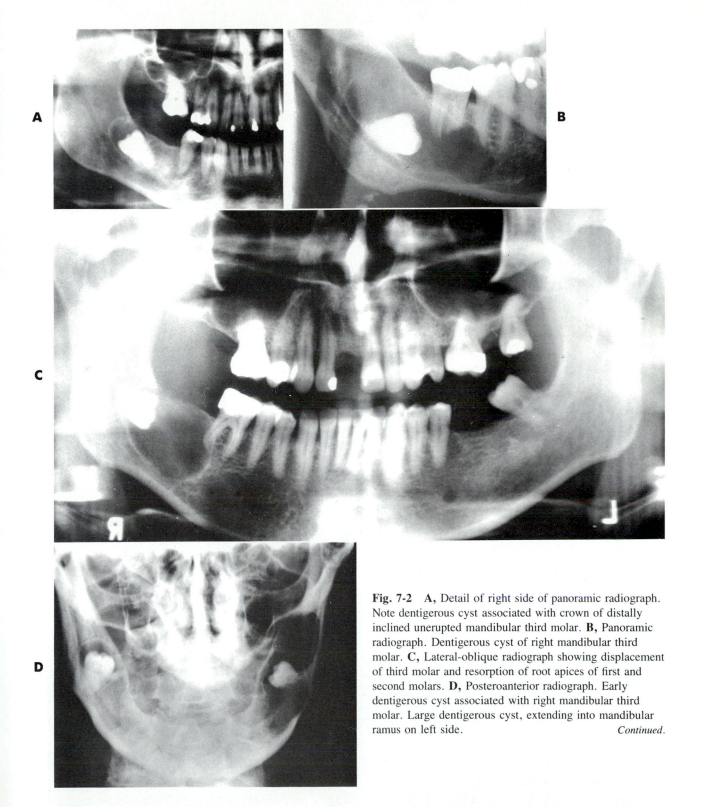

Fig. 7-2 **A,** Detail of right side of panoramic radiograph. Note dentigerous cyst associated with crown of distally inclined unerupted mandibular third molar. **B,** Panoramic radiograph. Dentigerous cyst of right mandibular third molar. **C,** Lateral-oblique radiograph showing displacement of third molar and resorption of root apices of first and second molars. **D,** Posteroanterior radiograph. Early dentigerous cyst associated with right mandibular third molar. Large dentigerous cyst, extending into mandibular ramus on left side. *Continued.*

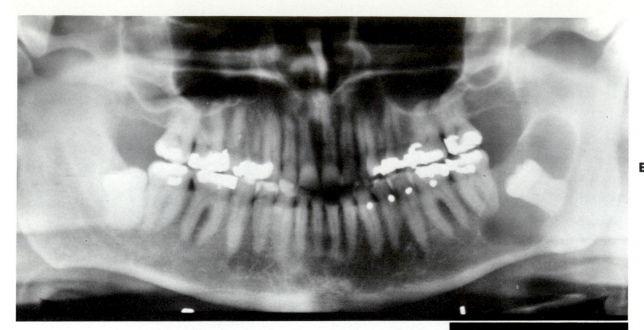

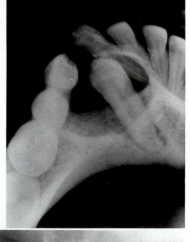

Fig. 7-2, cont'd. **E,** Panoramic radiograph. Large dentigerous cyst in left side of mandible. Note expansion into body and ramus of mandible. **F,** Topographic occlusal radiograph showing dentigerous cyst of right mandibular canine. Note displacement of adjacent teeth. **G,** Panoramic radiograph. Dentigerous cyst of left mandibular canine causing displacement of adjacent teeth and resorption of overlying teeth.

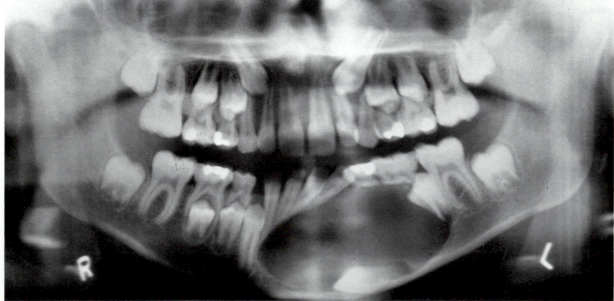

Continued.

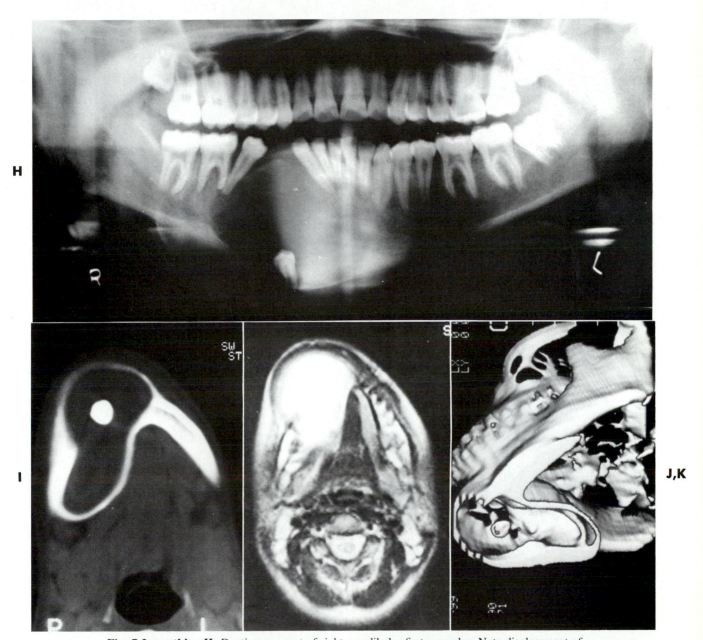

Fig. 7-2, cont'd.   H, Dentigerous cyst of right mandibular first premolar. Note displacement of teeth and expansion of jaw. **I,** Computed tomographic view demonstrating buccal and lingual expansion of mandible and position of affected tooth in same patient as in **H. J,** In the same patient, 0.5 Tesla T2-weighted MR image shows a strong positive response in the region of the fluid-filled dentigerous cyst. **K,** Three-dimensional CT reconstructed showing relation of impacted first premolar tooth to the jaw-deforming dentigerous cyst in the patient in **H.**

Continued.

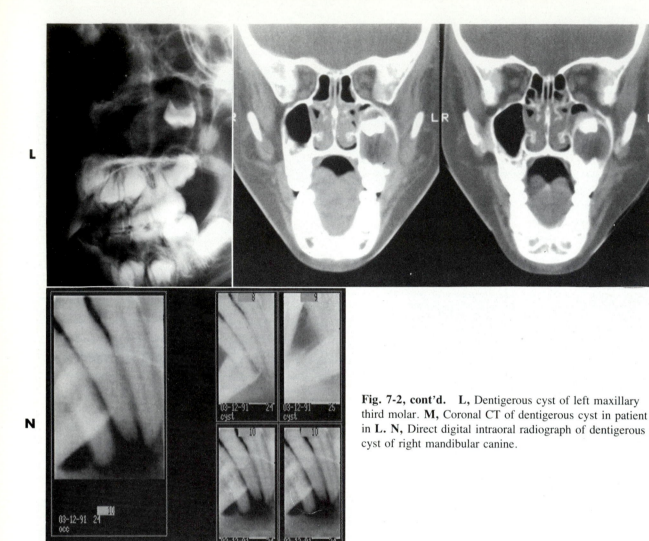

Fig. 7-2, cont'd.   L, Dentigerous cyst of left maxillary third molar. **M,** Coronal CT of dentigerous cyst in patient in **L. N,** Direct digital intraoral radiograph of dentigerous cyst of right mandibular canine.

the mandible and maxilla and the maxillary canine regions. In addition, these teeth are the most frequently impacted. The highest incidence of detection is in the second and third decades of life, with a greater frequency in males by a ratio of 1.6:1.

Signs and symptoms: Symptoms are generally absent, with late eruption or noneruption being an indicator of possible cyst formation. A dentigerous cyst may achieve significant size, with eventual bone expansion. As with other cysts, the dentigerous cyst tends to expand the outer plate more extensively than the lingual cortex. The cyst may involve many teeth as it enlarges, and it may be difficult to determine which was the offending tooth. If the cortex thins, there may be a crackling or crepitation on palpation.

RADIOLOGIC FEATURES

Cardinal Signs

Well-defined unilocular radiolucency associated with the crown of an unerupted tooth, with well-defined and sharp bony margins

Symmetric envelopment of the crown of unerupted tooth

Lateral radiolucencies possible representing region of least resistance to cyst expansion (In the mandible the radiolucency can extend up the ramus and along the body of the mandible.)

Displacement of the affected tooth and adjacent teeth

Resorption of the apices of overlying teeth not infrequent

Demarcation between the lucency of the cyst and the surrounding bone generally obvious

Ancillary Signs

Occasionally trabeculations are seen overlying the cystic area with erroneous impression of multilocularity.

Loss of the bony cortex from the margin of a cyst thought to be dentigerous suggests the presence of suppuration or malignancy.

With larger cysts the lamina dura around the affected tooth is sometimes not visible on the radiograph.

Differential Diagnosis

Ameloblastoma

Envelopmental keratocyst

Adenomatoid odontogenic tumor

Ameloblastic fibroma

KERATOCYST

Overview

Definition: A keratocyst is an odontogenic cyst lined by keratinizing epithelium, with an aggressive biologic behavior. Histologically it is characterized by a keratinized surface, a uniform six-cell to ten-cell thick epithelium with a prominent palisaded polarized basal layer of cells, relatively high mitotic figures, and no rete pegs.

Pathogenesis: The origin of keratocysts is thought to be the proliferation of dental lamina remnants in the mandible and maxilla.

Clinical Features

Demographics: Patients with keratocysts range widely in age, with a peak incidence for detection in the second and third decades of life. There is a male-to-female ratio of 1.3:1, with the average age of male patients being almost 1 decade older than female patients. The chief site of involvement is the mandible, which is affected twice as frequently as the maxilla. In the mandible the cyst occurs mostly in the posterior portion of the body and ramus region. Maxillary cysts are noted chiefly in the third molar area. The cysts may be part of the basal cell nevus syndrome. Lesions found in children often reflect multiple odontogenic keratocysts as a component of this syndrome.

Signs and symptoms: Bone expansion is an infrequent sign, with maxillary lesions producing buccal rather than palatal expansion, and mandibular lesions showing buccal expansion in one half of the cases. However, bony expansion is considered a late sign, as the lesions generally grow along the marrow spaces first. Most are discovered fortuitously, as they are asymptomatic. Unexpected tooth movements associated with keratocysts may include tooth extrusion. Associated pain or discharge may be present if the cyst is secondarily infected.

Keratocysts tend to recur after inadequate surgery, with recurrence rates reportedly ranging from 0% to 62%. Most recurrences occur in the first 5 years after surgery, but they have also been reported 20 to 40 years after the initial operation. Recurrence is felt to be due to the high rate of proliferation of epithelium compared with that in other odontogenic cysts. Reports of malignant change in the epithelium are well documented but no more common than for other odontogenic cysts.

Special tests: Positive staining of specimens with carcinoembryonic antigen may reflect a more aggressive nature of this cyst. The keratocyst is different from other cysts in lumen contents in protein, immunoglobulin, and glycosaminoglycan. The lumen is often filled by keratin. A definitive diagnosis requires histopathologic analysis.

RADIOLOGIC FEATURES

Cardinal Signs

Well-circumscribed radiolucency with smooth margins and thin radiopaque borders is seen.

Unilocular lesions can have scalloped margins.

Multilocularity can be present and tends to be seen more frequently in larger lesions.

Multilocular lesions appear to be larger than unilocular lesions.

Most lesions are unilocular, with up to 40% noted adjacent to the crown of an unerupted tooth. Impeded eruption of underlying teeth or ingrowth into the follicular space around an unerupted tooth may produce a dentigerous appearance.

Ancillary Signs

There may be extensive involvement of the body and ramus of the mandible before any expansion occurs.

Text continued on page 220.

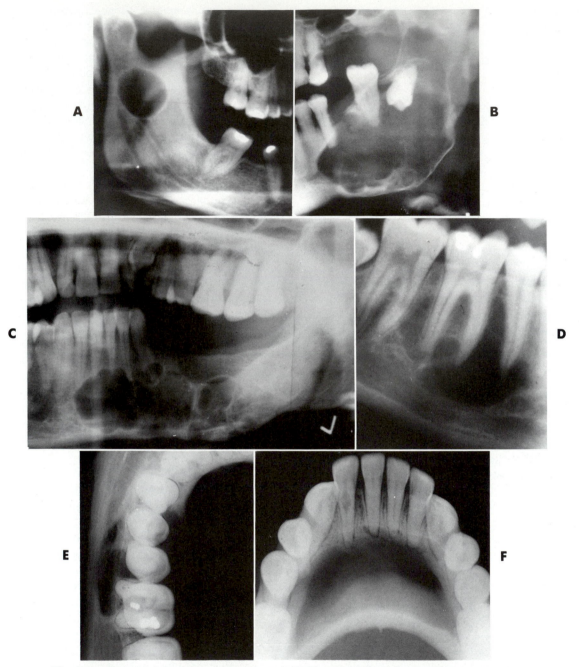

Fig. 7-3 A, Detail from panoramic radiograph. Unilocular keratocyst in right mandibular ramus. **B,** Detail from panoramic radiograph. Crenated keratocyst in left mandibular third molar region, enveloping that tooth. **C,** Detail from panoramic radiograph. Multilocular keratocyst. Note that this relatively large lesion causes relatively little bony expansion. **D,** Detail from panoramic radiograph. Keratocyst involving roots of second premolar and first molar. **E,** True occlusal radiograph of patient in **D.** Note the lack of buccal cortical plate expansion. **F,** Topographic occlusal radiograph. Large odontogenic keratocyst occupying anterior mandible. Note relative lack of displacement or resorption of adjacent teeth. (The internal resorption of the right lateral incisor was considered an unrelated process.)   *Continued.*

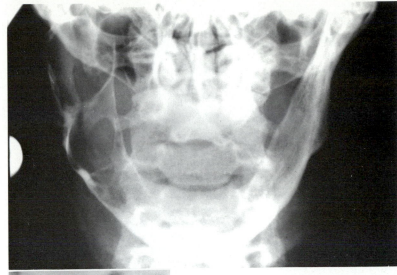

G

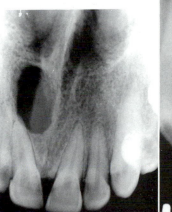

H,I

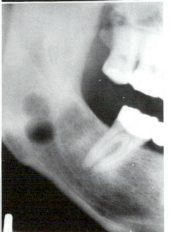

Fig. 7-3, cont'd. **G,** Posteroanterior radiograph. Multilocular keratocyst of the right side of the mandible. Expansion of the afflicted jaw is seen as a late finding. **H,** Unilocular keratocyst in anterior maxilla. Note that this lesion does not cross the midline and has neither displaced nor caused resorption of the adjacent central incisor. **I,** Recurrent odontogenic keratocyst in right mandibular third molar and angle region. **J,** Panoramic radiograph. Keratocyst subjacent to mandibular first permanent molar.

J

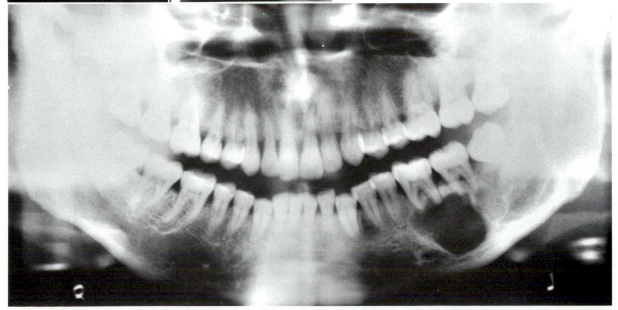

Continued.

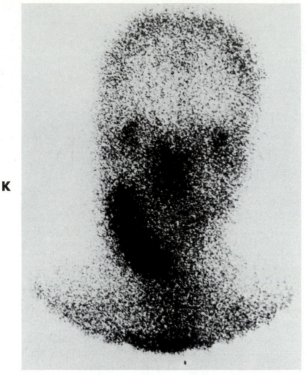

Fig. 7-3, cont'd.   K, Technetium 99m pertechnetate scintigraphy showing increased uptake in mandible in site of keratocyst.

Displacement and resorption of teeth are sometimes present in long-standing lesions. Resorption of teeth, however, is rare.

Differential Diagnosis
Dentigerous cyst
Ameloblastoma
Calcifying odontogenic cyst
Ameloblastic fibroma
Adenomatoid odontogenic tumor
Traumatic bone cyst

LATERAL PERIODONTAL CYST

Overview

Definition: The lateral periodontal cyst may be defined as a nonkeratinized, noninflammatory, developmental intraosseous cyst occurring adjacent or lateral to the root of a tooth. It is directly associated with the periodontal membrane.

Pathogenesis: The origin of lateral periodontal cysts is related to the proliferation of rests of odontogenic epithelium from the dental lamina or Hertwig root sheath.

Clinical Features

Demographics: Most lateral periodontal cysts occur in the mandibular premolar and canine regions, with fewer in the incisor area. Most occur toward the facial aspect of the alveolus. There is a distinct male predilection, with a 2:1 male-to-female ratio. The age range reported is 20 to 85 years, with a predominance for detection in the fifth and sixth decades of life.

Signs and symptoms: The clinical course is insidious. Most lateral periodontal cysts are asymptomatic and found incidentally on radiographic examination. Peripheral lesions (the so-called gingival cyst of adults) can appear as a small soft tissue swelling in or inferior to the interdental papilla, with a slightly bluish discoloration.

RADIOLOGIC FEATURES

Cardinal Signs

Well-delineated radiolucency with an opaque margin along the lateral surface of the tooth root

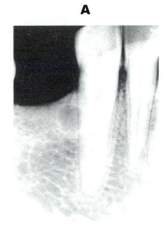

A

Fig. 7-4 **A,** Periapical radiograph showing unilocular lateral periodontal cyst distal to right mandibular canine. **B,** Panoramic radiograph demonstrating bilateral lateral periodontal cysts between the mandibular canines and first premolars. **C,** Periapical radiograph. Lateral periodontal cyst anterior to left mandibular first molar. **D,** Periapical radiograph. Multilocular (botryoid) lateral periodontal cyst between the left mandibular first and second premolars.

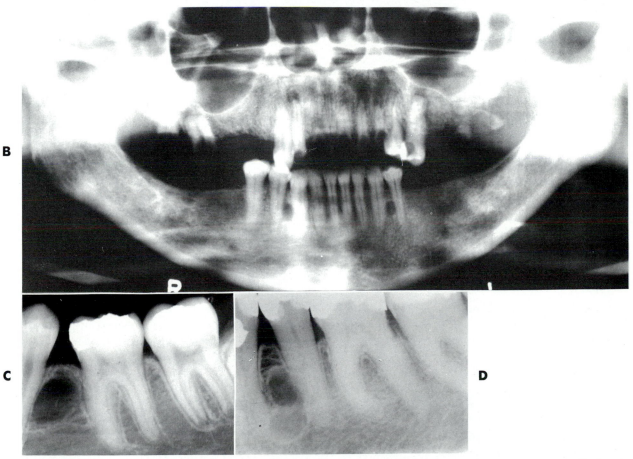

B

C

D

Continued.

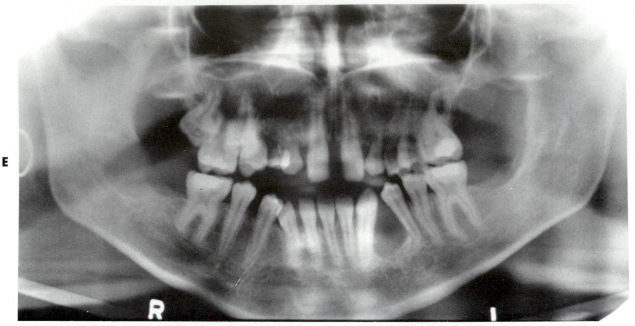

Fig. 7-4, cont'd.   E, Panoramic radiograph showing large unilocular lateral periodontal cyst between left mandibular canine and first premolar.

Differential Diagnosis

Cyst forming secondary to severe periodontitis
Lateral radicular cyst (inflammatory origin)
Keratocyst
Any radiolucent odontogenic tumor
Central mucoepidermoid tumor

RADICULAR CYST

Overview

Definition: A radicular cyst is an inflammatory cyst that derives its epithelial lining from proliferation of small odontogenic epithelial residue of Malassez rest in the periodontal ligament.

Pathogenesis: The radicular cyst develops in a preexisting periapical granuloma. Stimulation of the epithelial rests is caused by the inflammatory process in the periapical granuloma, with resultant cyst formation as the epithelial elements proliferate beyond the size that can be supported by the surrounding vasculature. Remnants of cellular debris are found in the cyst lumen, which increases the osmotic pressure and allows transport of fluid across the epithelial lining. This ingress of fluid results in cyst enlargement.

Clinical Features

Demographics: The radicular cyst is by far the most common cyst of the oral and perioral regions. In most large series of cysts, the radicular cyst constitutes one half to three quarters of the total. The age distributions for discovery peak is the third to sixth decades of life. Most occur in men.

Signs and symptoms: Most radicular cysts are asymptomatic and are often discovered incidentally. They rarely produce bone expansion, but if they do, the expansion is slow. Long-standing cysts may be destructive. By definition the presence of a nonvital tooth is required for the diagnosis of a radicular cyst.

Special test: Pulp test of the involved tooth usually shows it to be nonvital.

RADIOLOGIC FEATURES

Cardinal Signs

No distinct radiographic differences between a radicular cyst and a periapical granuloma
Round to ovoid radiolucency with narrow opaque margin that is continuous with the lamina dura of the involved tooth

Ancillary Signs

    Root resorption in long-standing lesions

    Window in periosteum

    Displaced anatomic structures such as the mandibular canal

    Cysts differentiated from granulomas on the basis of computed tomographic findings indicating greater radiolucency for the former

Differential Diagnosis

    Periapical granuloma

    Surgical defect

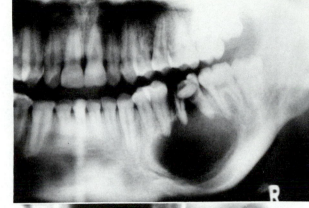

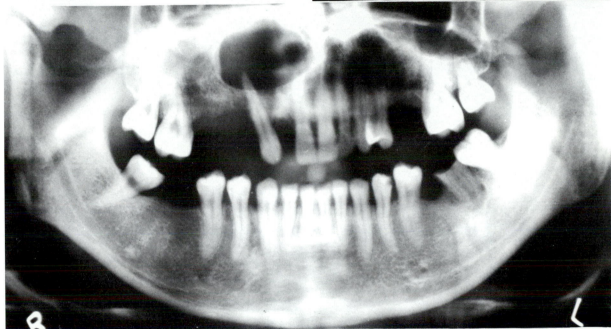

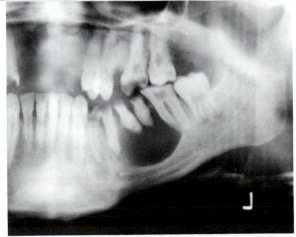

Fig. 7-5 A, Detail from panoramic radiograph. Radicular cyst associated with grossly carious mandibular first molar. Note the continuity between the cystic lesion and the periodontal ligament space of the affected tooth. **B,** Panoramic radiograph. Radicular cyst from right maxillary lateral incisor, incidentally superimposed over root of adjacent canine. Note upward displacement of the floor of the maxillary sinus on the side affected by the cyst. **C,** Detail of panoramic radiograph showing radicular cyst on left mandibular first molar.

Continued.

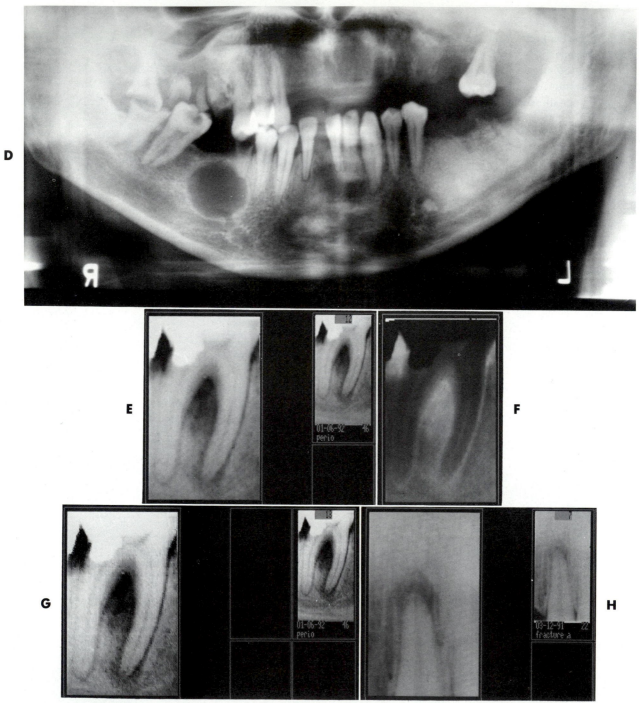

Fig. 7-5, cont'd.   D, Panoramic radiograph showing radicular cyst of right mandibular second premolar. **E,** Direct digital image of tooth with radicular cyst (mesial root) and periodontal disease. **F,** Same patient as in **E,** using negative mode. **G,** Same patient as in **E,** with computed edge enhancement. **H,** Direct digital image of early radicular cyst.

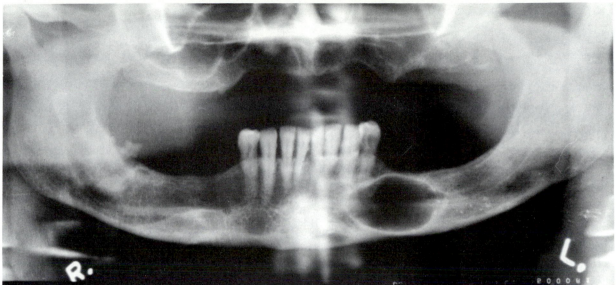

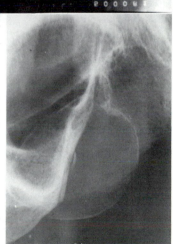

Fig. 7-6 A, Panoramic radiograph demonstrating residual radicular cyst in left mandibular premolar region. **B,** Periapical radiograph. Residual cyst in right maxillary premolar and canine region.

Early periapical cemental dysplasia
Traumatic bone cyst
Metastatic disease

RESIDUAL CYST

Overview

Definition: Residual cysts are cysts that are left behind after a tooth is removed. Most commonly they are radicular cysts initially.

Pathogenesis: A residual cyst develops in a preexisting periapical granuloma. Stimulation of the epithelial rests relates to the inflammatory process in the periapical granuloma, with resultant cystification as the epithelial elements proliferate. Remnants of cellular debris are found in the cyst lumen, which increases the osmotic pressure and allows transport of fluid across the epithelial lining. This ingress of fluid results in cyst enlargement.

Clinical Features

Demographics: Most residual cysts occur in the mandibular premolar region in older age groups.

Signs and symptoms: Residual cysts are usually related to a previous inflammatory periapical lesion. A missing tooth may be a sign. Large lesions are associated with jaw expansion.

RADIOLOGIC FEATURES

Cardinal Signs

Except for missing tooth, no distinct differences between a residual cyst and a periapical granuloma

Round to ovoid radiolucency with narrow opaque margin

Differential Diagnosis

Healing granuloma
Surgical defect
Traumatic bone cyst
Keratocyst
Metastatic disease

TRAUMATIC BONE CYST

Overview

Definition: A traumatic bone cyst is a bone cavity in the mandible not lined by epithelium. It is, therefore, not a true cyst. It may be a normal variant rather than a disease process. This cyst is also known as a *simple, solitary,* or *hemorrhagic* bone cyst.

Pathogenesis: The etiology and pathogenesis of traumatic bone cysts are unknown. The various names that have been applied suggest speculation as to the possible etiology of the lesion.

Clinical Features

Demographics: Traumatic bone cysts have been detected in patients with widely ranging ages (2 to 75 years); however, most are found during the second decade of life. They occur in the mandible with almost equal frequency in the body and vertical ramus. There is no gender predilection.

Signs and symptoms: Traumatic bone cysts are almost always asymptomatic. Swelling has been recorded in about 25% of the reported cases, and pain occurs in about 10%. The lesions are not infrequently bilateral. They can involute without treatment. Recurrence has also been reported after surgical intervention, albeit rarely.

RADIOLOGIC FEATURES

Cardinal Signs

Homogeneous radiolucency

Smooth outline usually not markedly corticated

Scalloping of margins especially likely to be prominent for superior margin interdigitating with overlying tooth roots

Margin cortication generally more noticeable for inferior margin; superior cortex often not readily discernible radiographically

Periodontal space of adjacent teeth generally traceable; however, resorption of lamina dura and tooth roots sometimes evident

Growth along the jaw, with expansion of jaw unusual

Generally above mandibular canal

Ancillary Signs

Sometimes associated with fibroosseous lesions, such as florid osseous dysplasia

Differential Diagnosis

Keratocyst

Central giant cell granuloma

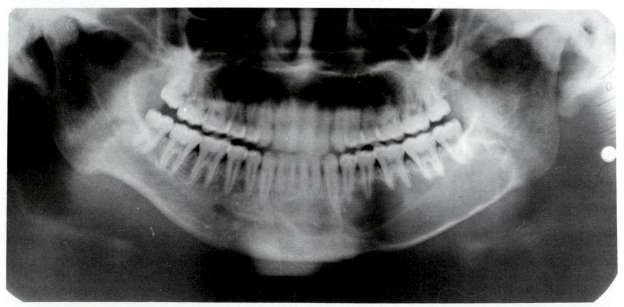

A

Fig. 7-7   A, Panoramic radiograph. Typical traumatic bone cyst of left side of mandible. Note scalloped margins between tooth roots and lack of jawbone expansion.

Continued.

Fig. 7-7, cont'd.   B, True occlusal radiograph of mandible showing traumatic bone cyst extending from right second premolar to left canine. Note lack of bone expansion. **C,** Axial CT view of traumatic bone cyst showing slight expansion of mandible in affected region. **D,** Axial CT view of patient in **C** at more superficial level shows less expansion of the jaw at the level of the molar roots. **E,** Detail from panoramic radiograph showing multilocular traumatic bone cyst in right mandibular region. Such a lesion needs surgical intervention and biopsy to rule out other pathoses. Note lack of expansion of jaw. **F,** Detail from panoramic radiograph showing traumatic bone cyst with partial loss of lamina dura around the dental roots.

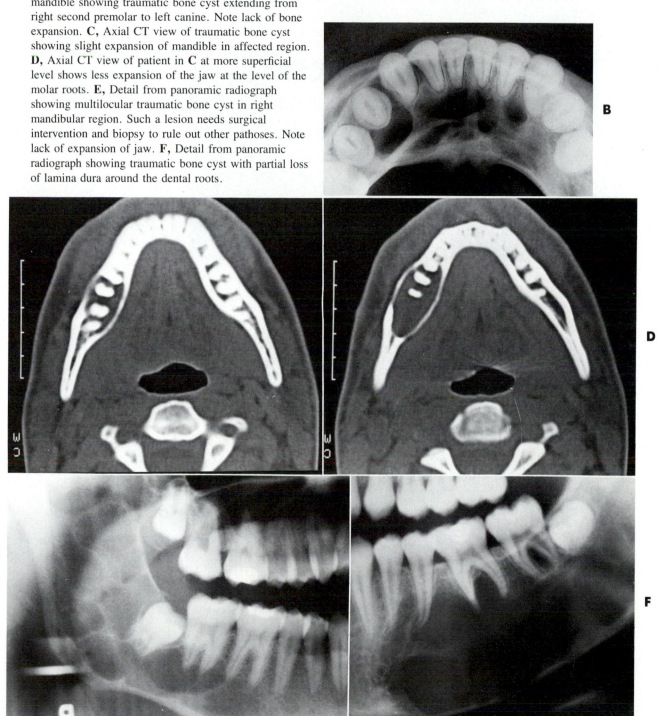

Continued.

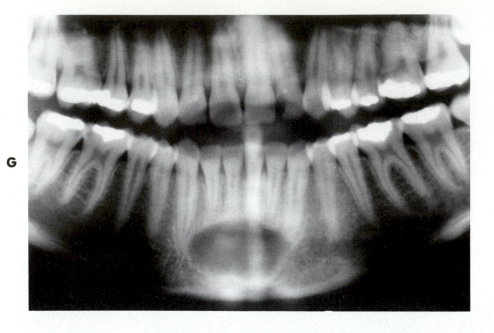

G

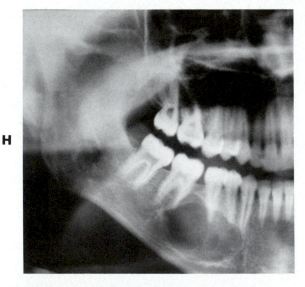

H

Fig. 7-7, cont'd. **G,** Panoramic radiograph showing traumatic bone cyst in midline of mandible. **H,** Detail from panoramic radiograph showing traumatic bone cyst in right mandibular premolar region.

ANEURYSMAL BONE CYST

Overview

Definition: An aneurysmal bone cyst is a nonneoplastic lesion of bone consisting of several cavities filled with blood and without an endothelial or epithelial lining.

Pathogenesis: The cause of aneurysmal bone cysts is uncertain, but they might arise as primary or secondary lesions. Alternatively they may develop as a consequence of an arteriovenous anomaly, local trauma, or degeneration of a preexisting neoplasm.

Clinical Features

Demographics: The aneurysmal bone cyst constitutes only 1% of all nonodontogenic, nonepithelial cysts of the jaws. Only about 1% of all aneurysmal bone cysts occur in the jaws. They most commonly occur in the long bones and spine. Almost all lesions in the jaws affect the mandible, especially the posterior body and vertical ramus. They are found predominantly in young persons, rarely manifesting after the third decade of life. There is no gender predilection.

Signs and symptoms: Aneurysmal bone cysts appear clinically as a swelling of overlying soft tissues caused by bony expansion. Perforation of the cortex is possible. Pain and tenderness to palpation are reported.

Text continued on page 231.

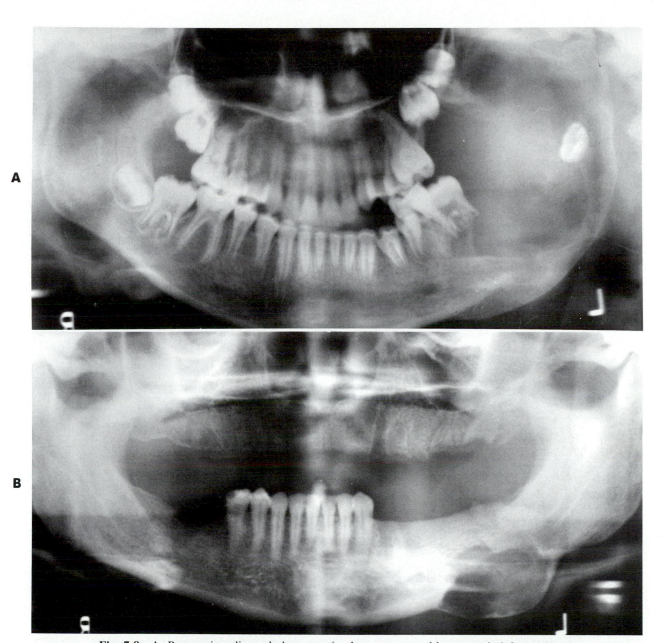

Fig. 7-8 **A,** Panoramic radiograph demonstrating large aneurysmal bone cyst in left mandibular ramus. The lesion envelops a developing mandibular third molar and has caused displacement of the ipsilateral mandibular and maxillary molar. **B,** Panoramic radiograph showing aneurysmal bone cyst of left mandibular body, causing expansion of lower cortical plate.

Continued.

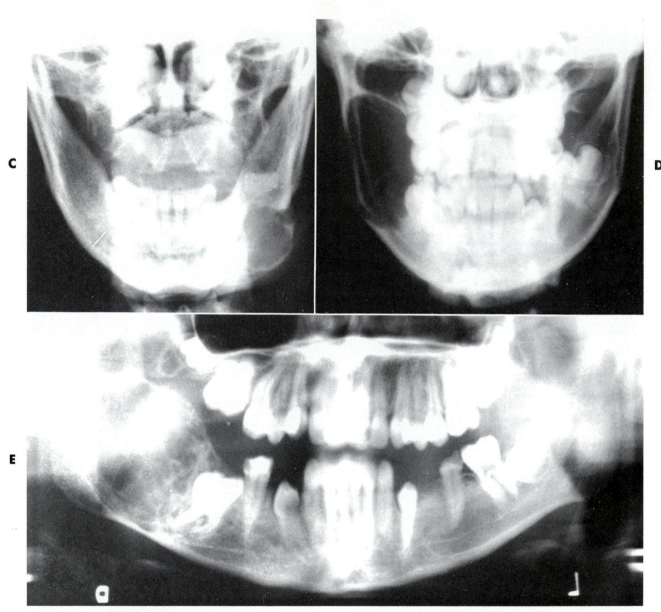

Fig. 7-8, cont'd.   C (above), Posteroanterior view showing buccal cortical expansion in patient in **B. D,** Posteroanterior view showing aneurysmal bone cyst of right mandibular ramus.
E, Panoramic radiograph of patient in **D.** This lesion shows expansion of the upper cortex and multilocularity. **F (opposite page),** Axial CT view of patient in **D** demonstrating the expansile nature of this lesion. Note that the cortex is nevertheless intact. **G,** Axial MR image using 0.5 Tesla and T2 weighting for patient in **D.** The lesion produces a homogenously strong signal.
H, Coronal MR image of patient in **D.** Note buccal and lingual expansion of the mandible.

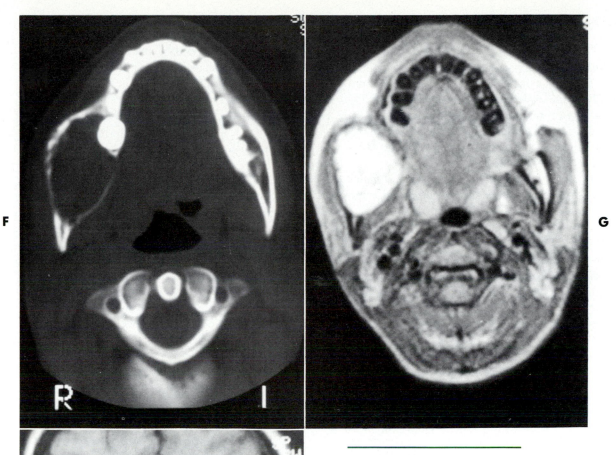

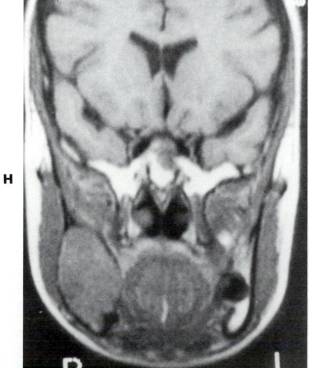

Fig. 7-8, F–H

RADIOLOGIC FEATURES

Cardinal Signs

Radiolucent expansile mass

Border well defined and well corticated in most instances; however, overlying cortex possibly effaced when gross ballooning of the jaw is
present

Multiloculation common

Reactive bone formation producing a mixed radiolucent and radiopaque lesion not uncommon

Ancillary Signs

Displacement of mandibular canal without erosion
of canal cortex

Vascularity demonstrated on angiography

Lesion generally positive on technetium 99m
pertechnetate bone scan scintigraphy

Differential Diagnosis

Ameloblastoma

Giant cell granuloma

Odontogenic myxoma

NASOPALATINE DUCT CYST

Overview

Definition: A nasopalatine duct cyst is a nonodontogenic cyst in the incisive canal area, arising from epithelial residue of the nasopalatine ducts. Practically speaking, there is no need to distinguish this cyst from cysts in the palatal midline from epithelial inclusions resulting from development of that site as the treatment and prognosis are identical.

Pathogenesis: Presumably inflammatory stimulus initiates nasopalatine duct cysts. The precise etiology, however, is not known.

Clinical Features

Demographics: Nasopalatine duct cysts constitute approximately 4% of all cysts in the oral cavity treated surgically; they are the most common form of nonodontogenic cyst, occurring in about 1% of the population. They are most frequently detected in patients between the second and fifth decades of life and are seldom found in children. Males are almost twice as frequently affected as females.

Signs and symptoms: Nasopalatine duct cysts are usually asymptomatic in patients from developed countries. They can manifest as a symmetric oral swelling in the anterior palate. Rarely a through-and-through fluctuant mass is visible between the palate and labial alveolus. Tooth displacement is quite common when the lesions are large. Adjacent teeth are generally vital to pulp testing. Pain is rare in the absence of secondary infection.

RADIOLOGIC FEATURES

Cardinal Signs

Well-circumscribed radiolucency in or close to the midline, with a well-defined cortical border

Radiolucencies less than 6 mm in diameter probably large incisive fossae; if more than 6 mm in diameter, nasopalatine duct cyst suspected

Usually unilocular and round, ovoid, or "pear shaped"; can be bilobed or "heart shaped" because of bilateral nature of nasopalatine ducts

Almost always cross the midline

Usually displace teeth rather than causing tooth resorption

Differential Diagnosis

Large incisive fossa

Residual radicular cyst

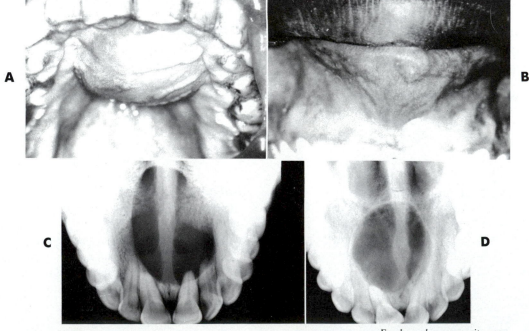

Fig. 7-9, A–D   *For legend see opposite page.*

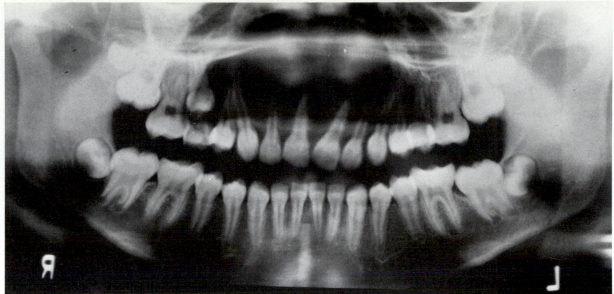

E

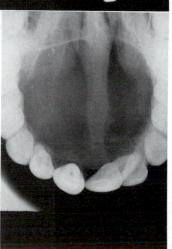

F

Fig. 7-9 A (opposite page), Large nasopalatine duct cysts can result in noticeable swelling in the midline of the anterior maxilla. B, Occasionally sublabial swelling is found with large nasopalatine cysts. C, Topographic occlusal view of ovoid-shaped nasopalatine duct cyst. D, Topographic occlusal view of round nasopalatine duct cyst. E (above), Panoramic radiograph demonstrating large nasopalatine duct cyst in midline of maxilla. F, Topographic occlusal radiograph of large nasopalatine duct cyst causing tooth displacement.

NASOLABIAL CYST

Overview

Definition: A nasolabial cyst is a soft tissue developmental fissural cyst characteristically occurring as a swelling in the nasolabial fold at the base of the alae.

Pathogenesis: The pathogenesis of nasolabial cysts is uncertain. They may arise from epithelial enclavements, possibly from the anterior portion of a developing nasolacrimal duct. Cyst formation may also be caused by inflammatory stimulus of epithelial rests.

Clinical Features

Demographics: Nasolabial cysts are rare lesions, comprising less than 1% of all jaw cysts. The peak time for discovery is the fourth and fifth decades of life. The reported age range is 4 months to 76 years. The female-to-male ratio is 4:1. These cysts are also more common in blacks than in other ethnic groups.

Signs and symptoms: The chief clinical sign is soft tissue swelling in the canine region of the upper jaw. The cyst occurs in the nasal vestibule, expanding laterally and causing elevation of the ipsilateral nasal ala. If the cyst is large enough, it can cause elevation and medial displacement of the anterior tip of the medial turbinate bone. The lesions are occasionally bilateral and can cause nasal obstruction and discomfort.

RADIOLOGIC FEATURES

Cardinal Signs

Osseous changes are late, representing minor saucerization and displacement of the "bracket-shaped line" of the anterior nasal spine and floor of the nasal fossae.

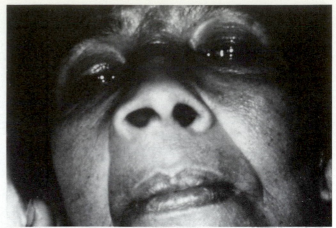

Fig. 7-10 **A,** Clinical features of nasolabial cyst. Note displacement of the ala. **B,** Panoramic radiograph of nasolabial cyst showing only minor displacement of the "bracket-shaped" line. **C,** Dimensions and position of the lesion can be illustrated by use of a radiopaque contrast medium.

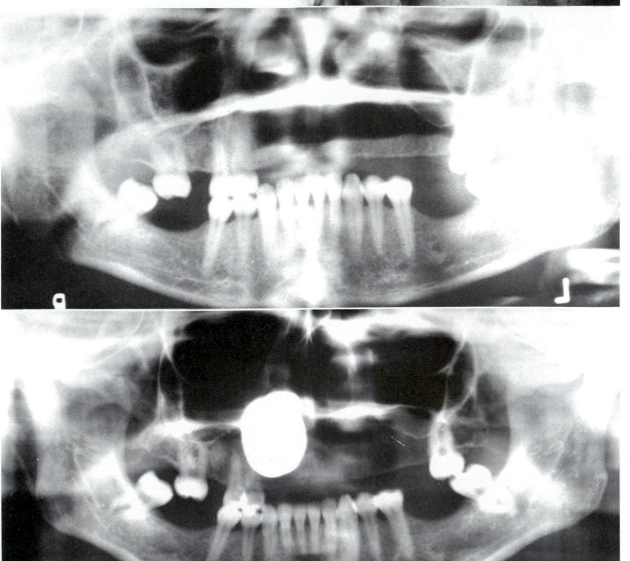

Continued.

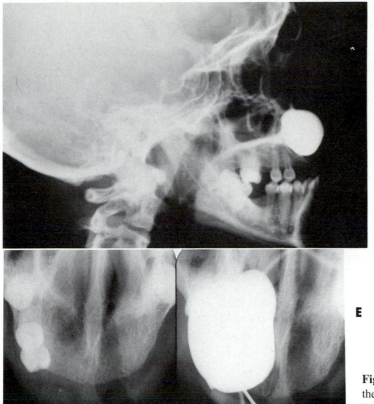

Fig. 7-10, cont'd.   D, Lateral view demonstrating the anteroposterior dimensions of the nasolabial cyst. **E,** Topographic occlusal view of nasolabial cyst before and after use of radiopaque dye.

Computed tomography and magnetic resonance imaging show an extraosseous fluid-filled sac overlying the maxillary canine region.

Ancillary Signs
Dimensions of the cyst can be established by introducing radiopaque contrast medium into the cyst lumen.

Differential Diagnosis
Minor salivary gland neoplasm

BIBLIOGRAPHY

Calcifying Odontogenic Cyst

Claman LJ, et al: Peripheral calcifying odontogenic cyst in a child: case report of an unusual lesion, *Pediatr Dent* 9:226, 1987.

El-Beialy RR, El-Mofty S, Refai H: Calcifying odontogenic cyst: case report and review of literature, *J Oral Maxillofac Surg* 48:637, 1990.

Kaugars CC, Kaugars GE, DeBiasi GF: Extraosseous calcifying odontogenic cyst: report of case and review of literature, *J Am Dent Assoc* 119:715, 1989.

Keszler A, Guglielmotti MB: Calcifying odontogenic cyst associated with odontoma: report of two cases, *J Oral Maxillofac Surg* 45:457, 1987.

Lello E, Makek M: Calcifying odontogenic cyst, *Int J Oral Maxillofac Surg* 15:637, 1986.

Mascres C, Donohue WB, Vauclair R: The calcifying odontogenic cyst: report of a case, *J Oral Maxillofac Surg* 48:319, 1990.

Regezi JA, Sciubba JJ: *Oral pathology—clinical pathologic correlations,* ed 1, Philadelphia, 1989, W.B. Saunders, p 554.

Scott J, Wood GD: Aggressive calcifying odontogenic cyst: a possible variant of ameloblastoma, *Br J Oral Maxillofac Surg* 27:53, 1989.

Shear M: *Cysts of the oral regions,* ed 1, Bristol, 1976, John Wright & Sons, p 170.

Slootweg PJ, Koole R: Recurrent calcifying odontogenic cyst, *J Maxillofac Surg* 8:143, 1980.

Soames JV: A pigmented calcifying odontogenic cyst, *Oral Surg Oral Med Oral Pathol* 53:395, 1982.

Swan RH, Houston GD, Moore SP: Peripheral calcifying odontogenic cyst (Gorlin Cyst), *J Periodontol* 56:240, 1985.

Tanimoto S, et al: Radiographic characteristics of the calcifying odontogenic cyst, *Int J Oral Maxillofac Surg* 17:29, 1988.

Wright BA, Bhardwaj AK, Murphy D: Recurrent calcifying odontogenic cyst, *Oral Surg Oral Med Oral Pathol* 58:579, 1984.

Dentigerous Cyst

Chretien PB, et al: Squamous carcinoma arising in a dentigerous cyst, *Oral Surg Oral Med Oral Pathol* 30:809, 1970.

Lapin R, et al: Squamous cell carcinoma arising in a dentigerous cyst, *J Oral Maxillofac Surg* 31:354, 1973.

Leis DA, Skinner RL, Weir JC: Cysts of the oral regions, *Arkansas Dent J* 56:13, 1985.

Regezi JA, Sciubba JJ: *Oral pathology—clinical pathologic correlations,* Philadelphia, 1989, W.B. Saunders, p 554.

Shear M: *Cysts of the oral regions,* Bristol, 1976, John Wright & Sons, p 170.

Worth HM: *Principles and practices of oral radiologic interpretation,* ed 2, Chicago 1972, Year Book Medical, p 746.

Keratocyst

Banks PA, Orth D: Pathologically induced molar extrusion: report of an unexpected odontogenic keratocyst, *Br J Orthod* 17:119, 1990.

Haring JI, Van Dis ML: Odontogenic keratocysts: a clinical radiographic, and histopathologic study, *Oral Surg Oral Med Oral Pathol* 66:145, 1988.

Howell RE, et al: CEA immunoreactivity in odontogenic tumors and keratocysts, *Oral Surg Oral Med Oral Pathol* 66:576, 1988.

Kakarantza-Angelopoulou E, Nichlatou O: Odontogenic keratocyst: clinicopathologic study of 87 cases, *J Oral Maxillofac Surg* 48:593, 1990.

MacLeod RI, Soames JV: Squamous cell carcinoma arising in an odontogenic keratocyst, *Br J Oral Maxillofac Surg* 26:52, 1988.

Moos KF, Rennie JS: Squamous cell carcinoma arising in a mandibular keratocyst in a patient with Gorlin's syndrome, *Br J Oral Maxillofac Surg* 25:280, 1987.

Oikarinen VJ: Keratocyst recurrences at intervals of more than 10 years: case reports, *Br J Oral Maxillofac Surg* 28:47, 1990.

Scharffetter K, et al: Proliferation kinetics: study of the growth of keratocysts, *J Craniomaxillofac Surg* 17:226, 1989.

Regezi JA, Sciubba JJ: *Oral pathology—clinical pathologic correlations,* Philadelphia, 1989, W.B. Saunders, p 554.

Shafer WG, Hine MK, Levy BM: *A textbook of oral pathology,* ed 4, Philadelphia, 1983, W.B. Saunders, p 917.

Shear M: *Cysts of the oral regions,* Bristol, 1976, John Wright & Sons, p 170.

Voorsmit RACA, Stoelinga PJ, van Haelst UJGM: The management of keratocysts, *J Oral Maxillofac Surg* 9:228, 1981.

Lateral Periodontal Cyst

Angelopoulou E, Angelopoulos AP: Lateral periodontal cysts: review of the literature and report of a case, *J Periodontol* 61:126, 1990.

Buckley FM, Huntley P, Speight PM: A lateral periodontal cyst in association with a follicular cyst, *Br Dent J* 167:26, 1989.

DiFiore PM, Hartwell GR: Median mandibular lateral periodontal cyst, *Oral Surg Oral Med Oral Pathol* 63:545, 1987.

Greer RO, Johnson M: Botryoid odontogenic cyst: clinicopathologic analysis of ten cases with three recurrences, *J Oral Maxillofac Surg* 46:574, 1988.

Kaugars GE: Botryoid odontogenic cyst, *Oral Surg Oral Med Oral Pathol* 62:555, 1986.

Legunn KM: Bilateral occurrence of the lateral periodontal cyst: a case report, *Periodont Case Rep* 6:56, 1984.

Lynch DP, Madden CR: The botryoid odontogenic cyst: report of a case and review of the literature, *J Periodontal* 56:163, 1985.

Padayachee A, Van Wyk CW: Two cystic lesions with features of both the botryoid odontogenic cyst and central mucoepidermoid tumor: sialo-odontogenic cyst? *J Oral Pathol Med* 16:499, 1987.

Phelan JA, et al: Recurrent botryoid odontogenic cyst (lateral periodontal cyst), *Oral Surg Oral Med Oral Pathol* 66:345, 1988.

Regezi Ja, Sciubba JJ: *Oral pathology—clinical pathologic correlations,* Philadelphia, 1989, W.B. Saunders, p 554.

Wysocki GP, et al: Histogenesis of the lateral periodontal cyst and the gingival cyst of the adult, *Oral Surg Oral Med Oral Pathol* 50:327, 1980.

Radicular Cyst

Cassella EA, Pickett AB, Chamberlain JH: Unusual management problems in the treatment of a long-standing destructive periapical cyst, *Oral Surg Oral Med Oral Pathol* 51:93, 1981.

Fergus HS, Savord EG: Actinomycosis involving a periapical cyst in the anterior maxilla: report of a case, *Oral Surg Oral Med Oral Pathol* 49:390, 1980.

Lavery K, et al: Squamous carcinoma arising in a dental cyst, *Br Dent J* 162:259, 1987.

Natkin E, Oswald RJ, Carnes LI: The relationship of lesion size to diagnosis, incidence, and treatment of periapical cysts and granulomas, *Oral Surg Oral Med Oral Pathol* 57:82, 1984.

Regezi JA, Sciubba JJ: *Oral pathology—clinical pathologic correlations,* Philadelphia, 1989 W.B. Saunders, p 554.

Shear M: *Cysts of the oral regions,* Bristol, 1976, John Wright & Sons, p 170.

Stockdale CR, Chandler NP: The nature of the periapical lesion: a review of 1108 cases, *J Dent* 16:123, 1988.

Trope M, et al: Differentiation of radicular cyst and granulomas using computerized tomography, *Endod Dent Traumatol* 5:69, 1989.

Worth HM: *Principles and practices of oral radiologic interpretation,* ed 2, Chicago, 1972, Year Book Medical, p 746.

Residual Cyst

High AS, Hirschmann PH: Age changes in residual radicular cysts, *J Oral Pathol Med* 15:524, 1986.

Molyneux GS: Observations on the structure and growth of periodontal and residual cysts, *Oral Surg Oral Med Oral Pathol* 18:80, 1964.

Natkin E, Oswald RJ, Carnes LI: The relationship of lesion size to diagnosis, incidence, and treatment of periapical cysts and granulomas, *Oral Surg Oral Med Oral Pathol* 57:82, 1984.

Oehlers FAC: Periapical lesions and residual dental cysts, *Br J Oral Maxillofac Surg* 8:103, 1970.

Regezi JA, Sciubba JJ: *Oral pathology—clinical pathologic correlations,* Philadelphia, 1989, W.B Saunders, p 554.

Weine FS, Silverglade LB: Residual cysts masquerading as periapical lesions: three case reports, *J Am Dent Assoc* 106:833, 1983.

Worth HM: *Principles and practices of oral radiologic interpretation,* ed 2, Chicago, 1963, Year Book Medical, p 746.

Traumatic Bone Cyst

Cowan CC: Traumatic bone cysts of the jaws and their presentation, *Int J Oral Maxillofac Surg* 9:287, 1980.

Feinberg SE, et al: Recurrent "traumatic" bone cysts of the mandible, *Oral Surg Oral Med Oral Pathol* 57:418, 1984.

Freedman GL, Beigleman MB: The traumatic bone cyst: a new dimension, *Oral Surg Oral Med Oral Pathol* 59:616, 1985.

Horner K, Forman GH: Atypical simple bone cysts of the jaws. II. A possible association with benign fibro-osseous (cemental) lesions of the jaws, *Clin Radiol* 39:59, 1988.

Patrikiou A, Sepheriadou-Mavropoulou T, Zambelis G: Bilateral traumatic bone cyst of the mandible, *Oral Surg Oral Med Oral Pathol* 51:131, 1981.

Precious DS, McFadden LR: Treatment of traumatic bone cyst of the mandible by injection of autogenic blood, *Oral Surg Oral Med Oral Pathol* 58:137, 1984.

Regezi JA, Sciubba JJ: *Oral pathology—clinical pathologic correlations,* Philadelphia, 1989, W.B. Saunders, p 554.

Sapp JP, Stark ML: Self-healing traumatic bone cysts, *Oral Surg Oral Med Oral Pathol* 69:597, 1990.

Aneursymal Bone Cyst

Carmichael F, Malcolm AJ, Ord RA: Aneurysmal bone cyst of the zygomatic bone, *Oral Surg Oral Med Oral Pathol* 68:558, 1989.

Dahlin DC, McLeod RA: Aneurysmal bone cyst and other nonneoplastic conditions, *Skeletal Radiol* 8:243, 1982.

El Deeb M, Sedano HO, Waite DE: Aneurysmal bone cyst of the jaws, *Int J Oral Maxillofac Surg* 9:301, 1980.

Karabouta I, Tsodoulos S, Trigonidis G: Extensive aneurysmal bone cyst of the mandible: surgical resection and immediate reconstruction, *Oral Surg Oral Med Oral Pathol* 71:148, 1991.

Nadimi H, Toto HD, McReynolds HD: Co-existent aneurysmal bone cysts with ameloblastomas: a histologic survey, *J Oral Pathol* 41:242, 1986.

Robinson PD: Aneurysmal bone cyst: a hybrid lesion? *Br J Oral Maxillofac Surg* 23:220, 1985.

Steidler NE, Cook PM, Reade PC: Aneurysmal bone cyst of the jaws: a case report and review of the literature, *Br J Oral Maxillofac Surg* 16:254, 1978-79.

Struthers PJ, Shear M: Aneurysmal bone cyst of the jaws. I Clinicopathologic features, *Int J Oral Maxillofac Surg* 13:85, 1984.

Struthers PJ, Shear M: Aneurysmal bone cyst of the jaws. II Pathogenesis, *Int J Oral Maxillofac Surg* 13:92, 1984.

Toljanic JA, et al: Aneurysmal bone cysts of the jaws: a case study and review of the literature, *Oral Surg Oral Med Oral Pathol* 64:72, 1987.

Zachariades N, et al: Aneurysmal bone cyst of the jaws: review of the literature and report of 2 cases, *Int J Oral Maxillofac Surg* 15:534, 1986.

Nasopalatine Duct Cyst

Allard RH: Naso-palatine duct cyst, *Int J Oral Maxillofac Surg* 10(suppl 1):131, 1981.

Allard RH, Van der Kwast WA, Van der Wall I: Nasopalatine duct cyst: review of the literature and report of 22 cases, *Int J Oral Maxillofac Surg* 10:447, 1981.

Bodin I, Isacsson G, Julin P: Cysts of the nasopalatine duct, *Int J Oral Maxillofac Surg* 15:696, 1986.

Hertzanu Y, Cohen M, Mendelsohn DB: Nasopalatine duct cyst, *Clin Radiol* 36:153, 1985.

Nortjé CJ, Wood RE: The radiologic features of the nasopalatine duct cyst: an analysis of 46 cases, *Dentomaxillofac Radiol* 17:129, 1988.

Regezi JA, Sciubba JJ: *Oral pathology—clinical pathologic correlations,* Philadelphia, 1989, W.B. Saunders, p 554.

Nasolabial Cyst

Adams A, Lovelock DJ: Nasolabial cyst, *Oral Surg Oral Med Oral Pathol* 60:118, 1985.

Allard RH: Nasolabial cyst: review of the literature and report of 7 cases, *Int J Oral Maxillofac Surg* 11:351, 1982.

Cohen MA: Huge growth potential of the nasolabial cyst, *Oral Surg Oral Med Oral Pathol* 59:441, 1985.

Karmody CS, Gallagher JC: Nasoalveolar cysts, *Ann Otol* 81:278, 1972.

Kutiloff DB: The nasolabial cyst-nasal hamartoma, *Otolaryngol Head Neck Surg* 96:268, 1987.

Regezi JA, Sciubba JJ: *Oral pathology—clinical pathological considerations,* Philadelphia, 1989, W.B. Saunders, p 554.

8

BENIGN TUMORS OF THE JAWS

ODONTOGENIC TUMORS

AMELOBLASTOMA

Overview

Definition: Ameloblastoma is a benign, locally aggressive epithelial odontogenic neoplasm. According to Regezi, Kerr, and Courtney, it accounts for approximately 11% of all odontogenic tumors.

Clinical Features

Demographics: The average age at diagnosis is in the fourth decade, but ameloblastoma can occur at any age. It occurs equally in males and females. The vast majority of ameloblastomas occur in the mandible. Reports vary, but 81% - 98% are in the lower jaw. Of these, the majority occur in the molar and ramus areas. In the maxilla the most common site is the premolar-molar region.

Signs and symptoms: Over 80% of patients with ameloblastoma experience painless swelling of the affected site. Pain or local discomfort are less common. Lesions of longer duration and greater size produce more symptoms.

Histologic findings: Five classical histologic patterns of ameloblastoma are recognized: the follicular (most common), plexiform, acanthomatous, basal cell, and granular cell types. A unicystic type and more recently a desmoplastic variant have also been described. The classical types all have tall, columnar ameloblast-like cells, which form a peripheral palisading layer surrounding the neoplastic islands and sheets of cells.

RADIOLOGIC FEATURES

Shape

The shape may vary from unicystic to multilocular.

Periphery

The periphery is usually well defined, corticated, smooth, and curved. The periphery in the maxilla, especially when the tumor involves the antrum, may be ill defined.

Internal Structure

The small, unicystic lesions may be completely radiolucent. When the tumor is multilocular, the cystic portions commonly appear larger in the posterior and smaller in the anterior part of the mandible. The internal septa are most commonly coarse and curved in outline. Small lesions involving the alveolar process may have very faint septa. When the loculations are small and numerous, they show a honeycomb-like pat-

Text continued on page 243.

239

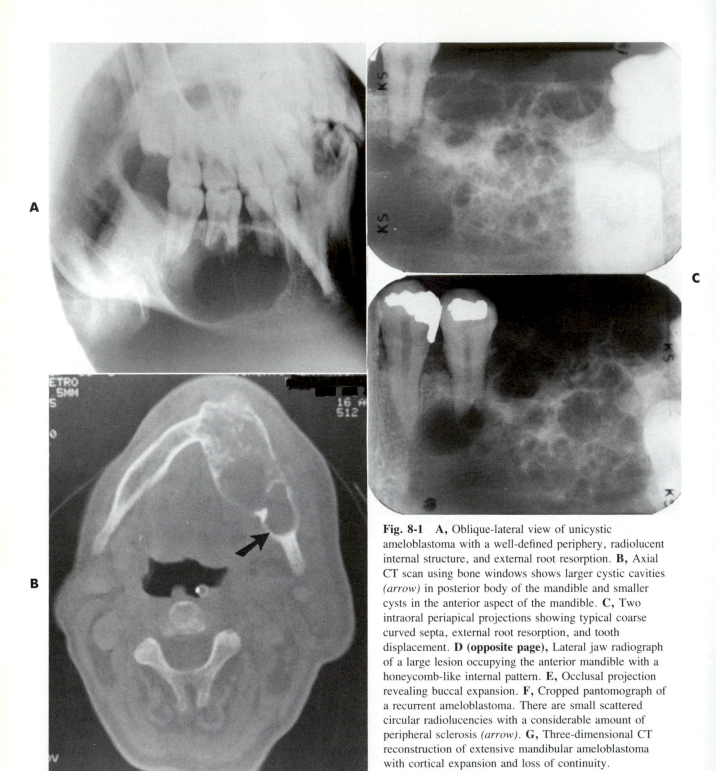

Fig. 8-1 **A,** Oblique-lateral view of unicystic ameloblastoma with a well-defined periphery, radiolucent internal structure, and external root resorption. **B,** Axial CT scan using bone windows shows larger cystic cavities *(arrow)* in posterior body of the mandible and smaller cysts in the anterior aspect of the mandible. **C,** Two intraoral periapical projections showing typical coarse curved septa, external root resorption, and tooth displacement. **D (opposite page),** Lateral jaw radiograph of a large lesion occupying the anterior mandible with a honeycomb-like internal pattern. **E,** Occlusal projection revealing buccal expansion. **F,** Cropped pantomograph of a recurrent ameloblastoma. There are small scattered circular radiolucencies with a considerable amount of peripheral sclerosis *(arrow).* **G,** Three-dimensional CT reconstruction of extensive mandibular ameloblastoma with cortical expansion and loss of continuity.

Continued.

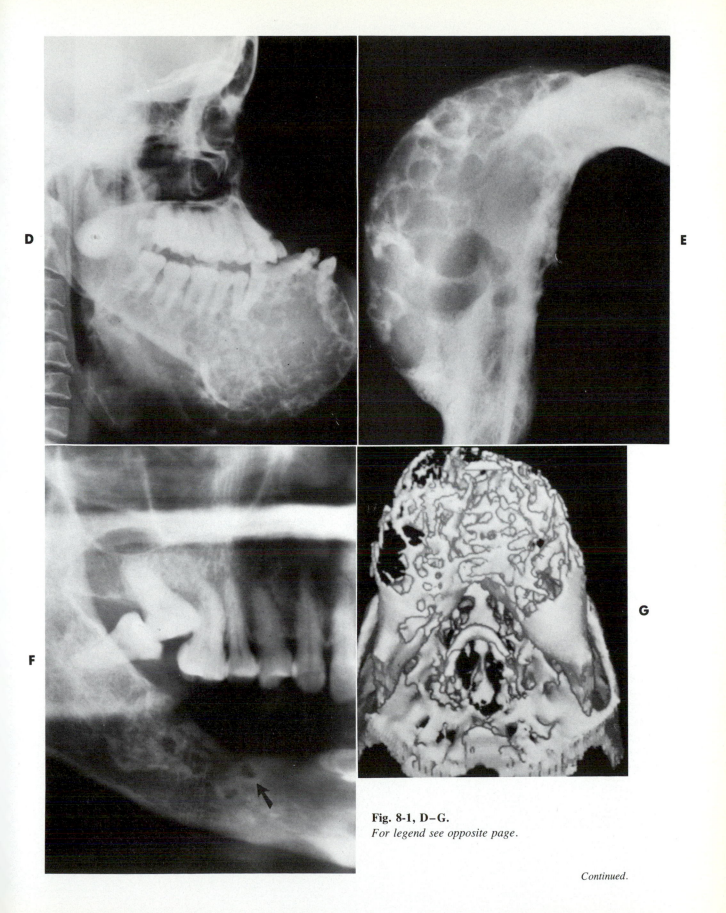

Fig. 8-1, D–G.
For legend see opposite page.

Continued.

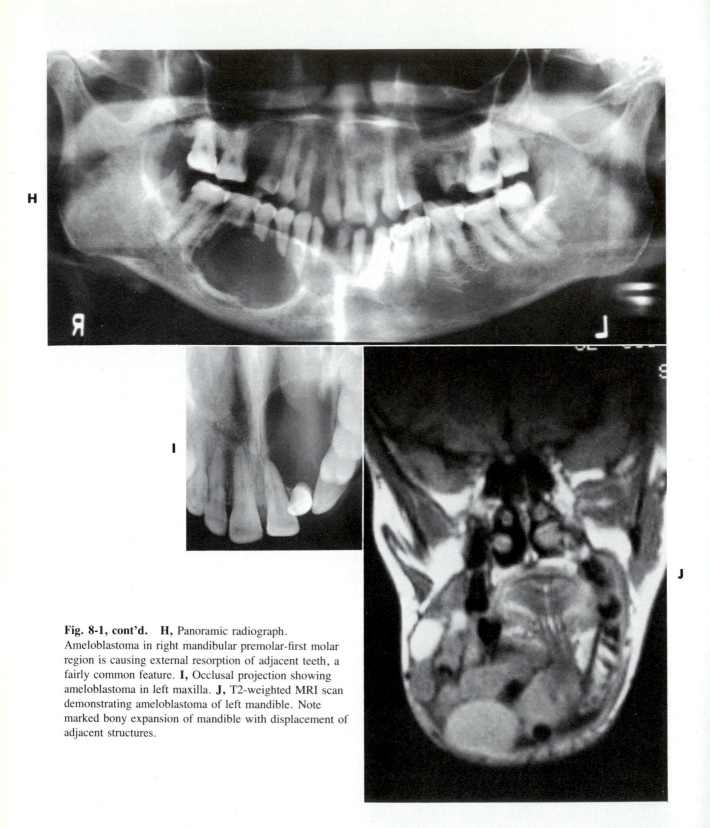

Fig. 8-1, cont'd. **H,** Panoramic radiograph. Ameloblastoma in right mandibular premolar-first molar region is causing external resorption of adjacent teeth, a fairly common feature. **I,** Occlusal projection showing ameloblastoma in left maxilla. **J,** T2-weighted MRI scan demonstrating ameloblastoma of left mandible. Note marked bony expansion of mandible with displacement of adjacent structures.

tern; this has been associated with the solid form as opposed to the cystic form of the tumor. Occasionally, strands of bony septa may appear to radiate from a common center.

Effects on Surrounding Structures

Ameloblastoma can displace teeth a considerable distance, often pushing the involved teeth apically. Root resorption, which may have an irregular shape, is commonly observed.

This tumor has considerable potential for bone expansion. It is worth noting that the cystic variety usually causes more expansion than is commonly seen in odontogenic keratocysts. The anterior boundary of the coronoid process is commonly lost in large tumors occupying the mandibular ramus.

Differential Diagnosis

Unicystic ameloblastoma is difficult to differentiate from follicular and odontogenic keratocysts. Tumors consisting of small locules may appear similar to giant cell granuloma.

Recurrent Tumors

Recurrent tumors are commonly associated with considerable sclerotic bone reaction. The appearance may be a collection of small cystlike spaces surrounded by a band of sclerotic bone. These spaces may be separated by what appears to be normal bone.

Other Radiologic Characteristics

The appearance on computed tomography (CT) is essentially the same as in plain films, except that the periphery and relationship to surrounding structures are better defined.

On magnetic resonance (MR) imaging, there may be intermediate to high signal on T1-weighted images and high signal on T2-weighted images. The solid type of tumor usually has a more uniform signal.

ADENOMATOID ODONTOGENIC TUMOR

Overview

Definition: Adenomatoid odontogenic tumor, formerly known as adenoameloblastoma, is a benign epithelial odontogenic neoplasm. It is relatively rare, accounting for approximately 3% of all odontogenic tumors.

Clinical Features

Demographics: Adenomatoid odontogenic tumor occurs in the young; the average age at diagnosis is in the second decade of life. Over 70% of cases occur in patients 20 years of age or less. There is a definite female predilection, with a male:female ratio of 2:3.

Approximately 65% of cases occur in the maxilla. The anterior segments appear to be more commonly affected. Over 70% of these tumors are found in association with an unerupted tooth, most commonly the cuspid.

Signs and symptoms: The most common symptom is an intraoral swelling.

Histologic findings: The tumor is composed of sheets and islands of epithelial cells with formation of rosettes, ductlike spaces, and whorls. Cystic spaces are common, as are foci of calcification. An enamel matrixlike material is often seen. Usually, a thick fibrous connective capsule surrounds the tumor cells.

RADIOLOGIC FEATURES

Shape

The lesion usually has curved borders, which may give it a cystlike appearance. An association with the coronal aspect of a tooth such as a cuspid may simulate the shape of a follicular cyst.

Periphery

Many tumors are well defined and appear to have a peripheral cortex, whereas others are ill defined.

Internal Structure

Some tumors have a totally radiolucent center; others have punctate calcifications sprinkled throughout or in clusters, giving a cloudlike appearance.

Effects on Surrounding Structures

The tumor can displace or prevent the eruption of teeth, especially the canine. Root resorption is rarely encountered. Considerable expansion of the jaw may be seen.

Differential Diagnosis

The appearance may be similar to that of calcifying odontogenic cyst, ameloblastic fibro-odontoma, and calcifying epithelial odontogenic tumor. The strong association with an unerupted canine is usually helpful.

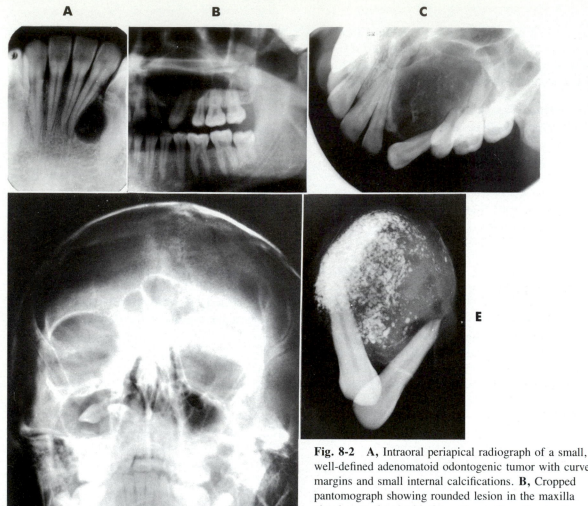

Fig. 8-2 **A,** Intraoral periapical radiograph of a small, well-defined adenomatoid odontogenic tumor with curved margins and small internal calcifications. **B,** Cropped pantomograph showing rounded lesion in the maxilla closely associated with the canine and causing tooth displacement and resorption. **C,** Lateral occlusal projection of lesion depicted in **B.** Note the rounded outline and internal calcifications. **D,** Posteroanterior projection with Waters modification to demonstrate well-delineated radiolucent adenomatoid odontogenic tumor. **E,** Radiograph of gross adenomatoid odontogenic tumor specimen showing fine, ribbonlike calcifications within.

CALCIFYING EPITHELIAL ODONTOGENIC TUMOR

Overview

Definition: Calcifying epithelial odontogenic tumor is a rare benign neoplasm, accounting for less than 1% of all odontogenic tumors.

Clinical Features

Demographics: The average age at diagnosis is 40 years; however, the tumor can occur at any age. It occurs equally in males and females. Approximately two thirds of cases are reported to occur in the mandible.

Most cases occur in the premolar-molar area and are commonly associated with an unerupted tooth.

Signs and symptoms: When symptomatic, the tumor is a painless, slowly enlarging mass.

Histologic findings: Calcifying epithelial odontogenic tumor has a very characteristic appearance. Sheets of polyhedral cells with well-defined eosinophilic cytoplasm and hyperchromatic nuclei are featured. Amyloid and ringlike calcifications may also be present.

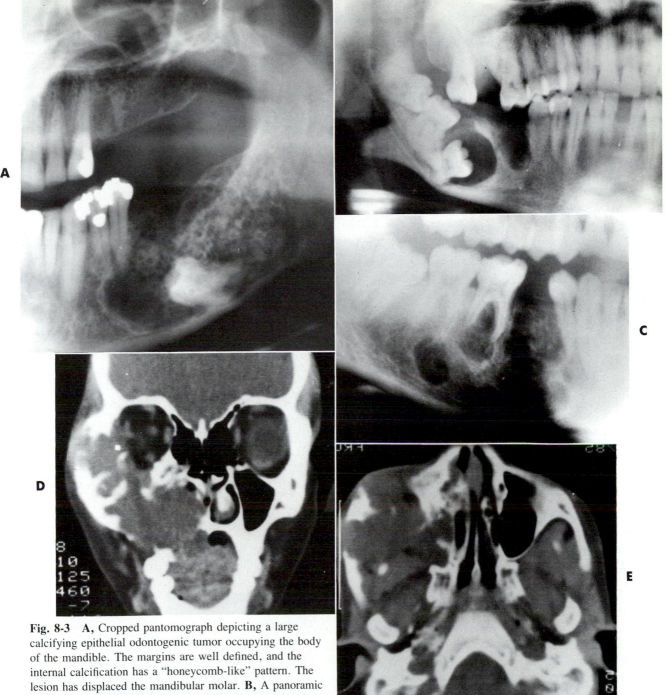

Fig. 8-3 **A,** Cropped pantomograph depicting a large calcifying epithelial odontogenic tumor occupying the body of the mandible. The margins are well defined, and the internal calcification has a "honeycomb-like" pattern. The lesion has displaced the mandibular molar. **B,** A panoramic radiograph showing calcifying epithelial odontogenic tumor distal to right mandibular second premolar. Tumor has caused displacement of ipsilateral first permanent molar. **C,** Mixed radiolucency-radiopacity in right mandibular premolar and molar region proved to be a calcifying epithelial odontogenic tumor. **D,** CT view of large calcifying epithelial odontogenic tumor affecting right maxilla. Note expansion and destruction. **E,** Axial view of patient in **C.**

RADIOLOGIC FEATURES

Shape

The tumor may be irregular or, in some cases, cystic.

Periphery

Cystic lesions may be well defined and corticated, whereas others appear ill defined.

Internal Structure

Many patterns have been described. Small unilocular lesions may have a completely radiolucent center. Others may have variable amounts of small flecks of calcification scattered throughout. Larger tumors may have a multilocular or honeycomb appearance.

Effects on Surrounding Structures

The tumor can displace and often prevent the eruption of teeth.

Differential Diagnosis

Radiographically the tumor may be very similar to calcifying odontogenic cyst, adenomatoid odontogenic tumor, and ameloblastic fibroodontoma.

AMELOBLASTIC FIBROMA

Overview

Definition: Ameloblastic fibroma is a benign, mixed epithelial-mesenchymal neoplasm that has been reported to represent approximately 2% of all odontogenic tumors.

Clinical Features

Demographics: Ameloblastic fibroma occurs in the young, with the peak incidence in the second decade of life. Over 70% of cases occur in patients younger than 20 years. There is no sex predilection. The vast majority of cases (over 80%) occur in the mandible, most in the posterior. Some small unilocular lesions may appear in a pericoronal position. Occasionally lesions may occupy the most superior aspect of the alveolar process.

Signs and symptoms: Over 50% of tumors cause either swelling, pain, or failure of tooth eruption. Seventeen percent are incidental radiographic findings. They are often associated with an unerupted tooth, most commonly the mandibular first molar.

Histologic findings: Both epithelial and mesenchymal components are present. The odontogenic epithelium occurs in strands and budding islands in a loose, dental papilla–like fibrous connective tissue stroma.

RADIOLOGIC FEATURES

Shape

Some small lesions may be very similar to a follicular cyst. Larger lesions are characteristically multilocular.

Periphery

Usually the periphery is well defined and appears corticated and similar to ameloblastoma. When the tumor occupies a superior position in the alveolar process, the periphery may be extremely delicate and difficult to identify.

Internal Structure

The internal aspect often is completely radiolucent; in multilocular cases there may be fine, curved trabeculae.

Effects on Surrounding Structures

Often the tumor prevents the eruption of one or more teeth. Tooth displacement and, very rarely, tooth resorption may occur. Larger lesions cause bone expansion.

Differential Diagnosis

Small lesions may be confused with dentigerous cyst, and larger lesions are very similar to ameloblastoma.

ODONTOMA

Overview

Definition: Odontomas are generally considered to represent hamartomas rather than true neoplasms. They are composed of all the components of dental hard and soft tissues. They are relatively common lesions and have been reported to represent approximately two thirds of all odontogenic tumors.

Clinical Features

Demographics: Odontoma occurs in a young age group, with the average age of diagnosis in the second decade of life. However, it has been reported in all age groups, with no significant sex predilection.

Text continued on page 250.

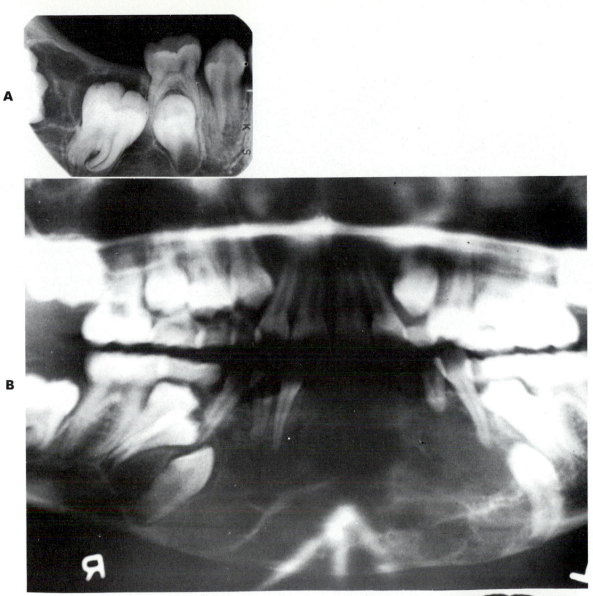

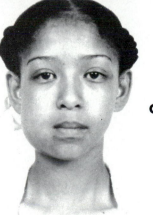

Fig. 8-4 **A,** Intraoral periapical view of an ameloblastic fibroma occupying the superior portion of the alveolar process. The lesion has a delicate multilocular appearance and has prevented the eruption of the first mandibular molar. **B,** Cropped pantomograph. Tumor has caused bone expansion and tooth displacement. The internal septa result in a multilocular appearance. **C,** Clinical feature of facial asymmetry in patient with large ameloblastic fibroma.

Continued.

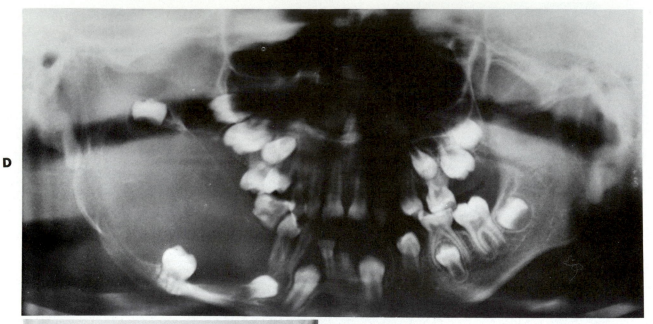

D

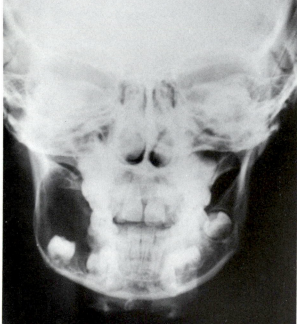

E

Fig. 8-4, cont'd. **D,** Panoramic radiograph of patient in **C.** The features are similar to ameloblastoma, but the lesion is generally found in a younger group. **E,** Posteroanterior radiograph of patient in **C.**

Fig. 8-5 **A (opposite page),** Cropped pantomograph showing a large complex odontoma into the maxillary sinus. The periphery is well defined with a thin radiolucent soft tissue band and a thin cortical line. The internal structure is profoundly radiopaque and homogeneous. **B,** Cropped pantomograph showing the internal structure of a complex odontoma. The lesion is considerably more radiopaque than the surrounding bone. **C,** Intraoral periapical projection reveals a compound odontoma associated with the crown of a mandibular canine. There appear to be three "denticles" within the lesion, and the eruption of the canine has been impeded. **D,** Intraoral periapical film revealing a compound odontoma associated with the maxillary central incisor *(large arrow).* The lesion has prevented the eruption of both the central and lateral incisors, and is composed of several "denticles," one having the appearance of an inverted tooth *(small arrow).* **E,** Intraoral periapical film showing a large compound odontoma. There has been considerable displacement of the first premolar and first and second molars. **F,** Standard occlusal radiograph showing complex odontoma of right side of mandible. **G,** Panoramic radiograph showing an ameloblastic odontoma—a rare variant combining features both of odontoma and ameloblastoma. The lesion is treated as an ameloblastoma.

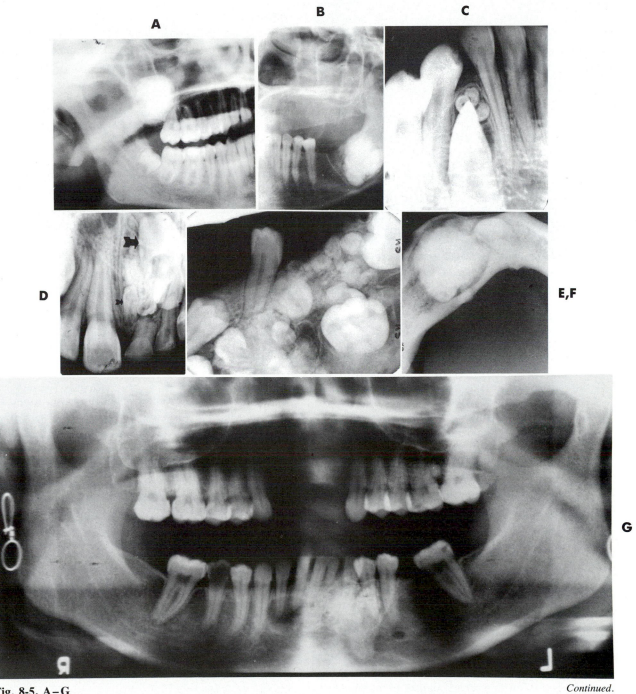

Fig. 8-5, A–G

Continued.

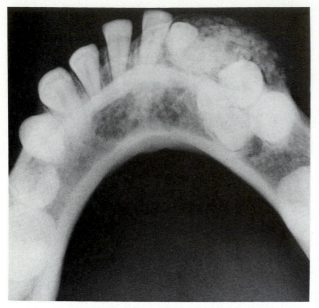

Fig. 8-5, cont'd. H, Occlusal radiograph of same patient as in **G.**

Odontoma occurs with equal frequency in the maxilla and mandible. The most common site is the anterior maxilla, with a predilection for the segment between the canines. Complex odontomas occur more commonly in the posterior portions of the jaws and compound odontomas in the anterior portions. As in ameloblastic fibroodontoma, younger patients tend to have lesions in the anterior regions of the jaws. About 50% of cases are associated with an unerupted tooth, and 27% are associated with a dentigerous cyst.

Signs and symptoms: Odontomas are almost always totally asymptomatic and discovered on routine radiographic examination. Failure of eruption of a permanent tooth may be the first presenting sign.

Histologic findings: Classically, two types of odontoma are recognized. Complex odontoma is composed of haphazardly arranged dental hard and soft tissue. Compound odontoma is composed of many small "denticles" with a greater degree of morphologic differentiation, so that the relationship of dentin, cementum, and enamel matrix is comparable to that of normal teeth. In some cases, termed *mixed odontomas,* both types can be found.

RADIOLOGIC FEATURES

Shape

Complex odontoma may have a roughly oval, round, or lobulated shape; compound odontoma is usually irregular.

Periphery

The lesions are well defined, often with a cortex surrounding an adjacent band of soft tissue of variable width.

Internal Structure

The internal aspect is characteristically very radiopaque compared to bone, which itself suggests the presence of tooth structure. The organization of complex odontoma is haphazard and may be so radiopaque as to give very little indication of any pattern. Compound odontoma appears more organized, composed of a variable number of unusually shaped toothlike structures (denticles). Often crude roots, root canals, and enamel-covered coronal portions can be identified.

Differential Diagnosis

The most common differential diagnosis would be a dense bone island (enostosis or osteosclerosis). However, the presence of a soft tissue capsule is very useful in differentiation. In some instances periapical cemental dysplasia may be considered. Cemental dysplasia is usually surrounded by a radiopaque band of sclerosis and positioned apical to surrounding teeth, whereas odontomas are commonly found occlusal to, or overlapping, the involved teeth.

AMELOBLASTIC FIBROODONTOMA

Overview

Definition: Ameloblastic fibroodontoma is a benign mixed odontogenic neoplasm characterized by a combination of the features of ameloblastic fibroma and odontoma. It accounts for 2% of odontogenic tumors.

Clinical Features

Demographics: Over 60% of ameloblastic fibroodontoma occur in the first decade of life; average age at

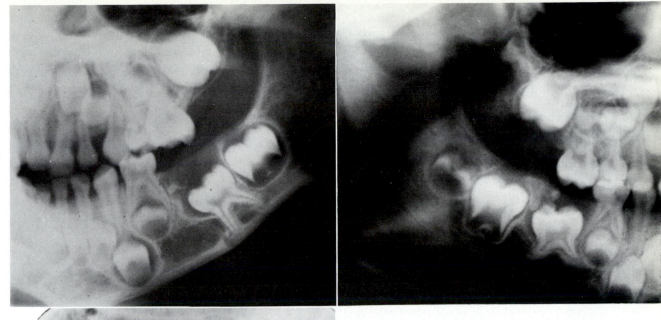

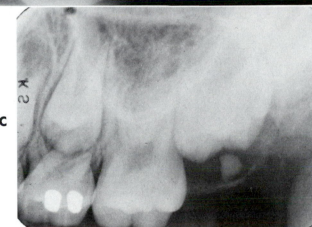

Fig. 8-6 **A,** Cropped pantomograph showing an ameloblastic fibroodontoma that has prevented the eruption of the primary second molar and eliminated a portion of the tooth follicle. A single calcification can be seen in the anterior aspect of the radiolucent lesion. **B,** Cropped pantomograph with a similar appearance to that in **A,** except that there are more calcifications in the internal aspect of the lesion. **C,** Intraoral periapical radiograph showing ameloblastic fibroodontoma in close association with the coronal portion of a permanent second molar. There is a single large calcification. **D,** Mixed radiolucency/radiopacity causing displacement of left mandibular canine and first premolar.

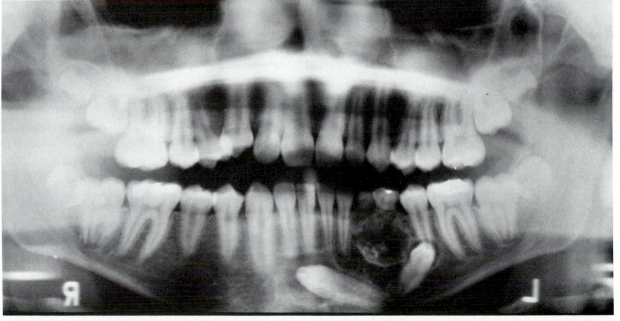

Continued.

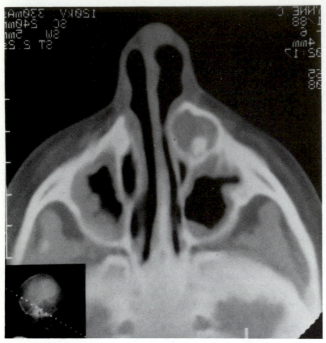

Fig. 8-6, cont'd. E, Axial CT scan showing ameloblastic fibroodontoma of left maxilla.

diagnosis is 8 years. The reported age range is 6 months to 39 years. There is a male-female ratio of 1.3:1. Most cases (62%) occur in the mandible, and of these the majority occur in the posterior aspect. Lesions in the anterior mandible tend to occur in younger patients. Often, the tumor may appear continuous with an adjacent tooth follicle.

Signs and symptoms: As with ameloblastic fibroma, the tumor may be asymptomatic or found because of a painless swelling of the affected jaw.

Histologic findings: Components of both ameloblastic fibroma and odontoma are seen. Dental hard tissues and enamel matrix in varying degrees of morphologic differentiation are seen, along with epithelial nests and branching elements in a dental papilla–like background stroma.

RADIOLOGIC FEATURES

Periphery
The tumor is usually well circumscribed, with apparent cortication of some segments.

Internal Structure
The internal aspect may have one fragment of tooth structure or may be composed of several small, irregular fragments of tooth material.

Effects on Surrounding Structures
Considerable bone expansion may be present. There may also be interference with tooth eruption and displacement of teeth.

Differential Diagnosis
The lesion may appear similar to calcifying epithelial odontogenic tumor, calcifying odontogenic cyst, or adenomatoid odontogenic tumor.

CEMENTOBLASTOMA

Overview
Definition: Cementoblastoma is a benign mesenchymal neoplasm composed of proliferating cementum tissue. It is reported to be very rare—representing less than 1% of odontogenic tumors—but this may underestimate its true occurrence.

Clinical Features
Demographics: Cementoblastoma is most commonly encountered in patients in their second and third decades, with an average age under 25 years. Age range is 7 to 72 years. There is a predilection for males, with a male:female ratio of 3:2. Cementoblastoma occurs more commonly in the mandible than the maxilla (3:2); the molar and premolar regions are most often affected.

Signs and symptoms: Pain is a significant symptom, occurring in approximately 50% of the cases. Swelling and tooth displacement are also fairly common.

Histologic findings: On gross examination, cementoblastoma consists of a round mass of hard tissue attached to the root of the affected tooth. Microscopically, sheets of hard tissue are seen to be intermingled with a very vascular and cellular fibrous connective tissue. The hard tissue has the appearance of cementum. It usually exhibits prominent resting and reversal lines with plump, hyperchromatic cementoblasts. These active cells, which may be quite numerous, give the appearance of a malignancy even though mitotic figures are absent. The morphologic pattern of

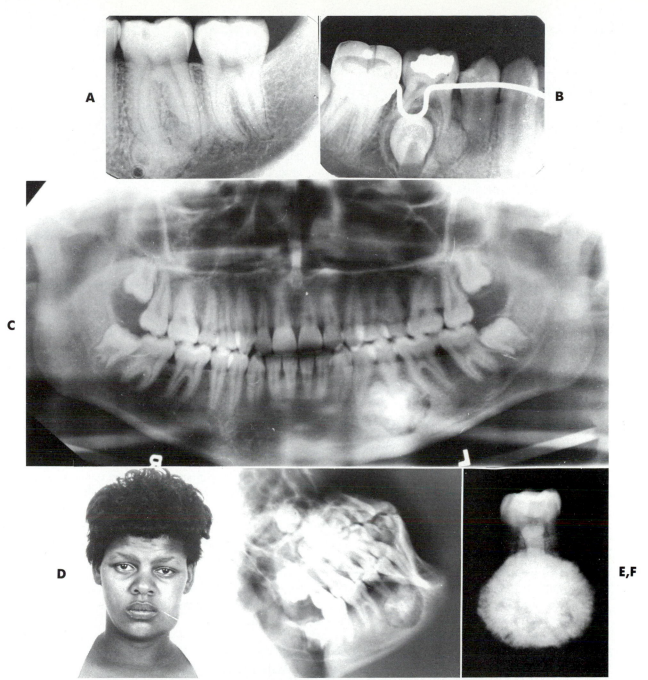

Fig. 8-7 A, Intraoral periapical radiograph showing cementoblastoma associated with the roots of the first molar. There appears to be a direct connection to the partially resorbed distal root. The periphery is well defined by a thin, rather uniform radiolucent line, and the internal aspect is densely calcified but without a characteristic pattern. **B,** Intraoral periapical radiograph with a similar appearance to that in **A,** except that it is unusual to see cementoblastoma associated with a second primary molar. **C,** Cementoblastoma of left second premolar. A large round radiopaque mass attached to a tooth root and surrounded by a radiolucent "capsule" is pathognomonic. **D,** Clinical features of the patient in **C.** The facial asymmetry is a late feature. **E,** Lateral oblique projection of the patient in **D. F,** Fine radiating trabelculations are seen in radiograph of a cementoblastoma specimen.

the hard tissue may be radiating trabeculae, especially at the periphery.

RADIOLOGIC FEATURES

Shape

Lesions are usually circular in shape.

Periphery

Tumors are well defined by a radiopaque band of reactive bone formation next to a band with the density of soft tissue. This may be of variable width but is usually uniformly thin.

Internal Structure

Most of the internal aspect is radiopaque, with the greatest density at the center of the lesions. There is sometimes a "spoked-wheel" pattern of density extending from the most central aspect; otherwise no specific pattern may be discernible. It is usually difficult to see the external surface of the tooth root embedded in the central portion.

Effects on Surrounding Structures

External resorption of the involved tooth root is common. Considerable expansion can occur, but outer cortical plates are usually maintained; perforation has been rarely reported. The inferior alveolar nerve canal may be displaced in an inferior direction.

Differential Diagnosis

The most difficult radiographic differential diagnosis would be periapical cemental dysplasia. Characteristics useful for differentiation are the presence of root resorption, attachment to the root, and internal spoked-wheel pattern.

Periapical sclerosing osteitis may appear similar but does not have the soft band at the periphery. Finally, the development of dense bone islands (enostosis or osteosclerosis) and external root resorption of the mandibular first molar may appear similar.

In considering the histopathologic appearance, the differential diagnosis includes osteoblastoma and well-differentiated osteogenic sarcoma. In these cases, radiologic interpretation becomes most important.

OSSIFYING AND CEMENTIFYING FIBROMA

Overview

Definition: We believe that ossifying and cementifying fibroma of the jaws represent histologic variants of the same underlying process: a benign fibroosseous neoplasm composed of varying amounts of immature hard tissues (osteoid, bone, and cementum) in a background of fibrovascular connective tissue.

Clinical Features

Demographics: Ossifying and cementifying fibroma occur most commonly in the third and fourth decades of life. An age range of 5 to 71 years has been reported. Females are affected much more commonly than males, with a reported ratio as high as 4:1. The mandible is more commonly affected than the maxilla. Seventy-five to eighty-five percent of lesions have been reported to occur in the lower jaw. Interestingly, multiple lesions have been reported.

Signs and symptoms: Ossifying and cementifying fibromas are generally asymptomatic. Unless they become large enough to produce enlargement of the affected site, they are usually found on routine radiographic examination.

Histologic findings: The histologic appearance is quite variable. Various amounts of hard tissue are seen in a very cellular fibrovascular connective tissue. The hard tissue may range in composition from total bone to total cementum; most lesions, however, are composed of bone and cementum. The hard tissue may be represented by irregular trabeculae of woven bone, rimmed on some surfaces with plump cells or globules of cementum or varying amounts of each. The amount of hard tissue varies from small foci to large, coalescing trabeculae of bone or sclerotic cemental masses.

RADIOLOGIC FEATURES

Shape

Most tumors are irregular, although some may have a roughly round or oval shape.

Periphery

The periphery may sometimes be ill defined and blend in with the surrounding bone, but usually it is well defined.

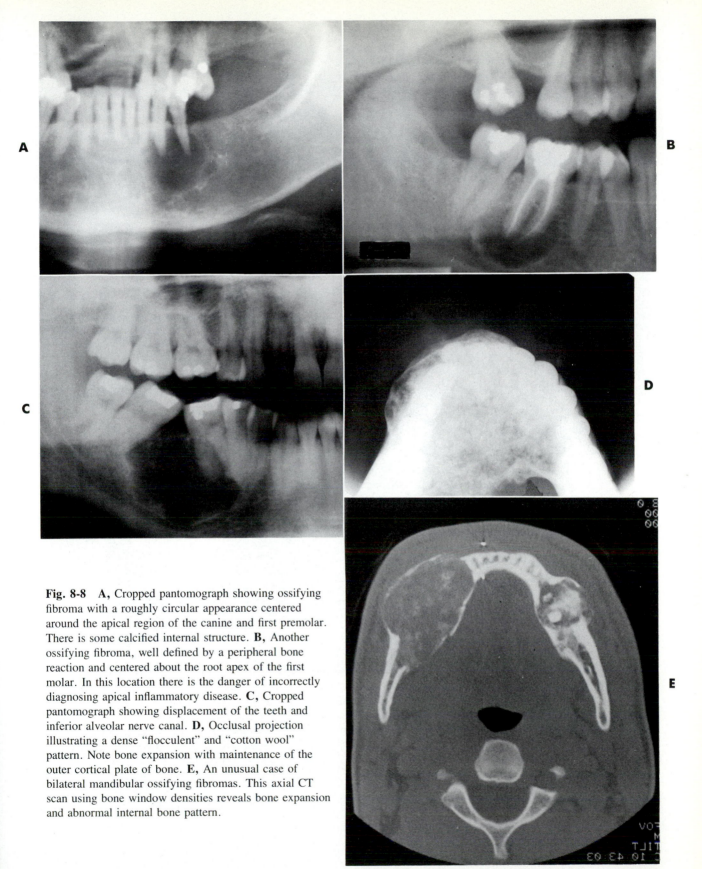

Fig. 8-8 **A,** Cropped pantomograph showing ossifying fibroma with a roughly circular appearance centered around the apical region of the canine and first premolar. There is some calcified internal structure. **B,** Another ossifying fibroma, well defined by a peripheral bone reaction and centered about the root apex of the first molar. In this location there is the danger of incorrectly diagnosing apical inflammatory disease. **C,** Cropped pantomograph showing displacement of the teeth and inferior alveolar nerve canal. **D,** Occlusal projection illustrating a dense "flocculent" and "cotton wool" pattern. Note bone expansion with maintenance of the outer cortical plate of bone. **E,** An unusual case of bilateral mandibular ossifying fibromas. This axial CT scan using bone window densities reveals bone expansion and abnormal internal bone pattern.

Continued.

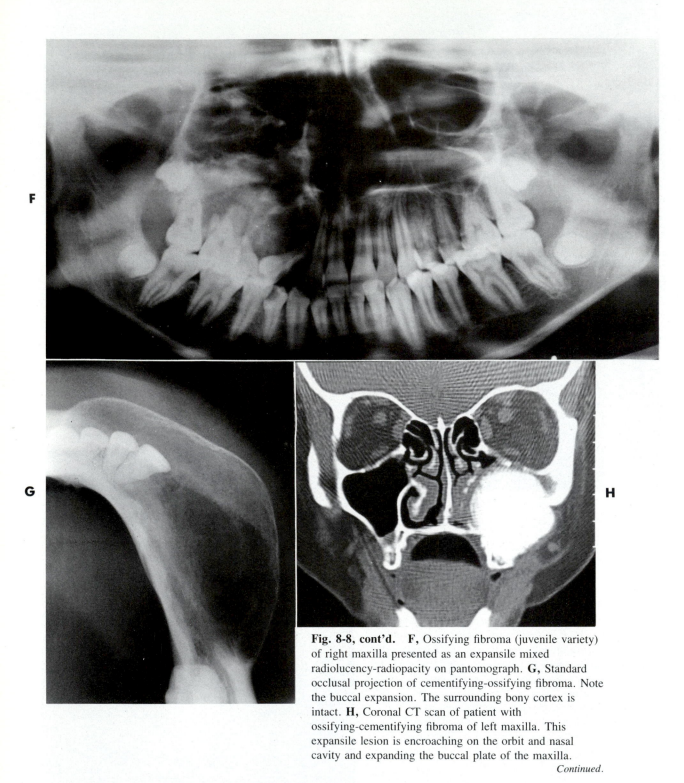

Fig. 8-8, cont'd.   F, Ossifying fibroma (juvenile variety) of right maxilla presented as an expansile mixed radiolucency-radiopacity on pantomograph. **G,** Standard occlusal projection of cementifying-ossifying fibroma. Note the buccal expansion. The surrounding bony cortex is intact. **H,** Coronal CT scan of patient with ossifying-cementifying fibroma of left maxilla. This expansile lesion is encroaching on the orbit and nasal cavity and expanding the buccal plate of the maxilla.

Continued.

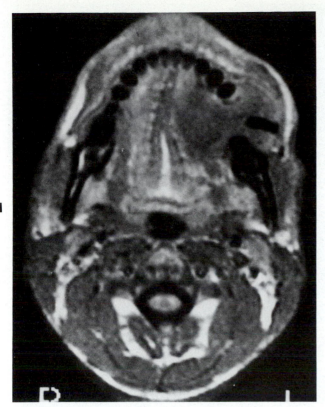

Fig. 8-8, cont'd. I, Axial MR image showing mandibular ossifying-cementifying fibroma of left mandible.

Internal Structure

The internal aspect is a mixture of radiolucent and radiopaque tissue, with a predominance of calcified material. Internal patterns vary greatly from granular to "cotton wool" to flocculent to "ground glass." These patterns are at times indistinguishable from fibrous dysplasia. Round or oval densities resembling cementum-like structures are occasionally present. The organization of the granular pattern may suggest the presence of thick granular septa similar to those seen in a giant cell granuloma. These septa may give a multilocular appearance. Very rarely the lesions may appear as "cystlike" structures with a radiolucent center.

Effects on Surrounding Structures

The tumors commonly displace teeth, but root resorption is rarely observed. The lamina dura is usually altered into the granular pattern of the tumor. There is the potential for considerable expansion of the jaws. The tumor will displace the inferior alveolar canal and floor of antrum.

Differential Diagnosis

The most difficult differentiation to make is with fibrous dysplasia; on occasion this distinction may be impossible. If the lesion is well defined and has a localized "cystlike" expansion, it is probably a cementifying or ossifying fibroma. The tumor may sometimes be difficult to differentiate from giant cell granuloma.

ODONTOGENIC MYXOMA

Overview

Definition: Odontogenic myxoma is a benign mesenchymal neoplasm that has been reported to represent approximately 3% of all odontogenic tumors.

Clinical Features

Demographics: An age range of 1 to 76 years has been reported. The tumor is most common in the second and third decades of life. There is a slight female predilection, with a female: male ratio of 1.3:1. Odontogenic myxoma occurs more commonly in the mandible than in the maxilla, by a ratio of 1.5:1. In the mandible, the molar and ramus regions are the most common sites. In the maxilla, the premolar-first molar region is most often affected.

Signs and symptoms: Lesions are usually seen as painless, slowly enlarging swellings. Pain, displacement of teeth, and paresthesia are rare presenting symptoms.

Histologic findings: The tumor is composed of a very loose fibrillar connective tissue interspersed with varying numbers of stellate fibroblasts. Islands of odontogenic epithelium are occasionally encountered.

RADIOLOGIC FEATURES

Shape

The form of the tumor is usually irregular; however, a minority of small lesions appear cystic.

Text continued on page 260.

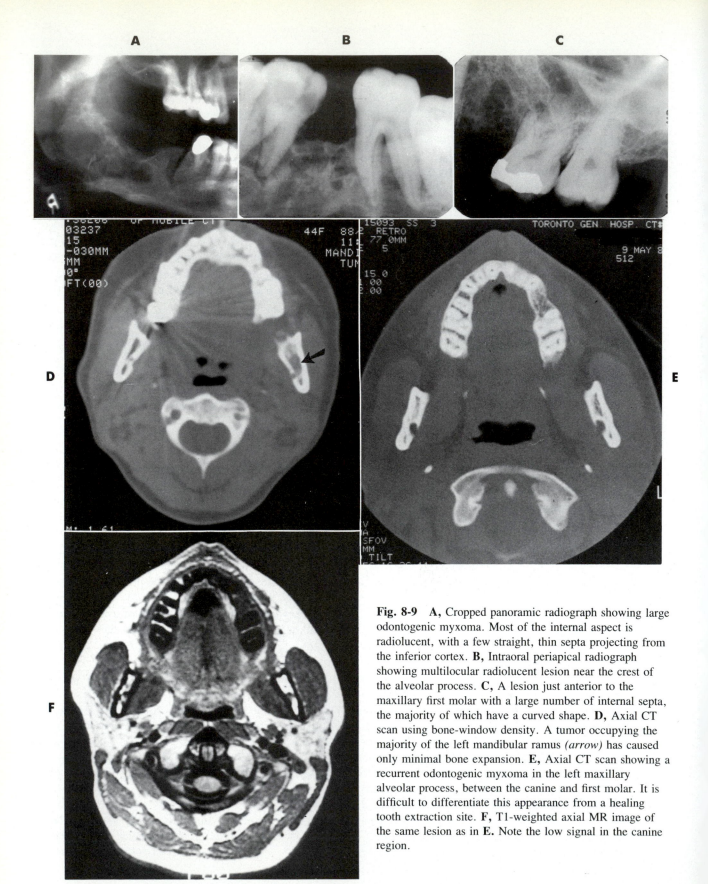

Fig. 8-9 **A,** Cropped panoramic radiograph showing large odontogenic myxoma. Most of the internal aspect is radiolucent, with a few straight, thin septa projecting from the inferior cortex. **B,** Intraoral periapical radiograph showing multilocular radiolucent lesion near the crest of the alveolar process. **C,** A lesion just anterior to the maxillary first molar with a large number of internal septa, the majority of which have a curved shape. **D,** Axial CT scan using bone-window density. A tumor occupying the majority of the left mandibular ramus *(arrow)* has caused only minimal bone expansion. **E,** Axial CT scan showing a recurrent odontogenic myxoma in the left maxillary alveolar process, between the canine and first molar. It is difficult to differentiate this appearance from a healing tooth extraction site. **F,** T1-weighted axial MR image of the same lesion as in **E.** Note the low signal in the canine region.

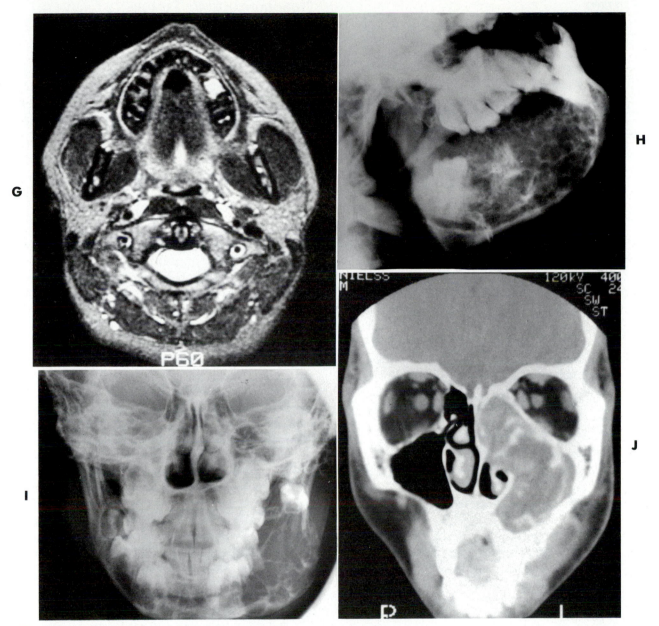

Fig. 8-9, cont'd.   G (above), T2-weighted axial MR image of same lesion as in **E.** Note that the premolar region now has a higher signal than bone marrow, indicating the presence of tumor. **H,** Lateral-oblique projection of odontogenic myxoma showing angular septa within the lesion. **I,** Posteroanterior projection showing buccal expansion of the mandible and angular septa within an odontogenic myxoma. Expansion is a late finding. **J,** Coronal CT scan showing odontogenic myxoma of left maxilla extending into nasal cavity and displacing floor of orbit.

Periphery

Odontogenic myxoma may have well- or ill-defined borders; the latter are more common, perhaps because of the lack of bone reaction. If there is expansion beyond the borders of the affected bone, the straight internal trabeculae may have a "sun ray" spiculated appearance.

Internal Structure

The internal aspect is usually a mixture of radiolucency and septa, which can result in a multilocular appearance. However, on close inspection some fine, straight septa can be seen among the curved septa. These straight septa are characteristically thin with an etched appearance. Usually, thicker curved trabeculae are also present.

Effects on Surrounding Structures

Odontogenic myxoma can displace teeth, but it can also grow around them with little movement. It very rarely causes any root resorption, and there is usually less bone expansion than in other benign tumors. In some cases, the tumor tends to grow along the bone with little expansion. Extremely rare is a granular appearance similar to a fibroosseous lesion.

Other Radiologic Characteristics

Because the periphery of the tumor is ill defined, advanced imaging studies such as CT or MR should be used to define the margins before surgery.

This lesion has a medium signal strength on T1-weighted MR images, which in cases of recurrent tumor can make differentiation from fibrous tissue difficult. An intense signal on T2-weighted images usually makes differentiation possible.

CT using the soft tissue window may reveal an internal multilocular pattern, even in the absence of bony septa.

Differential Diagnosis

Radiographic differentiation from ameloblastoma may be difficult; the lack of expansion and the presence of straight, fine trabeculae may be important criteria. The same characteristics may be used to differentiate giant cell granuloma.

NONODONTOGENIC TUMORS

OSTEOBLASTOMA

Overview

Definition: Osteoblastoma is a rare benign neoplasm of bone composed of functional osteoblasts and their products. It represents only 1% of all primary bone tumors.

Clinical Features

Demographics: Osteoblastomas are diagnosed at the average age of 17 years, with an age range of 5 to 37 years. Osteoblastoma occurs twice as often in males as females. Most tumors have a central location, but a number appear to have a periosteal location. The central form can occur in the maxilla or mandible, with a slight predominance in the mandible. The alveolar process appears to be a common location; however, some reported cases may not have been differentiated from benign cementoblastomas.

Signs and symptoms: Pain and swelling are common symptoms. The enlarged area may be tender to palpation. The adjacent teeth may be sensitive to percussion; they may also be mobile or exhibit root resorption.

Histologic findings: Osteoblastoma is composed of rows of plump osteoblasts producing abundant trabeculae of osteoid and immature bone, which are seen in varying stages of calcification. Numerous osteoclasts are also present. The trabeculae tend to form in the pattern of an anastomosing network. The supporting connective tissue is remarkable for its high degree of vascularity. The dense cellularity of the osteoblasts may mimic the osteoblastic variant of osteosarcoma. Mitoses and atypia are not present.

RADIOLOGIC FEATURES

Shape

The overall shape may be irregular or round to oval if growth is not resisted by surrounding structures.

Periphery

Tumors are usually well delineated by a bone reaction, seen radiographically as a variably wide band of bone sclerosis. This reaction is less pro-

Text continued on page 262.
Text continued on page 262.

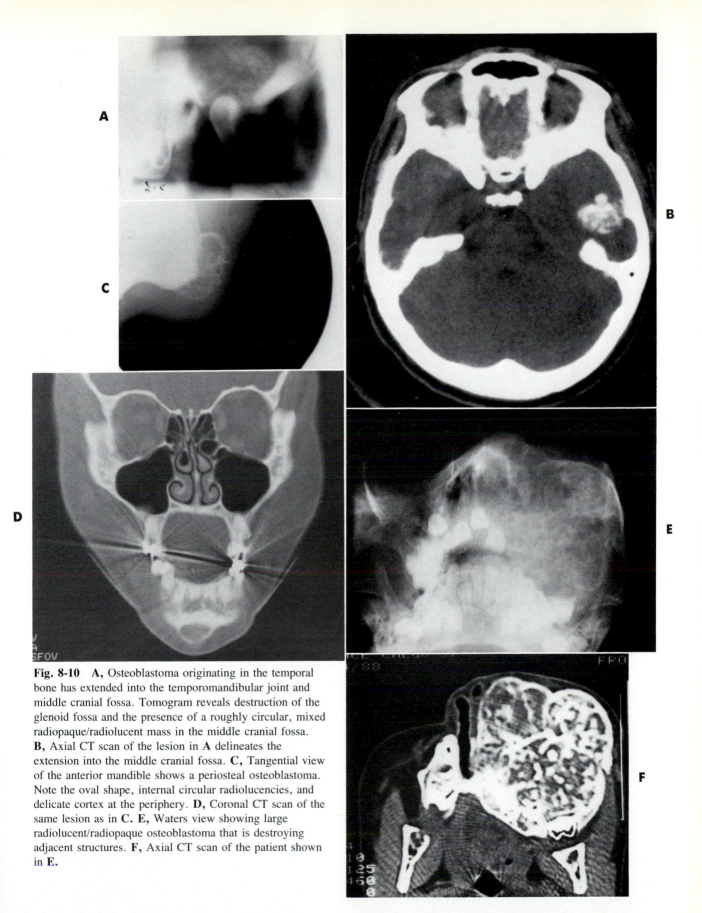

Fig. 8-10   A, Osteoblastoma originating in the temporal
bone has extended into the temporomandibular joint and
middle cranial fossa. Tomogram reveals destruction of the
glenoid fossa and the presence of a roughly circular, mixed
radiopaque/radiolucent mass in the middle cranial fossa.
B, Axial CT scan of the lesion in **A** delineates the
extension into the middle cranial fossa. **C,** Tangential view
of the anterior mandible shows a periosteal osteoblastoma.
Note the oval shape, internal circular radiolucencies, and
delicate cortex at the periphery. **D,** Coronal CT scan of the
same lesion as in **C. E,** Waters view showing large
radiolucent/radiopaque osteoblastoma that is destroying
adjacent structures. **F,** Axial CT scan of the patient shown
in **E.**

found than that seen in osteoid osteoma. In some cases the border of the tumor may be composed of an irregular radiolucent band directly adjacent to the reactive bone.

Internal Structure

Young immature tumors may have a radiolucent center. Most have a variable amount of irregular bone formation, resulting in a mixed radiolucent-radiopaque pattern. The bone may have a granular texture, which may form circular radiopaque regions or suggest the presence of thick, coarse trabeculae. A pattern of irregular bone that contains roughly circular radiolucent regions has also been described. The radiographic appearance may suggest a sequence of maturity, with a relatively radiopaque center and less bone formation at the periphery, seen as a radiolucent band.

Effects on Surrounding Structures

The tumor appears to be capable of considerable growth, which is reflected in significant expansion of the involved bone. Evidence of maintenance of a portion of the outer cortical bone is usually present. Tooth movement, resorption, and destruction of the lamina dura have been reported.

Other Radiologic Characteristics

Osteoblastomas characteristically show intense uptake on technetium scans. Computed tomography is usually the most accurate means of defining the extent of the tumor.

Differential Diagnosis

For lesions in the alveolar process, the possibility of a benign cementoblastoma should be considered. The histopathologic findings of some lesions are very similar to those of well-differentiated osteogenic sarcomas and can be identical to those of osteoid osteoma.

OSTEOMA

Overview

Definition: Osteoma is a benign lesion of bone characterized by a bony protuberance of mature lamellar or woven bone that usually arises in membranous bones. These lesions are usually considered to represent hamartomas or reactive lesions secondary to low-grade inflammation. When they occur centrally within bone, they are endosteal in origin; when they occur on the peripheral surface of bone, they are subperiosteal in origin.

Clinical Features

Demographics: The reported age range for osteomas of the head and neck is 16 to 74 years, with patients in their sixth decade being most commonly affected. There is a female predominance, with a ratio of 3:1. The most common locations are the mandibular condyle and near the angle of the mandible. Other notable sites are the coronoid notch and the lateral aspect of the ramus. Osteomas are common in the frontal sinuses, but they are rare in the maxillary sinus.

Signs and symptoms: The lesions are usually painless, slowly enlarging, and discovered incidentally on radiographs. When large, they may produce asymmetry, headaches, or symptoms related to sinus obstruction.

Histologic findings: Two types of osteoma are classically recognized. The compact, or ivory, osteoma is composed of dense lamellar bone with few small medullary spaces. The trabecular, or spongy, osteoma is composed of trabeculae of bone with varying amounts of fatty, hematopoietic marrow and loose connective tissue in large medullary spaces.

RADIOLOGIC FEATURES

Shape

The tumor is usually round or oval and attached by a broad base or more rarely by a stalk to the parent bone.

Periphery

The external surface is usually smooth, well defined, and well corticated.

Internal Structure

The more common compact variety has a homogeneous radiopaque appearance, sometimes with a granular texture. The cancellous type usually has a normal-appearing trabecular pattern.

Effects on Surrounding Structures

There appears to be no effect on the parent bone. The outer cortex is contiguous with the cortical

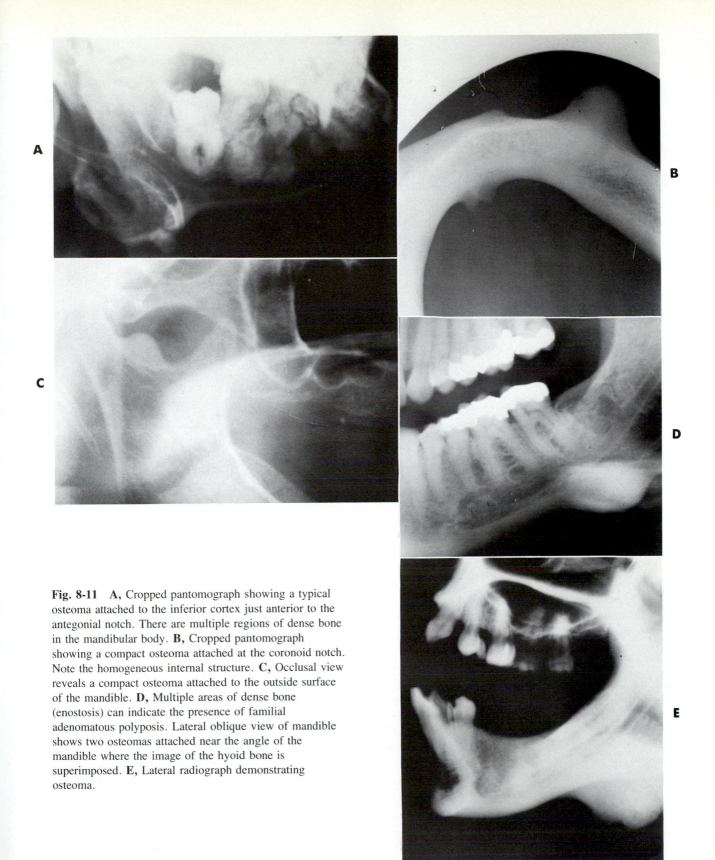

Fig. 8-11 **A,** Cropped pantomograph showing a typical osteoma attached to the inferior cortex just anterior to the antegonial notch. There are multiple regions of dense bone in the mandibular body. **B,** Cropped pantomograph showing a compact osteoma attached at the coronoid notch. Note the homogeneous internal structure. **C,** Occlusal view reveals a compact osteoma attached to the outside surface of the mandible. **D,** Multiple areas of dense bone (enostosis) can indicate the presence of familial adenomatous polyposis. Lateral oblique view of mandible shows two osteomas attached near the angle of the mandible where the image of the hyoid bone is superimposed. **E,** Lateral radiograph demonstrating osteoma.

boundary of the osteoma. This lesion may cause displacement of the surrounding soft tissue and displacement of the mandibular condyle when associated with it. Remodeling of the articular eminence and fossa to accommodate the osteoma may also be present.

Differential Diagnosis

The appearance may be difficult to differentiate from that of osteochondroma and an area of hyperostosis. Irregular outlines seen at muscle attachment sites (e.g., the masseter muscle attachment to the ramus) may have a similar appearance, as may large osteophyte attached to the anterior aspect of the condyle. Periosteal forms of osteogenic sarcoma and osteoblastoma may also be considered.

Gardner syndrome and familial adenomatous polyposis may be associated with multiple osteomas. Multiple areas of dense bone islands (enostosis or osteosclerosis) may be also seen.

NEURAL TUMORS OF THE JAWS

Overview

Definition: Benign nerve sheath neoplasms of Schwann cells originating in the nerves have been described as neurofibromas or neurilemomas based on histologic differences. Neurofibroma may occur as a solitary lesion or as a component of the syndrome of neurofibromatosis. Neurilemmoma may occur sporadically in neurofibromatosis but is usually a solitary lesion. Rarely, both may occur centrally within bone, although neurilemoma does so more frequently.

Clinical Features

Demographics: Neural tumors occur in a broad age range of 2 to 65 years. Mean age has been reported to be 29 years, with over 80% of cases occurring before the age of 45. There is a female predilection for the central jaw lesions, with a female:male ratio of 2:1.

Sites vary according to tumor type:

1. Neurofibroma—Common soft tissue sites include the cheek, palate, tongue and lips; central tumors occur in the mandible more often than the maxilla. The inferior alveolar canal and mental foramen are common sites.

2. Neurilemmoma—Neurilemmomas are most common in the inferior alveolar canal and rare in the maxilla and soft tissue.

3. Neurofibromatosis—Common sites include the posterior mandible and the premolar region. Attempts can be made to differentiate between soft tissue and intraosseous sites; however, many lesions in the facial region include simultaneous intraosseous and soft tissue locations. Less commonly, some lesions may have a subperiosteal location.

Signs and symptoms: Pain and swelling are the most common symptoms. Paresthesia may also occur.

Histologic findings: Solitary neurofibroma is a well-circumscribed but nonencapsulated neoplasm composed of spindle-shaped fibroblasts in a delicate matrix of collagen fibrils in a loose, myxomatous ground substance. The appearance of neurofibromatosis varies from large hyperplastic nerves (plexiform neurofibroma) to a very dense connective tissue with occasional Meissner corpuscle–like structures. Neurilemmoma is encapsulated and is composed of two types of tissue in varying proportions. Antoni A tissue is composed of closely packed Schwann cells arranged in rows with palisaded nuclei (Verocay bodies). Antoni B tissue is a mixture of Schwann cells and fibroblasts in a loose myxoid connective tissue. Vacuolization and microcystic spaces are prominent.

RADIOLOGIC FEATURES

The radiographic characteristics of lesions of neurofibromatosis, neurilemmoma, or neurofibroma may be identical.

Fig. 8-12   **A (opposite page),** Lateral-oblique film of the mandible showing a neurilemmoma that has caused significant expansion of the inferior alveolar nerve canal and tooth resorption. **B,** Cropped pantomograph shows a roughly oval expansion of the inferior alveolar nerve canal with cortical margins caused by the presence of a neurofibroma. **C,** A case of neurofibromatosis with displacement of teeth, enlarged coronoid notch, decreased mandibular angle, and lowered mandibular foramen *(arrow).* **D,** Neurofibromatosis. Significant changes to the left side are displaced maxillary and mandibular teeth, irregular inferior mandibular cortex, enlarged coronoid notch, enlarged inferior alveolar nerve canal, and increased bone density.

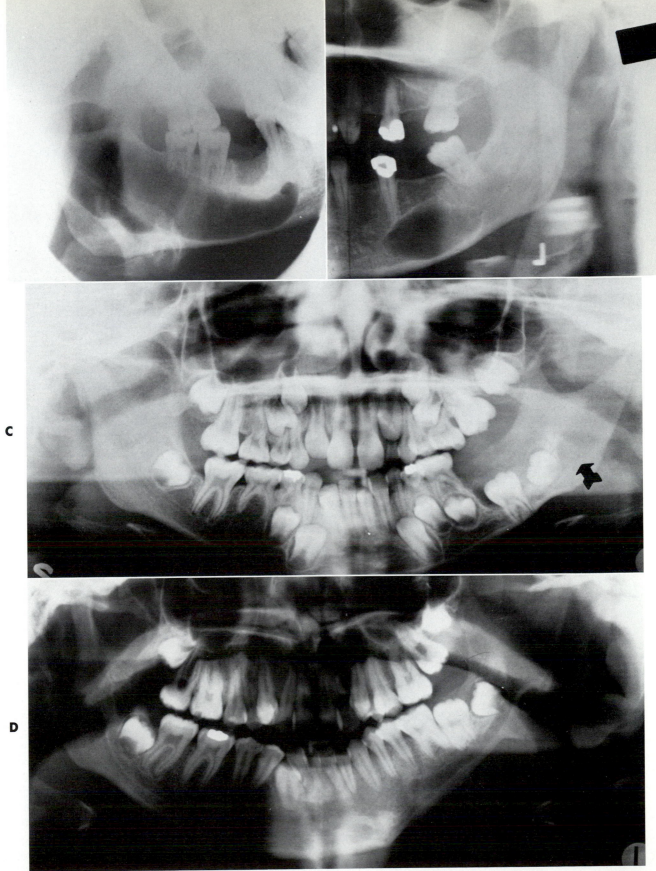

Fig. 8-12, A–D.

Continued.

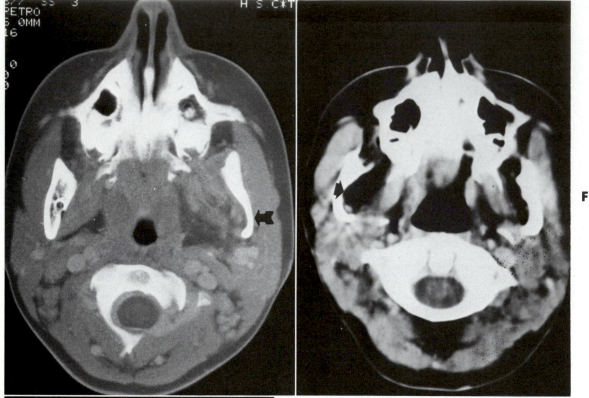

E

F

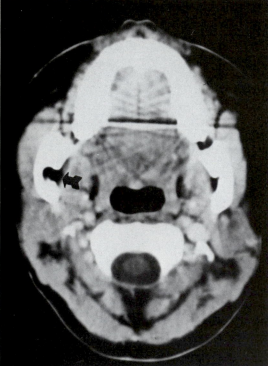

G

Fig. 8-12, cont'd.   **E (above),** Axial CT scan (bone window) of patient with neurofibromatosis revealing lateral bowing of the ramus *(arrow)* and thinning of the mediolateral width of the ramus. **F,** Axial CT scan (soft tissue window) of patient with neurofibromatosis showing tissue with the density of fat immediately adjacent to the medial aspect of the deformed ramus *(arrow).* **G,** Axial CT scan (soft tissue window) of patient with neurofibromatosis showing enlargement of the mandibular foramen.

Shape

Lesions starting within the canal usually have a smooth fusiform or oval shape. *Rarely* they may have a multilocular appearance; these lesions, especially in neurofibromatosis, usually have an irregular shape.

Periphery

Lesions originating within the canal are well defined and may be corticated. Others, especially in neurofibromatosis, may be ill defined. The margins are not invasive but hard to define. This may also be true of the soft tissue margins as seen in CT scans.

Internal Structure

Central osseous lesions usually do not have any discernible internal structure.

Effects on Surrounding Structures

Teeth—Tumors adjacent to teeth may cause tooth resorption with smooth margins. Displacement and suppression of eruption may also be seen, especially in neurofibromatosis. The follicular space may be enlarged and appear cystic.

Inferior alveolar canal—Tumors may cause enlargement of the girth of the inferior alveolar canal with maintenance of the peripheral cortex. It is noteworthy that in large neurofibromas, especially those with a soft tissue component, the enlarged canal will have ill-defined margins. This is common in neurofibromatosis.

Bone—Adjacent bone may be enlarged or decreased in size or deformed.

Mandible—Specific deformities may include the following: ribbonlike, irregular shape to the inferior cortex; loss of the angle of the mandible, increase in the depth and width of the coronoid notch and deformity of the mandibular condyle; thin, elongated coronoid process; bowing of the ramus with the convexity toward the lateral aspect of the face; and enlargement of the mandibular foramen with a lower position of the foramen on the affected side. Notably, deformity and increase in the size of the mandibular foramen may not result from direct pressure effects from the tumor. In many instances soft tissue CT scans reveal tissue with the density of fat within the foramen or immediately adjacent to the deformed medial aspect of the ramus.

MELANOTIC NEUROECTODERMAL TUMOR OF INFANCY

Overview

Definition: The melanotic neuroectodermal tumor of infancy is a rare, benign pigmented neoplasm arising from remnants of the neural crest.

Clinical Features

Demographics: The vast majority (over 95%) occur under the age of 1 year. There is no sex predilection. Approximately 70% of tumors occur in the anterior maxilla. Other sites include the mandible, epididymis, thigh, mediastinum, zygoma, shoulder, skull, brain, and other tissues.

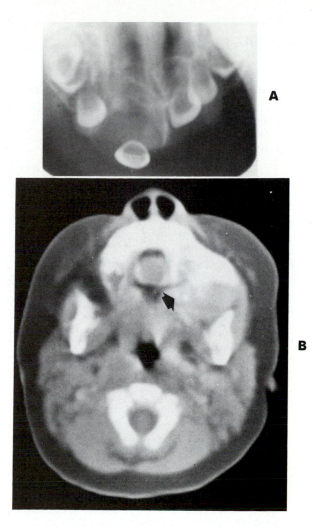

Fig. 8-13 **A,** Occlusal radiograph of infant with melanotic neuroectodermal tumor showing irregular destruction of anterior maxilla and significant displacement of the developing teeth. **B,** Axial CT scan (soft tissue window) revealing a large tumor causing destruction of the posterior maxilla *(arrow)*.

Signs and symptoms: In the maxilla, there is usually a pigmented swelling with displacement of the deciduous central incisors.

Histologic findings: The neoplasm is composed of two main cell types, an epithelial-like cell that occurs in strands and cords adjacent to sheets of small, round dark cells that resemble lymphocytes. Varying amounts of melanin pigment are present, especially in association with the larger epithelial-like cells.

RADIOLOGIC FEATURES

Shape

The shape is usually irregular, although some tumors may cause a circular expansion of the maxilla.

Periphery

The periphery is ill defined on plain radiographs because of the lack of a perceptible bone reaction. The border may appear similar to that of a malignant tumor; it appears better defined on soft tissue CT scans.

Effects on Surrounding Structures

Lesions appear very destructive with no perceptible bone reaction. It is common to see a developing deciduous incisor tooth displaced in a buccal-inferior direction. The follicular cortex is usually destroyed.

HEMANGIOMA

Overview

Definition: Central hemangioma of bone is considered to be a benign proliferation of endothelium-lined vascular channels. It has been reported to represent approximately 1% of all primary bone tumors.

Clinical Features

Demographics: The reported age range for jaw hemangiomas is 5 to 74 years; they are most common in the second decade. Hemangioma of the jaw is twice as common in males as females. Hemangiomas occur approximately twice as often in the mandible as in the maxilla.

Signs and symptoms: The lesions may be asymptomatic or present as an enlargement of the affected bone. There may be pericoronal oozing, displacement of teeth, hyperemia of the area, swelling of the adjacent soft tissue, pain, or pulsation.

Histologic findings: Classically, two histologic patterns are described. The cavernous type is composed of numerous large, dilated thin-walled channels lined with a layer of flattened endothelial cells. These spaces are often filled with blood. The capillary type is composed of numerous small vessels lined with plump endothelial cells in a background of cellular granulation-like tissue. Often, these cellular areas are arranged in a lobular pattern.

RADIOLOGIC FEATURES

These characteristics of hemangioma may also be seen in arteriovenous (AV) malformations.

Shape

Many central lesions have an ill-defined, irregular shape. If the lesion originates within the inferior alveolar canal, the deformed cortical boundaries of the canal will give the lesion a serpiginous shape. Some lesions, especially AV aneurysms, may have a cystic or occasionally a multilocular shape.

Periphery

The periphery is defined by the amount of remaining bone; hence extensive intraosseous lesions are ill defined and may actually appear invasive and very similar to malignant tumors. Other lesions originating within the alveolar nerve canal and those composed of large vascular channels (e.g., AV aneurysms) may have a well-defined cortical boundary.

Internal Structure

The internal aspect of hemangiomas may be more radiolucent or radiopaque than the surrounding bone, depending on the amount of remaining bone and the ability to stimulate new bone formation. A completely radiolucent appearance may result from the presence of a large vascular channel or numerous vascular channels with little or no intervening bone. In the latter case the internal aspect may have multiple circular, non-corticated radiolucencies. This appearance is the most likely to be confused with a malignant lesion. In other cases enough bone remains to produce a radiopaque pattern. Vascular channels traveling in the same direction as the x-ray beam will appear as circular radiolucencies with cortical boundaries.

Occasionally, remaining bone septa may appear to emanate from a central point, resulting in a "spoked wheel" pattern. Internal septa have been described as thickened and coarse with straight or curved paths. Many curved septa may give a multilocular appearance. In some radiographs, the internal aspect may be projected to overlap the outer boundary of the affected bone, especially if the lesion has caused expansion. In these cases, internal straight septa may mimic

Text continued on page 272.

Fig. 8-14 **A,** Cropped pantomograph of patient with central hemangioma, which has ill-defined margins and multiple small circular radiolucencies and has caused extrusion of the second molar. This appearance may be falsely interpreted as a malignant lesion. **B,** Intraosseous hemangioma affecting both sides of the mandible, the left side to a greater degree. The inferior alveolar nerve (mandibular) canal has been widened and its course has been altered, but its peripheral cortex is intact. **C,** Hemangioma with both a soft tissue and a hard tissue component that has caused enlargement of the left mandible. Also note the increased number of trabeculae in the left mandible. A large hemangioma in the cheek has displaced the teeth in a lingual direction.

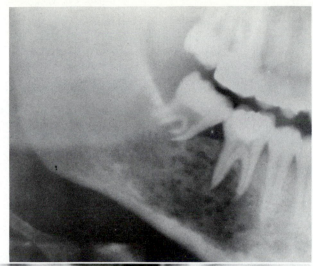

A

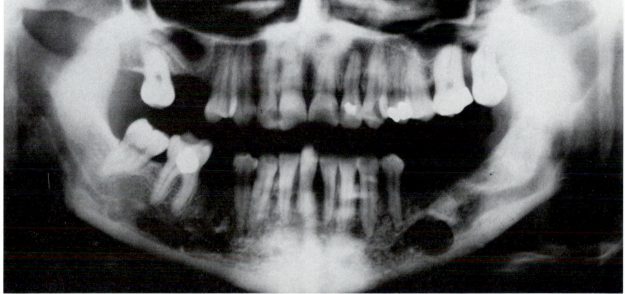

B

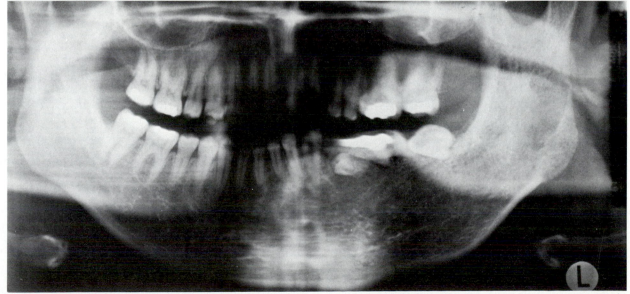

C

Continued.

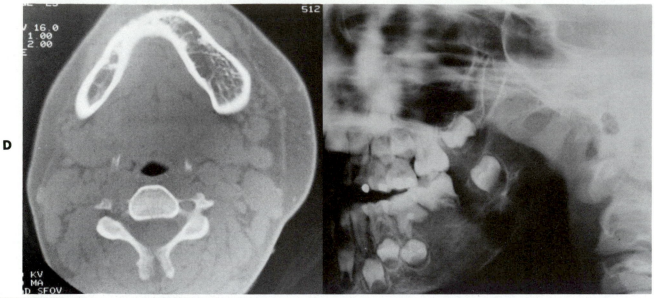

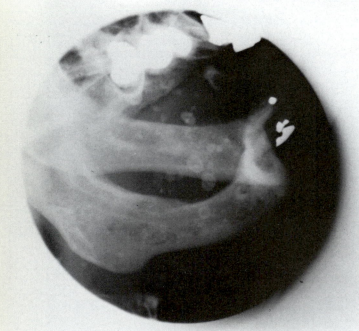

Fig. 8-14, cont'd.   D, Axial CT scan (bone window) of the same patient as in **C** shows the enlargement of the left mandible and numerous coarse trabeculae within the affected region of the bone. **E,** Intraosseous hemangioma that has caused root resorption and extrusion of the second primary and first permanent molar. Furthermore, there is enlargement of the body of the mandible and part of the follicle of the second permanent molar. The internal aspect is essentially radiolucent. **F,** A soft tissue hemangioma with multiple phleboliths. Note the round to oval shape and the more radiopaque appearance of the peripheral rim.

Fig. 8-14, cont'd.   G (opposite page), Pantomograph showing central hemangioma of the mandible. **H,** Axial MRI of hemangioma affecting structures on left side. **I,** Sagittal MRI of hemangioma.

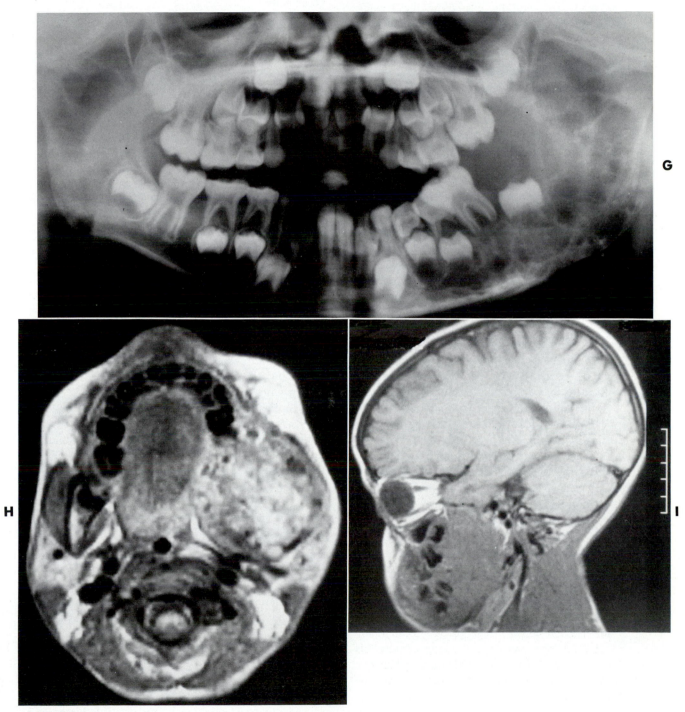

Fig. 8-14, G–I.

the appearance of the "sun ray" spiculation seen in osteogenic sarcoma. The differentiation may be made by carefully examining the leading edge of these septa for a right-angle trabecular, which will give a shape roughly similar to a capital T. This is characteristic of a benign lesion.

Some lesions are composed of a few widely spaced vessels with a considerable amount of intervening normal bone. This particular variation may result in an area of very sclerotic bone that is otherwise normal except that it is punctuated by small, well-defined, circular radiolucencies. This appearance may be very similar to that of osteomyelitis.

Effects on Surrounding Structures

Vascular lesions may cause either resorption or formation of the involved bone. Soft tissue vascular lesions may cause enlargement of the adjacent bone and increase the number and width of trabeculae. This occurs to a greater degree if the bone is next to a vascular lesion during the period of normal growth. Also, the outer cortex lying in intimate contact with the vascular lesion may be thickened or indented with an erosion.

Resorption of tooth roots has been reported. Involved teeth may be elevated out of their sockets, increasing the width of the periodontal ligament space. The development of adjacent teeth may also be affected. The teeth may be larger and more mature in their development and may erupt earlier than adjacent uninvolved teeth.

The inferior alveolar nerve canal may be wider than normal, and its path may be altered (e.g., serpiginous route).

Other Radiological Characteristics

The presence of phleboliths within the soft tissues indicates the diagnosis. These are calcified bodies of round, oval, or cigar shape. Occasionally the calcifications may appear laminated about a radiolucent center. Computed tomography should be done after contrast administration; this will will make vascular lesions more radiopaque than the surrounding soft tissues, enhancing their identification. This is useful unless a large clot has temporarily prevented the flow of blood. The lesions have a low to intermediate signal similar to that of muscle on T1-weighted MR images, but they usually show a high signal on T2-weighted images.

CENTRAL GIANT CELL GRANULOMA

Overview

Definition: Central giant cell granuloma of the jaws is considered to be a fairly common benign reactive rather than neoplastic lesion. It is characterized by the presence of numerous multinucleated giant cells. Its nature is somewhat controversial, but there is support for the contention that it represents the same lesion as the giant cell tumor of long bones.

Clinical Features

Demographics: Central giant cell granuloma most commonly affects young people; over 50% of cases occur in the first two decades of life. The average age of occurrence is 21 years, with a range of 3 to 68 years. Females are affected slightly more commonly than males in a ratio of 1.4:1.

The mandible is affected in two thirds of cases, with the anterior segments being affected more often than the posterior. However, the tumor can definitely occur posterior to the first molars. A slightly greater incidence in the mandible has been reported in the literature, but the anterior maxilla is also a common site.

Signs and symptoms: The tumor usually presents as a painless, enlarging mass with either mobile or displaced teeth.

Histologic findings: Central giant cell granuloma consists of a very cellular connective tissue stroma with little intercellular matrix. Numerous multinucleated giant cells are dispersed throughout. Hemorrhage and hemosiderin pigment are common findings. Osteoid production and inflammation may also be found.

RADIOLOGIC FEATURES

Shape

The shape is usually irregular and may appear undulating as the result of uneven expansion of bone. A few multilocular-shaped lesions have been noted.

Periphery

The borders of the tumor are commonly ill defined and in some circumstances can appear invasive, similar to a malignant tumor. This aggressive appearance is most commonly seen in the maxilla. Another appearance is that of an indistinct boundary, similar to the appearance of a simple bone cyst.

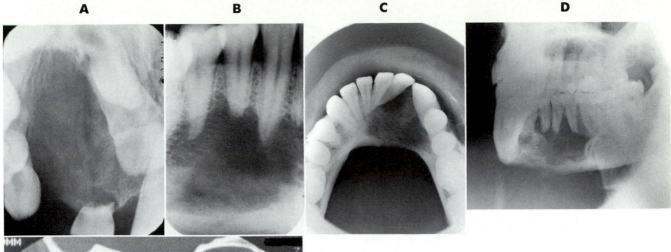

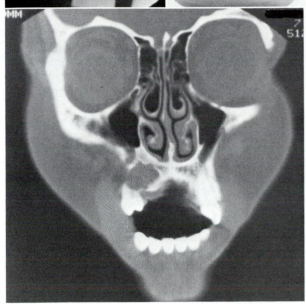

Fig. 8-15 A, Periapical radiograph reveals an ill-defined central giant cell granuloma in the anterior maxilla with displacement of teeth and root resorption. There appeared to be a fine granular bone pattern within the lesion. **B,** Mandibular tumor characterized by indistinct boundaries and appearing to interdigitate between the tooth roots in a similar fashion to a simple bone cyst. Note the root resorption of the first premolar on this periapical radiograph. **C,** Occlusal projection showing a thinned and expanded cortex. The cortex is slightly undulating with thick septa extending at right angles from the cortex. It is directed towards the contact point between the two premolars. **D,** Lateral-oblique view showing a mandibular tumor that has caused irregular root resorption of the adjacent teeth. **E,** Coronal CT scan (bone window) of a recurrent central giant cell granuloma. The lesion has caused considerable root resorption of the first premolar and destroyed the lateral cortex of the alveolar process.

Internal Structure

Some tumors, especially small ones, may be completely radiolucent. Others may have a slight suggestion of the presence of bone; this is seen as a barely detectable radiopaque granular haze. This granular pattern may be organized to form wide, ill-defined septa. A rather straight septum, which appears to project at a right angle from the undulating expanded cortex, is a very distinctive characteristic.

Effects on Surrounding Structures

The tumor usually destroys the lamina dura and causes displacement of teeth. It may lie in intimate contact with the teeth, causing very few changes; in other cases it may cause extensive root resorption. This root resorption is usually irregular and leaves a ragged surface, in contrast to the smooth resorption seen in association with cysts.

The outer cortex may show irregular, undulating expansion, giving the appearance of a double cortical boundary on a tangential view of the affected cortex. In rare circumstances, perforation of the outer cortex may be seen. This is more common in recurrent lesions (especially in the maxilla), which take on a more malignant appearance, with invasive margins, significant bone destruction, widening of the periodontal ligament space, and invasion into developing dental follicles.

Differential Diagnosis

If there is considerable expansion, the lesion may have radiographic appearance similar to that of an aneurysmal bone cyst. Small lesions may appear similar to simple bone cysts, and multilocular lesions can appear similar to ameloblastoma. There may also be a resemblance to early fibrous dysplasia, which appears radiolucent before a significant amount of bone has been laid down.

EOSINOPHILIC GRANULOMA

Overview

Definition: Eosinophilic granuloma of the jaws is a benign lytic lesion of bone characterized by the proliferation of Langerhans cells. It may be a solitary lesion or part of a systemic condition (Langerhans cell granulomatosis or histiocytosis X), which may affect several bones as well as components of the reticuloendothelial system and skin.

Clinical Features

Demographics: Eosinophilic granuloma of the jaws affects younger individuals; over 50% of cases occur in the first two decades of life. An age range of 2 weeks to 53 years has been reported. Males predominate by a ratio of 4.7:1.

In the jaws, the mandible is affected in over 75% of cases. Of these, two thirds occur in the posterior segments. These lesions may be divided into those occurring in the alveolar process of the maxilla and mandible and those intraosseous lesions exclusive of the alveolar process. Multiple lesions tend to occur in the alveolar process and to be centered at the midroot or apical region of the teeth. These lesions also occur more commonly in the molar-bicuspid regions; it is extremely rare that they originate anterior to the cuspid. The most common sites outside of the alveolar process are the posterior body of the mandible and the ramus. In the ramus, lesions commonly affect the lateral cortical bone to a greater degree than the medial.

Signs and symptoms: Patients may have pain, swelling, or loose teeth.

Histologic findings: The lesion is characterized by sheets of histiocytic-appearing cells with large vesicular nuclei and ill-defined cytoplasmic boundaries. Varying numbers of eosinophils are scattered throughout. Secondary inflammation is common and often misrepresents the underlying picture.

RADIOLOGIC FEATURES

Shape

Small lesions in the alveolar process have a round or oval shape and may look like "scooped-out" defects (an appearance of bone destruction in which a shelf of bone still extends from the superior margin of the alveolar process, partially covering the lesion). In other regions of the mandible, small or medium-sized lesions have a round or oval shape, whereas large lesions have an irregular shape.

Periphery

The periphery is usually ill defined except when there is remaining cortical bone or periosteally derived new bone. The ill-defined border often simulates that which is seen with malignant neoplasms.

Internal Structure

The majority of the lesions are totally radiolucent.

Effects on Surrounding Structures

Destruction of bone, including the lamina dura around erupted teeth, is commonly observed with very little effect on the teeth themselves. This leaves the teeth without osseous support. There may be some root resorption, but it is usually very mild. The lesions very commonly provoke a profound periosteal reaction, which is seen radiographically as new bone production. This may occur a considerable distance from the apparent border of the lytic lesions. Some displacement of the remaining cortical bone, and hence apparent expansion of the bone structure, may also be present. The cortical bone or cortical boundaries of other structures, such as the maxillary antrum or inferior alveolar canal, may be partially or totally destroyed. When developing teeth are affected, the follicular cortex may be destroyed and the tooth displaced from its crypt in an occlusal direction. In some cases, lesions of the alveolar process may be surrounded by a sclerotic bone reaction; this may result from a superimposed infection.

Other Radiologic Characteristics

Technetium bone scans may reveal a considerable amount of bone reaction and thus play an impor-

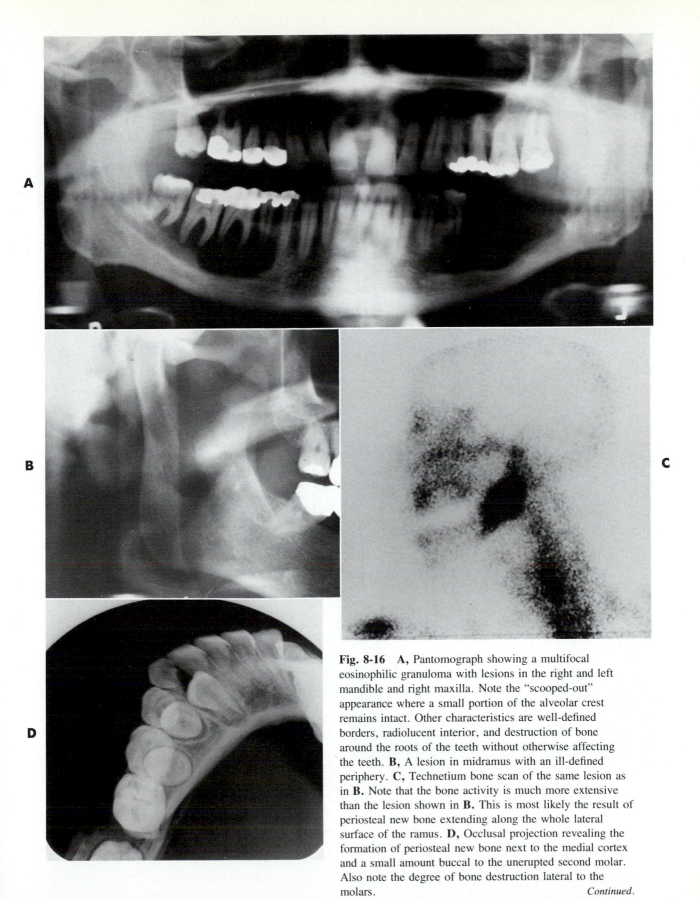

Fig. 8-16 A, Pantomograph showing a multifocal eosinophilic granuloma with lesions in the right and left mandible and right maxilla. Note the "scooped-out" appearance where a small portion of the alveolar crest remains intact. Other characteristics are well-defined borders, radiolucent interior, and destruction of bone around the roots of the teeth without otherwise affecting the teeth. **B,** A lesion in midramus with an ill-defined periphery. **C,** Technetium bone scan of the same lesion as in **B.** Note that the bone activity is much more extensive than the lesion shown in **B.** This is most likely the result of periosteal new bone extending along the whole lateral surface of the ramus. **D,** Occlusal projection revealing the formation of periosteal new bone next to the medial cortex and a small amount buccal to the unerupted second molar. Also note the degree of bone destruction lateral to the molars. *Continued.*

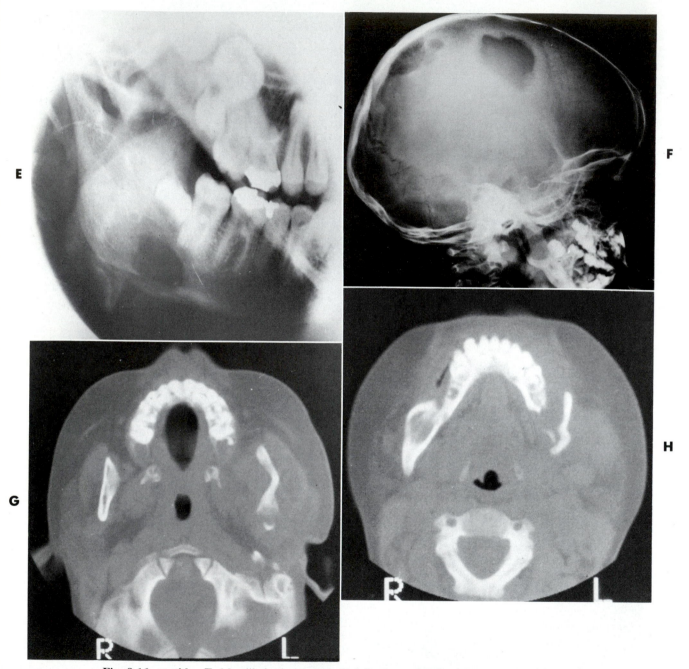

Fig. 8-16, cont'd.   E, Mandibular lesion with ill-defined margins that has caused considerable bone destruction. Note the faint new periosteal bone formation along the inferior aspect and the destruction of the follicular cortex of the third molar. The developing third molar has been extruded in an occlusal direction. **F,** Lateral skull radiograph showing two eosinophilic granulomas in the calvarium. **G,** Axial CT scan showing eosinophilic granuloma of the left mandibular ramus. **H,** Axial CT scan showing eosinophilic granuloma of the right mandibular body.

tant role in the ultimate diagnosis. This bone activity is usually quite extensive in area compared to the lesion and most likely represents periosteal new bone formation. Computed tomography can provide more detail regarding the amount of osseous involvement and aid in determining appropriate biopsy sites.

Differential Diagnosis

Radiologic investigation plays an important role in the diagnosis, because in many cases the histopathologic findings may be obscure or misleading. It may be very difficult to obtain an adequate biopsy of small intraosseous lesions, and lesions in the alveolar process may be secondarily infected, complicating or obscuring the true histopathologic nature of the disease. Nonspecific inflammatory lesions such as periodontal disease may be considered. Radiographically, lesions may mimic periodontal disease; malignant diseases; and metastatic disease, specifically multiple myeloma.

BIBLIOGRAPHY

Ameloblastoma

Cohen MA, Hertzanu Y, Mendelsohn DB: Computed tomography in the diagnosis and treatment of mandibular ameloblastoma, *J Oral Maxillofac Surg* 43:796, 1985.

Heffez L, Mafee MF, Vaiana J: The role of magnetic resonance imaging in the diagnosis and management of ameloblastoma, *Oral Surg Oral Med Oral Pathol* 65:2, 1988.

Kameyama Y, et al: A clinicopathological study of ameloblastomas, *Int J Oral Maxillofac Surg* 16:706, 1987.

Regezi JA, Kerr DA, Courtney RM: Odontogenic tumors: analysis of 706 cases, *J Oral Surg* 36:771, 1978.

Small IA, Waldron CA: Ameloblastomas of the jaws, *Oral Surg Oral Med Oral Pathol* 8:281, 1955.

Ueno S, Nakamura S, Mushimoto K, et al: A clinicopathologic study of ameloblastoma, *J Oral Maxillofac Surg* 44:361, 1986.

Worth HM: *Principles and practice of oral radiologic interpretation,* Chicago, 1963, Year Book Medical, pp 476-488.

Yamane GM, et al: Noninductive epithelial odontogenic tumors: clinico-pathologic study of 48 cases, *J Oral Med* 39:104, 1984.

Adenomatoid Odontogenic Tumor

Cina MT, Dahlen DC, Gares RJ: Ameloblastic adenomatoid tumors, *Am J Clin Pathol* 39:59, 1936.

Courtney RM, Kerr DA: The odontogenic adenomatoid tumor, *Oral Surg Oral Med Oral Pathol* 39:424, 1975.

Giansanti JS, Someren A, Waldron CA: Odontogenic adenomatoid tumor, *Oral Surg Oral Med Oral Pathol* 30:69, 1969.

Yamane GM, et al: Noninductive epithelial odontogenic tumors: clinico-pathologic study of 48 cases, *J Oral Med* 39:104, 1984.

Calcifying Epithelial Odontogenic Tumor

Franklin CD, Pindborg JJ: The calcifying epithelial odontogenic tumor, *Oral Surg Oral Med Oral Pathol* 42:753, 1976.

Ameloblastic Fibroma

Hansen LS, Ficarra G: Mixed odontogenic tumors: an analysis of 23 new cases, *Head Neck Surg* 10:330, 1988.

Shafer WG, Hine MK, Levy BM: *A textbook of oral pathology,* ed 4, Philadelphia, 1983, W.B. Saunders, pp 304-305.

Slootweg PJ: An analysis of the interrelationship of the mixed odontogenic tumors—ameloblastic fibroma, ameloblastic fibro-odontoma and the odontomas, *Oral Surg Oral Med Oral Pathol* 51:266, 1981.

Trodahl JM: Ameloblastic fibroma, *Oral Surg Oral Med Oral Pathol* 33:547, 1972.

Zallen RD, Preskar MH, McClary SA: Ameloblastic fibroma, *J Maxillofac Surg* 56:513, 1982.

Odontoma

Katz RW: An analysis of compound and complex odontomas, *J Dent Child* 56:445, 1989.

Kaugars GE, Miller ME, Abbey LM: Odontomas, *Oral Surg Oral Med Oral Pathol* 67:172, 1989.

Worth HM: *Principles and practice of oral radiologic interpretation,* Chicago, 1963, Year Book Medical, pp 420-438.

Ameloblastic Fibro-odontoma

Hooker SP: Ameloblastic odontoma: an analysis of 26 cases, *Oral Surg Oral Med Oral Pathol* 24:375, 1967 (abstract).

Miller AS, et al: Ameloblastic fibroodontoma, *Oral Surg Oral Med Oral Pathol* 41:354, 1976.

Shafer WG, Hine MK, Levy BM: *A textbook of oral pathology,* ed 4, Philadelphia, 1983, W.B. Saunders, pp 307-308.

Slootweg PJ: An analysis of the interrelationship of the mixed odontogenic tumors—ameloblastic fibroma, ameloblastic fibro-odontoma and the odontomas, *Oral Surg Oral Med Oral Pathol* 51:266, 1981.

Cementoblastoma

Abrams AM, Kirby JW, Melrose RJ: Cementoblastoma, *Oral Surg Oral Med Oral Pathol* 38:394, 1974.

Cherrick HM, et al: Benign cementoblastoma: a clinicopathologic evaluation, *Oral Surg Oral Med Oral Pathol* 37:54, 1974.

Corio RL, Crawford BE, Schaberg SJ: Benign cementoblastoma, *Oral Surg Oral Med Oral Pathol* 41:524, 1976.

Farman AG, et al: Cementoblastoma: report of case, *J Oral Surg* 37:198, 1979.

Langdon JD: The benign cementoblastoma—just how benign, *Br J Oral Surg* 13:239, 1976.

Larsson A, Forsberg O, Sjogren S: Benign cementoblastoma—cementum analogue of benign osteoblastoma, *J Oral Surg* 36:299, 1978.

Vindenes H, Nilsen R, Gilhuus-Moe O: Benign cementoblastoma, *Int J Oral Surg* 8:318, 1979.

Zachariades N, et al: Cementoblastoma: review of the literature and report of a case in a 7-year-old girl, *Br J Oral Maxillofac Surg* 23:456, 1985.

Ossifying and Cementifying Fibroma

Thoma K: Differential diagnosis of fibrous dysplasia and fibro-osseous neoplastic lesions of the jaws and their treatment, *J Oral Surg* 14:185, 1956.

Eversole LR, Merrell PW, Strub D: Radiographic characteristics of central ossifying fibroma, *Oral Surg Oral Med Oral Pathol* 59:522, 1985.

Hamner JE, Scofield HH, Cornyn J: Benign fibro-osseous jaw lesions of periodontal membrane origin: an analysis of 249 cases, *Cancer* 22:861, 1968.

Langdon JD, Rapidis AD, Patel MF: Ossifying fibroma—one disease or six? An analysis of 39 fibro-osseous lesions of the jaws, *Br J Oral Surg* 14:1, 1976.

Schmaman A, Smith I, Ackerman LV: Benign fibro-osseous lesions of the mandible and maxilla: a review of 35 cases, *Cancer* 25:303, 1970.

Waldron CA, Giansanti JS: Benign fibro-osseous lesions of the jaws: a clinical-radiologic-histologic review of sixty-five cases. Part II. Benign fibro-osseous lesions of periodontal ligament origin, *Oral Surg Oral Med Oral Pathol* 35:340, 1973.

Zachariades N, et al: Ossifying fibroma of the jaws: review of the literature and report of 16 cases, *Int J Oral Surg* 13:1, 1984.

Odontogenic Myxoma

Adekeye EO, et al: Advanced central myxoma of the jaws in Nigeria: clinical features, treatment and pathogenesis, *Int J Oral Surg* 13:177, 1984.

Farman AG, et al: Myxofibroma of the jaws, *Br J Oral Surg* 15:3, 1977.

Slootweg PJ, Wittkampf ARM: Myxoma of the jaws: an analysis of 15 cases, *J Oral Maxillofac Surg* 14:46, 1986.

Worth HM: *Principles and practice of oral radiologic interpretation,* Chicago, 1963, Year Book Medical, pp 518-522.

Osteoblastoma

Farman AG, Nortje CJ, Grotepass F: Periosteal benign osteoblastoma of the mandible: report of a case and review of the literature pertaining to benign osteoblastic neoplasms of the jaws, *Br J Oral Surg* 14:12, 1976.

Greer RO, Berman DN: Osteoblastoma of the jaws: current concepts and differential diagnosis, *J Oral Surg* 36:304, 1978.

Jaffe RH: Benign osteoblastoma, *Bull Hosp J Dis* 17:141, 1956.

Smith RA, et al: Comparison of the osteoblastoma in gnathic and extragnathic sites, *Oral Surg Oral Med Oral Pathol* 54:285, 1982.

Osteoma

Carl W, Sullivan MA: Dental abnormalities and bone lesions associated with familial adenomatous polyposis: report of cases, *J Am Dent Assoc* 119:137, 1989.

Shafer WG, Hine MK, Levy BM: *A textbook of oral pathology,* ed 4, Philadelphia, W.B. Saunders, p 163.

Worth HM: *Principles and practice of oral radiologic interpretation,* Chicago, 1963, Year Book Medical.

Neural Tumors

D'Ambrosio JA, Langlais RP, Young RS: Jaw and skull changes in neurofibromatosis, *Oral Surg Oral Med Oral Pathol* 66:391, 1988.

D'Ambrosio JA, Langlais RP, Young RS: Jaw skull changes in neurofibromatosis, *Oral Surg Oral Med Oral Pathol* 66:391, 1988.

Das Gupta TK, et al: Benign solitary schwannomas (neurilemmomas), *Cancer* 24:355, 1969.

DeLaMonte SM, et al: Intraosseous schwannoma: histologic features, ultrastructure and review of the literature, *Human Pathol* 15:551, 1984.

Ellis GL, Abrams AM, Melrose RJ: Intraosseous benign neural sheath neoplasms of the jaws, *Oral Surg Oral Med Oral Pathol* 41:731, 1977.

Eversole LR: Central benign and malignant neural neoplasms of the jaws: a review, *J Oral Surg* 27:716, 1969.

Fawcett KJ, Dahlin DC: Neurilemmoma of bone, *Am J Clin Pathol* 47:759, 1967.

Hunt JC, Puch DG: Skeletal lesions in neurofibromatosis, *Radiology* 76:1, 1961.

Pitt MJ, Mosher JF, Edeiken J: Abnormal periostium and bone in neurofibromatosis, *Pediatr Radiol* 103:143, 1972.

Polak M, et al: Solitary neurofibroma of the mandible: Case report and review of the literature, *J Oral Maxillofac Surg* 47:65, 1989.

Samter TG, Vellios F, Shafer WG: Neurilemmoma of bone, *Radiology* 75:215, 1960.

Shafer WG, Hine MK, Levy BM: *A textbook of oral pathology,* ed 4, Philadelphia, 1983, W.B. Saunders, pp 206-208.

Shapiro SD, et al: Neurofibromatosis: oral and radiographic manifestations, *Oral Surg Oral Med Oral Pathol* 58:493, 1982.

Swangsilpa K, Winther JE, Mybroe L: Neurilemmomas in the oral cavity, *J Dent* 4:237, 1976.

Worth HM: Principles and practice of oral radiologic interpretation, Chicago, 1963, Year Book Medical, pp 513-517.

Melanotic Neuroectodermal Tumor of Infancy

Borello ED, Gorlin RJ: Melanotic neuroectodermal tumor of infancy: a neoplasm of neural crestal origin, *Cancer* 19:196, 1966.

Cutler LS, Chaudry AP, Topazian R: The melanotic neuroectodermal tumor of infancy: an ultrastructural study, literature review and reevaluation, *Cancer* 48:257, 1981.

Stowens D, Lin T-H: Melanotic progonoma of the brain, *Hum Pathol* 5:105, 1974.

Hemangioma

Clay RC, Blalock A: Congenital A-V fistulas in the mandible, *Surg Gynecal Obstet* 90:543, 1950.

Gamey-Araujo JJ, Toth BB, Luna MA: Central hemangioma of the mandible and maxilla: review of a vascular lesion, *Oral Surg Oral Med Oral Pathol* 37:230, 1974.

Kaplan PA, Williams SM: Mucocutaneous and peripheral soft-tissue hemangiomas: MR imaging, *Radiology* 163:163, 1987.

Lund BA, Dahlin DC: Hemangiomas of the mandible and maxilla, *J Oral Surg* 22:234, 1964.

Macpherson RI, Letts RM: Skeletal diseases associated with angiomatosis, *J Can Assoc Radiol* 29:90, 1978.

Rappaport I, Rappaport J: Congenital arteriovenous fistula of the maxillofacial region, *Am J Surg* 134:39, 1977.

Schindel J, Edlan A, Abraham A: Central cavernous hemangioma of the jaws, *J Oral Surg* 36:803, 1978.

Sherman RS, Wilner D: The roentgen diagnosis of hemangioma of bone, *AJR* 86:1146, 1961.

Wallis LA, Maisel BW: Diffuse skeletal hemangiomatosis, *Am J Med* 37:545, 1964.

Worth HM: *Principles and practice of oral radiologic interpretation,* Chicago, 1963, Year Book Medical, pp 522-526.

Central Giant Cell Granuloma

Auclair PL, et al: A clinical and histomorphologic comparison of the central giant cell granuloma and the giant cell tumor, *Oral Surg Oral Med Oral Pathol* 66:197, 1988.

Austin LT, Dahlin DC, Royer RQ: Giant-cell reparative granuloma and related conditions affecting the jawbones, *Oral Surg Oral Med Oral Pathol* 12:1285, 1959.

Cohen MA, Hertzanu Y: Radiologic features, including those seen with computed tomography of central giant cell granulomas of the jaws, *Oral Surg Oral Med Oral Pathol* 65:255, 1988.

Jaffe HL: Giant-cell reparative granuloma, traumatic bone cyst, and fibrous dysplasia of the jawbones, *Oral Surg Oral Med Oral Pathol* 6:159, 1953.

Waldron CA, Shafer WG: The central giant cell reparative granuloma of the jaws, *Am J Clin Pathol* 45:437, 1966.

Worth HM: Principles and practice of oral radiologic interpretation, Chicago, 1963, Year Book Medical, pp 497-505.

Eosinophilic Granuloma

Artzi A, Gorsky M, Raviv M: Periodontal manifestations of adult onset histiocytosis X, *J Periodontol* 60:57, 1989.

Dagenais M, Pharoah MJ, Sikorski PA: *An analysis of the radiographic characteristics of histiocytosis X of the jaws,* thesis, Toronto, 1988, University of Toronto.

Hartman KS: Histiocytosis X: a review of 114 cases with oral involvement, *Oral Surg* 49:38, 1980.

McDonald JS, et al: Histiocytosis X: a clinical presentation, *J Oral Pathol* 9:342, 1980.

Rapidis AD, et al: Histiocytosis X: an analysis of 50 cases, *Int J Oral Surg* 7:76, 1978.

9

MALIGNANCIES AFFECTING THE JAWS

OSTEOGENIC SARCOMA

Overview

Definition: Osteogenic sarcoma is a primary malignant neoplasm of bone.

Pathogenesis: The precise cause of osteogenic sarcoma is unknown, although antecedent trauma, excess bone growth, genetic susceptibility, and viral pathogens may be implicated. Osteogenic sarcoma is also known to occur in association with Paget disease,[10] fibrous dysplasia, and in persons exposed to therapeutic ionizing radiation.

Clinical Features

Demographics: Osteogenic sarcoma is the most common malignancy of bone tissue, constituting 20% of all sarcomas. Most cases occur in the appendicular skeleton, where sarcomas are likely to be found in the metaphyseal region. The distal femur and proximal tibia are the most common sites. The neoplasm is rare in the jaws, where 7% of the lesions may be expected to be found. The overall incidence of osteogenic sarcoma of the jaws in the United States is 0.07 per 100,000 per year. There are variants including the parosteal, periosteal, and extraosseous forms.

The peak age of occurrence for osteogenic sarcoma of the facial bones is in the third to fourth decade of life, with an age range of 12 to 79 years. Maxillofacial lesions occur in a significantly older age group than do long bone lesions. This neoplasm is exceedingly rare in children. There is no racial predilection.

Males are more commonly affected than females, although some series have demonstrated a female predominance. Slightly more mandibular cases than maxillary cases have also been reported. Patients with mandibular lesions tend to be younger than patients with maxillary lesions.

Signs and symptoms: The signs and symptoms of osteogenic sarcoma include painless or painful mass that may be rapidly growing, toothache, proptosis, partial blindness, loose teeth, bleeding gingiva, soft tissue swelling, paresthesia, nasal obstruction or discharge, epistaxis, and mucosal ulceration. Dental extractions are often the first (and improper) treatment rendered. In many cases increased serum alkaline phosphatase levels are a useful marker of disease activity.

Text continued on page 285.

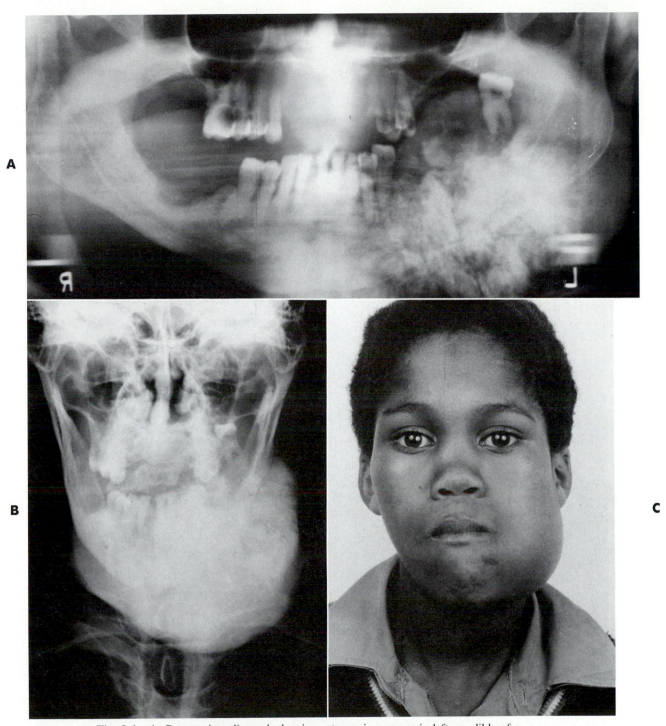

Fig. 9-1 A, Panoramic radiograph showing osteogenic sarcoma in left mandible of a 44-year-old man. Note destruction of mandible, including bone surrounding the molar. There is a deposition of abnormal new bone. **B,** Posteroanterior view of osteogenic sarcoma of lower jaw in same patient. **C,** Hard swelling of left cheek in a 14-year-old boy.

Continued.

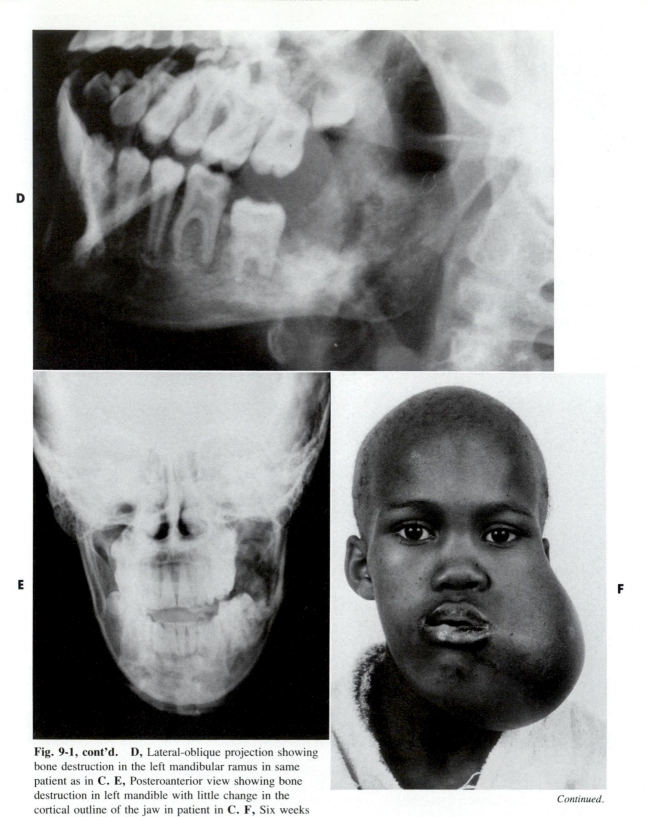

Fig. 9-1, cont'd.   D, Lateral-oblique projection showing bone destruction in the left mandibular ramus in same patient as in **C. E,** Posteroanterior view showing bone destruction in left mandible with little change in the cortical outline of the jaw in patient in **C. F,** Six weeks later the patient in **C** has noticeably larger swelling.

Continued.

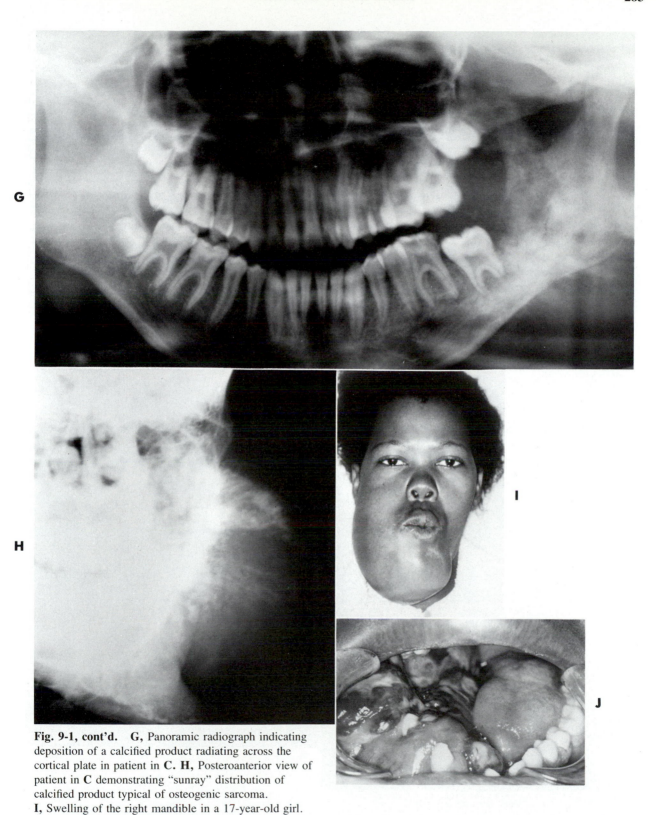

Fig. 9-1, cont'd. **G,** Panoramic radiograph indicating deposition of a calcified product radiating across the cortical plate in patient in **C. H,** Posteroanterior view of patient in **C** demonstrating "sunray" distribution of calcified product typical of osteogenic sarcoma.
I, Swelling of the right mandible in a 17-year-old girl.
J, Intraoral swelling in same patient as in **I.**

Continued.

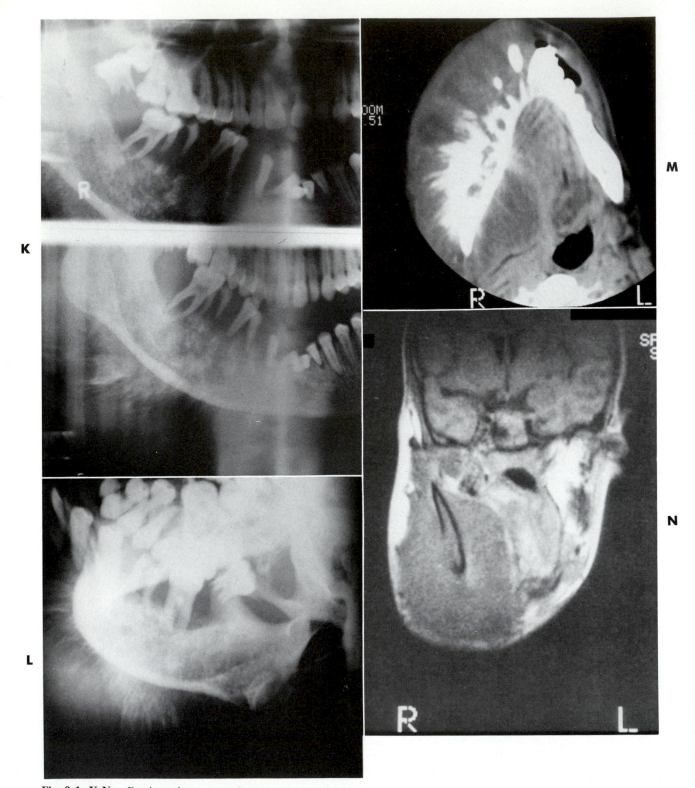

Fig. 9-1, K-N. *For legends see opposite page.*

RADIOLOGIC FEATURES

Cardinal Signs

Single, ragged, or ill-defined radiolucency not necessarily contacting teeth

Expansile jaw lesion or mass with or without a breach or defect in the overlying cortex

Short linear areas of radiolucency in the inferior cortical band in mandibular lesions

Discontinuity in the antral or nasal wall cortices in maxillary lesions

Ballooning of the inferior cortical band in mandibular lesions

Single, destructive radiolucent, mixed, or radiopaque lesion in either the maxilla or mandible; continuum of variable calcification usual

Granular- or sclerotic-appearing bone, "cotton wool" internal structure, or even honeycombed patterning, especially when accompanied by adjacent or contiguous bony destruction

New periosteal bone with associated destruction within it

New bone, perpendicular to the existing cortical plate (often destroyed), giving the appearance of a "sunray" or "hair on end"

Localized increased density of a cortical margin, especially when accompanied by adjacent bone destruction

Production of a typical Codman triangle

Parosteal lesions usually appearing as dense lobulated masses with broad-based attachment to the underlying bones

On computed tomography (CT), a nonsharply demarcated mass; on magnetic resonance (MR) imaging, usually a mass poorly demarcated from adjacent bone

Ancillary Signs

Symmetric widening of a periodontal ligament space shadow

Visible soft tissue mass associated with a destructive or productive osseous lesion

Loss of the lamina dura shadow on teeth adjacent the tumor

Irregular widening of the shadow of the mandibular canal with areas of narrowing and loss of fine parallel cortical margins

Loss of normal random cancellous bone pattern in the jaw

Rarely, laminar periosteal new bone

Cortex possibly merging with the tumor mass, although more often the cortex is completely transgressed

Occasionally, areas of destruction and malignant bone formation interspersed with areas of apparently normal bone

May show a radiographically identifiable capsule enveloping the bone with sparing of the medullary cavity

Differential Diagnosis

Chondrosarcoma

Osteoblastoma

Ossifying fibroma

Fibrous dysplasia

Myositis ossificans

Fibrosarcoma

Ewing sarcoma

Osteolytic metastases

Giant cell tumors

Osteomyelitis

Charcot joint mimicking mixed (opaque and lucent) lesions that affect the temporomandibular joint

Osteoblastic metastases

Carcinoma of the maxillary sinus and chronic sinusitis destroying maxillary cortical boundaries similar to osteogenic sarcoma but without internal calcifications

Fig. 9-1, cont'd.   K (opposite page), Panoramic radiograph of patient in I showing a destructive lesion with loss of tooth support and deposition of a calcified product. L, Lateral oblique radiograph of patient in I, demonstrating the typical "sunray" appearance of the osteogenic sarcoma. M, Computed tomographic view showing "sunray" trabeculation in patient in I. N, Magnetic resonance image of patient in I showing loss of continuity of the buccal cortical plate of the mandible and soft tissue proliferation.

CHONDROSARCOMA

Overview

Definition: Chondrosarcoma is a malignant cartilaginous tumor arising de novo in a bone or soft tissue or superimposed on a preexisting benign cartilaginous neoplasm. These lesions tend to maintain their essentially cartilaginous nature throughout their evolution.

Classification: Chondrosarcomas are classified as primary or secondary, depending on whether they arise from a preexisting benign cartilaginous neoplasm. They are further classified as central (arising inside bone) or peripheral (protruding from bone). They have been seen in association with fibrous dysplasia, Paget disease, and many other benign conditions. There are four subtypes, including clear cell, undifferentiated, myxoid, and mesenchymal.

Clinical Features

Demographics: Chondrosarcomas comprise 10% or less of primary malignant bone tumors and occur in patients ranging in age from 16 months to 81 years. The peak age of occurrence is in the third to fourth decade of life. In the jaws the peak incidence is in the third to fifth decades of life. Mesenchymal chondrosarcomas, which have a propensity for occurring in the craniofacial region, are found in a younger age group. Chondrosarcomas are rare in children.

Chondrosarcomas occur in males and females in equal proportions, although some authors suggest there is a male preponderance. There is no facial predilection. Extragnathically they occur in the pelvic bones, rib, femur, humerus, spine, scapula, sacrum, and sternum. Approximately 10% of chondrosarcomas arise in the craniofacial bones. The mandible and maxilla are probably affected in similar proportions with maxillary lesions favored in some series and mandibular lesions in others. In the maxilla anterior sites are favored, whereas in the mandible the symphysis, coronoid, and condylar processes are most likely affected.

Signs and symptoms: Presenting symptoms include swelling, pain, facial deformity, proptosis, nasal obstruction, visual disturbance, loose teeth, moved teeth, gingival bleeding, paresthesia, headache, and epistaxis. The mucosa is usually intact. There are no reliable laboratory tests that distinguish chondrosarcoma.

RADIOLOGIC FEATURES

Most chondrosarcomas have radiographic features that permit an interpretation of malignancy, but seldom is chondrosarcoma diagnosed from radiologic features alone.

Cardinal Signs

Mixed radiolucent/radiopaque lesion

Area of bone with a ground glass or granular appearance

Solitary radiopacity in or adjacent to bone, not necessarily contacting teeth

Periosteal new bone perpendicular to the original cortex (so-called sunray type or hair-on-end spicules)

Radiolucent lesion with rounded, speckled, mottled, or flocculent internal calcifications (Flocculent internal structures appear as multiple areas with central radiolucency and surrounding calcification.)

Ancillary Signs

Widening of the periodontal ligament space shadow is seen.

Opacification or dense calcification of a paranasal sinus is present.

On CT a nonenhancing mass may be seen. Flocculent calcifications may also be visible on CT. Computed tomography may show expansion of bony walls rather than frank destruction.

An area of osseous destruction may be present with an associated adjacent soft tissue mass. In such cases cortical destruction usually will be evident.

Areas of moth-eaten bone may alternate with islands of normal intervening bone.

Teeth may be separated. Root resorption and deep bone pocketing have also been reported.

Differential Diagnosis

Osteogenic sarcoma
Old bony infarct
Dental abscess
Osteoma
Ossifying fibroma
Sinusitis

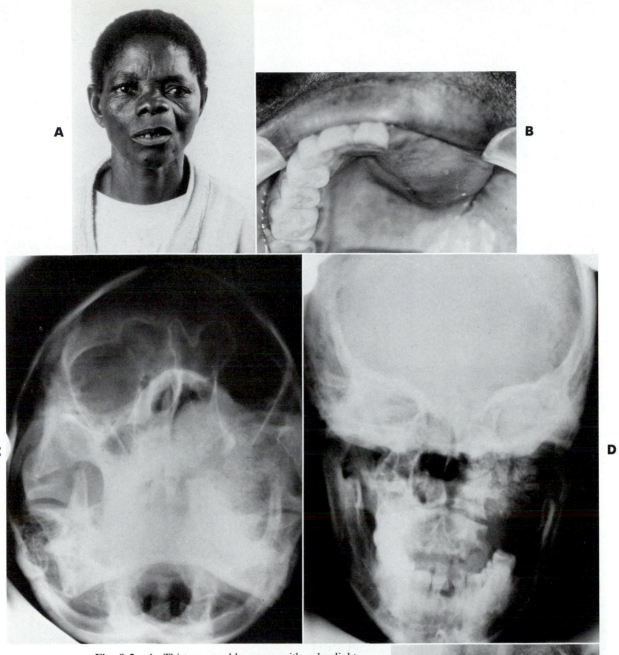

Fig. 9-2 **A,** Thirty-year-old woman with only slight swelling of left maxilla. **B,** In this patient swelling was evident in the left maxilla intraorally. **C,** Waters view of patient in **A** shows radiopacity occluding left maxillary sinus and extending into nasal cavity. Destruction of the left zygomatic arch is evident in this case of chondrosarcoma. **D,** In the same case mixed radiolucency/radiopacity fills the left maxillary sinus. **E,** "Sunray" appearance on topographic occlusal view of maxilla is evident in the patient in **A.**

Continued.

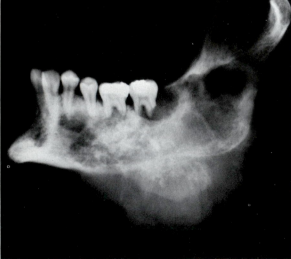

Fig. 9-2, cont'd. **F,** Computed tomography at level of mandibular condyle shows space occupying calcified lesion in left maxillary sinus in the same patient. **G,** Coronal CT in patient in **A** shows mixed radiolucent/radiopaque mass in left maxilla extending into adjacent nasal fossa and orbit. Chondrosarcoma is a productive/destructive lesion.
H (above), Chondrosarcoma of left mandibular body in a 24-year-old woman. Note destruction of bone and tooth roots, plus "sunray" deposition of calcified product on this panoramic radiograph. **I,** Radiograph of resected specimen from patient in **H** shows fine details of this destructive/productive malignant neoplasm.

RHABDOMYOSARCOMA

Overview

Definition and Demographics: Rhabdomyosarcoma is the most commonly encountered myogenic neoplasm of the head and neck. It is the second most prevalent malignant tumor of the head and neck region in children. Approximately one third of rhabdomyosarcomas involve the head and neck, and of these about one quarter affect the oral region. Most rhabdomyosarcomas arise in young children, with a peak incidence occurring between 4 and 9 years of age. Patients can range in age from birth to 80 years. Whereas some authors report no sex predilection, others report a male preponderance. Masson and Soule believe that more females are affected by head and neck embryonal rhabdomyosarcoma. The condition is rare in blacks.

Classification: There are four distinct histologic variants: pleomorphic, alveolar, embryonal, and botryoid. The embryonal form favors the head and neck. It may be defined as a malignant tumor of rhabdomyoblasts with a microscopic pattern resembling embryonic striated muscle.

Clinical Features

Clinical signs and symptoms are attributable to an enlarging mass. Pain is not usually an early feature. The mass is fairly rapidly growing, and patients tend to seek treatment soon after initial symptoms. Nerve involvement, otitis media, sinusitis, reactive or metastatic lymphadenopathy, proptosis, and rubor and calor of the overlying skin are common presenting symptoms.

RADIOLOGIC FEATURES

Cardinal Signs

Soft tissue swelling may be all that is evident.

Ancillary Signs

Premature loss of teeth from exfoliation

Displaced tooth buds in bone

Displacement of the forming tooth shadow in the follicle itself

Radiolucent region, ill defined in extent, with ragged borders

Disruption or attenuation of the shadow of the cortices of a forming tooth follicle

Radiolucency or erosive destruction of any portion of the jaws

Evidence of a radiographically discernible soft tissue mass with underlying bone erosion or frank destruction

Large lobulated soft tissue mass adjacent to bone

Spotty osteopenia present in bone underlying a soft tissue mass

Clouding or opacification of paranasal sinuses with or without destruction of sinus wall cortices

Soft tissue orbital mass with gross adjacent bone destruction

Increased uptake of technetium 99methylene diphosphonate in 76% of cases involving bone

Differential Diagnosis

Osteogenic sarcoma

Histiocytosis X

Neuroblastoma (This is usually seen in younger age groups, but it can produce similar radiographic features.)

Any malignancy adjacent to forming teeth disrupting and displacing tooth buds

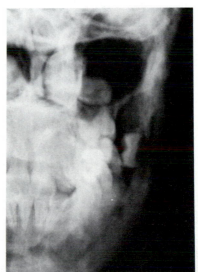

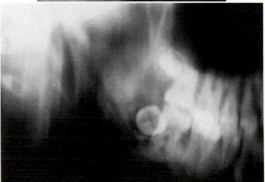

For legend see next page.
Continued.

C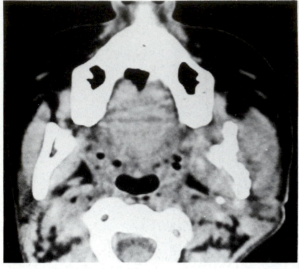

D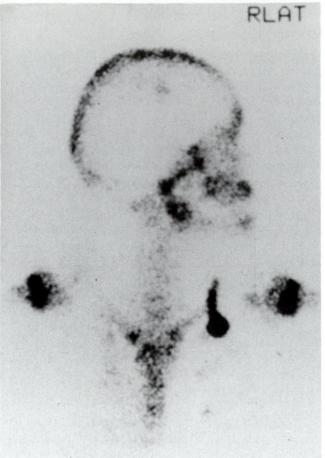

Fig. 9-3 **A (previous page),** Rhabdomyosarcoma affecting left masseter and adjacent tissues. Posteroanterior view shows erosion of mandibular ramus. **B,** Lateral tomograph of patient in **A** showing destruction of bone in the mandibular ramus. **C (above),** Axial CT view of patient in **A** showing swelling of left masseter and destruction of the outer cortical plate of the left ascending ramus of the mandible. **D,** Scintigraphy of patient in **A** showing positive uptake of technetium 99methylene diphosphonate in site of rhabdomyosarcoma.

MULTIPLE MYELOMA

Overview

Definition: Multiple myeloma is a multifocal plasma cell cancer of the osseous system.

Pathogenesis: The cell of origin is the primitive reticulum cell. The tumor itself is a monoclonal proliferation of B cells. The precise cause of myeloma is not known, but chronic inflammation, chronic myeloproliferative disorders, prolonged antigenic stimulus, karyotypic abnormalities, Gaucher disease, and Paget disease have all been implicated.

Clinical Features

Demographics: Multiple myeloma is the most common malignancy of bone. In one large series, it constituted 53% of all bone tumors. Myeloma most commonly affects men. It is associated with advanced age, rarely occurring in those younger than 30 years.

Most patients are 50 to 70 years of age.

Signs and symptoms: Multiple myeloma is characterized by widespread osteolytic bone destruction and is often associated with refractory anemia, hypercalcemia, renal dysfunction, and decreased ability to resist infections. Rarely the lesions are limited to one site, in which case they are termed *plasmacytoma.*

Clinically, myeloma is heralded by bone pain, anemia, pathologic fracture, obvious swelling, neurologic involvement, abnormal bleeding, fever, and weight loss. In the jaw, pain, swelling, expansion, numbness of the lip, mobility of the teeth, and hemorrhage are reported.

Laboratory tests: Tests frequently reveal a normochromic, normocytic anemia and an elevated sedimentation rate. Patients may also have leukopenia, thrombocytopenia, elevated serum calcium, hyperuricemia,

Text continued on page 294.

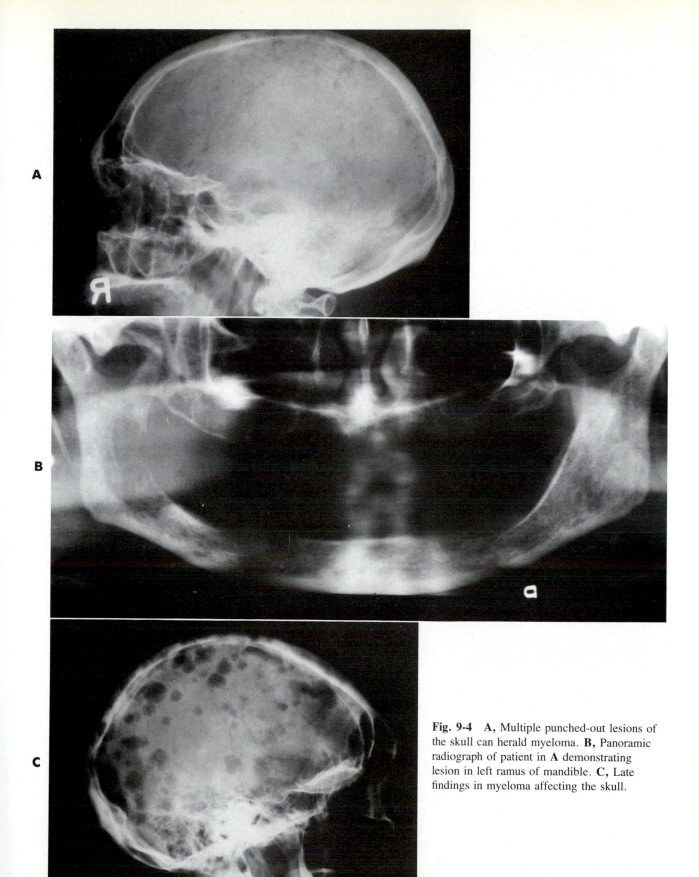

Fig. 9-4 **A,** Multiple punched-out lesions of the skull can herald myeloma. **B,** Panoramic radiograph of patient in **A** demonstrating lesion in left ramus of mandible. **C,** Late findings in myeloma affecting the skull.

Continued.

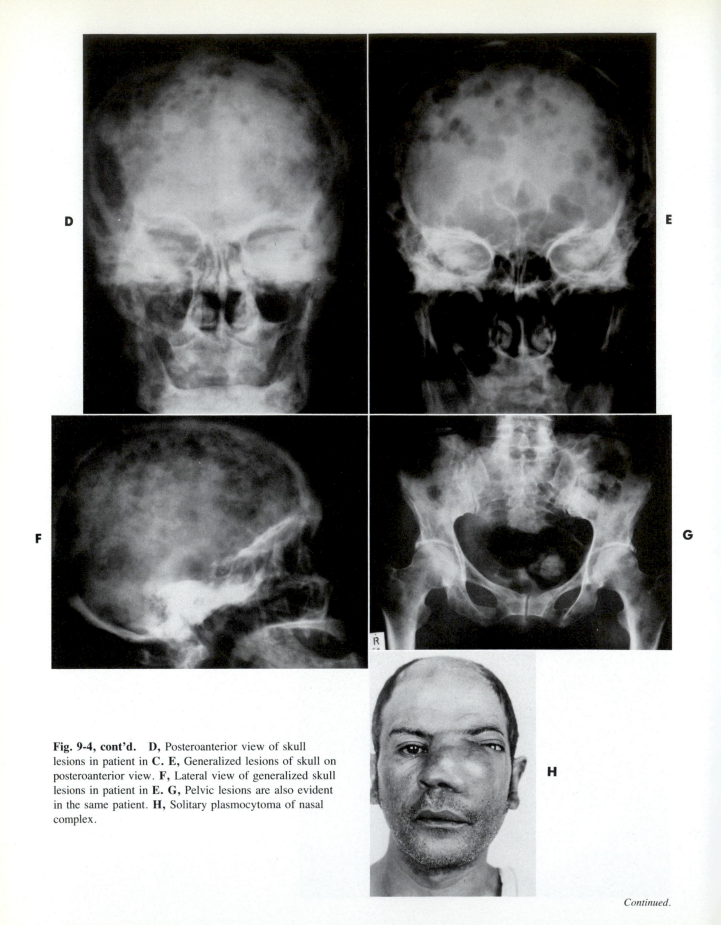

Fig. 9-4, cont'd. D, Posteroanterior view of skull lesions in patient in **C. E,** Generalized lesions of skull on posteroanterior view. **F,** Lateral view of generalized skull lesions in patient in **E. G,** Pelvic lesions are also evident in the same patient. **H,** Solitary plasmocytoma of nasal complex.

Continued.

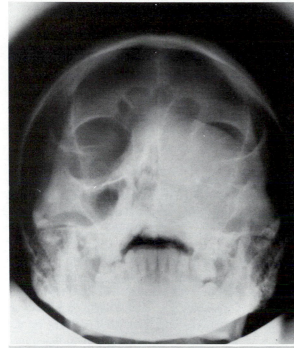

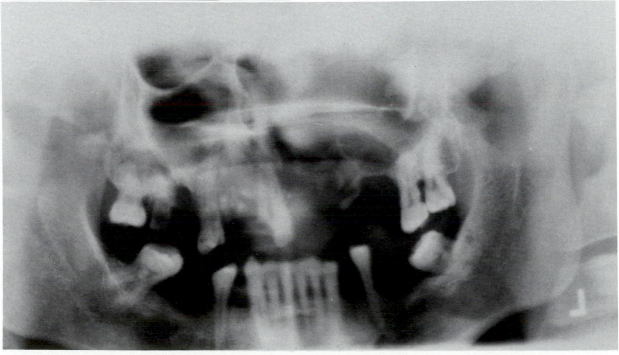

Fig. 9-4, cont'd. **I,** Waters view for paranasal sinuses in patient in **H** revealing large space occupying mass on left side, involving nasal passage and adjacent structures. **J,** Panoramic radiograph of patient in **H** showing loss of continuity of floor of maxillary sinus on left side in site of the plasmocytoma.

azotemia, increased total serum protein, and Bence Jones proteins in their urine.

RADIOLOGIC FEATURES

Cardinal Signs

Multiple punched-out (uncorticated periphery) radiolucencies in the skull and jaws involving the mandible more often than the maxilla

Lesion margins most often well defined but may occasionally appear ragged and infiltrative

Areas of scattered bone destruction separated by normal or nearly normal bone

Great variation in area size and overall lucency; may occasionally appear multilocular

Ancillary Signs

Loss of bone density so that teeth appear to stand out from the jaws, which appear quite radiolucent

Loss of lamina dura—generalized (This feature is not seen until late in the disease.)

Periapical radiolucency, single or multiple, possibly the first sign

Thinning of the mandibular inferior cortex and all cortices, which may appear narrower and "sharpened"

Pathologic fractures of the jaw rarely

Nasopharyngeal soft tissue density mass as the first sign of a plasmacytoma or multiple myeloma

Area of granular bone in the skull or hair-on-end calvarial density

Diffuse area of bone destruction

Occasionally no radiologic signs

In lesion extending to the edge of the bone, periosteal reactive bone deposition rarely (The lesion will usually be covered completely with a thin bony shell.)

Endosteal scalloping of the mandible

Very rarely wholly sclerotic lesions

Differential Diagnosis

Metastatic carcinoma
Hyperparathyroidism
Histiocytosis X
Lymphoma
Oxalosis
Ameloblastoma

LEUKEMIA

Overview

Definition: Leukemia is divided into two main subtypes: acute and chronic. Leukemias are neoplastic monoclonal proliferations of hematopoietic stem cells, characterized by a paucity of mature cells and an accumulation of leukocyte precursors.

Pathogenesis: Most leukemias are associated with nonrandom chromosomal abnormalities. They may result from a leukemogenic insult to hematopoietic cells, with resultant clonal expansion and uncontrolled proliferation of the leukemic cell population.

Clinical Features

Demographics: Acute leukemia is more common in young persons, and chronic leukemia is more common in those 25 to 60 years of age.

Signs and symptoms: Acute leukemias have an abrupt onset characterized by fever, bleeding episodes, lymphadenopathy, splenohepatomegaly, and bone pain. Patients with chronic leukemia also manifest fatigue, splenomegaly, and bone pain but do so over a longer period. Oral symptoms depend on the severity of the disease and include gingival inflammation and hyperplasia, oral bleeding, petechiae, loose teeth, and ulceration.

Laboratory tests: Changes associated with acute leukemias include anemia, presence of blast cells, thrombocytopenia, and pancytopenia. Chronic leukemias often cause a marked elevation in the white cell count and exhibit the Philadelphia chromosome.

RADIOLOGIC FEATURES

Radiologic changes are said to occur in 50% to 70% of children and 10% of adults. In adults changes are preferentially seen in the axial skeleton; in children the appendicular skeleton is most commonly involved. Overall 50% of patients show radiologic changes and 63% exhibit abnormalities on panoramic dental radiographs.

Cardinal Signs

Premature loss of teeth
Generalized absence of the lamina dura
Radiolucency of the crest of the periodontal bone
Periapical radiolucency simulating typical inflammatory periapical changes
Single, noncystlike radiolucency of the alveolar bone

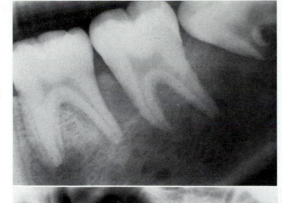

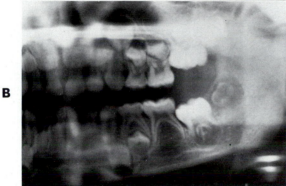

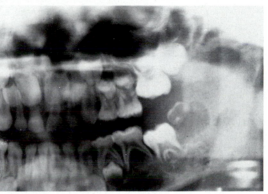

Fig. 9-5   A, Periapical film demonstrates general rarefaction and loss of lamina dura. Note periapical radiolucency on mesial root of vital first molar. **B,** In this case of acute leukemia there is some rarefaction surrounding the developing mandibular second permanent molar. The interradicular bone under the mandibular primary second molar is intact (incidentally there is congenital absence of the mandibular second premolar). **C,** Six weeks later in the same patient, the new panoramic radiograph demonstrates displacement of the developing mandibular second permanent molar tooth and loss of bone surrounding the mandibular primary second molar.

Generalized rarefaction of the jawbones, which may take the form of a reduction in the number of radiographically demonstrable trabeculae in the mandible or maxilla

Ancillary Signs

Cortical outline of the follicle wall of unerupted teeth absent

Multiple separate well-defined radiolucencies

Single layer of periosteal new bone possible on the inferior aspect of the mandible—most common in children with acute leukemia

Granular-appearing bone or multiple well-defined punched-out radiolucencies in the skull of children with leukemia

Bone sclerosis possible, although sclerosis in the jaw bones is excessively rare

Teeth, including those in crypts, displaced

Rarely, localized deposits of leukemia cells (chloromas) in the jaws (cannot be differentiated radiologically from osteolytic malignancies)

Differential Diagnosis

Hyperparathyroidism

Multiple myeloma

Neuroblastoma metastatic to bone

Renal osteodystrophy

EWING SARCOMA

Overview

Definition: Ewing sarcoma is a highly lethal round cell sarcoma of bone.

Pathogenesis: The pathogenesis of Ewing sarcoma is unknown, although it is associated with the unique characteristic of reciprocal translocation of a portion of the long arms of chromosome 11 and 22. The cell of origin may be the neuroectodermal cell, although this is not certain.

Clinical Features

Demographics: Any bone may be involved, but tubular bones are more likely to be affected than flat bones. Greenfield states that in patients younger than 20 years, tubular bone sites are more common, whereas in those older than 20 years, flat bones are most often affected.

The lesion arises in the medullary cavity and may spread to involve all the internal aspects of the bone. It is rarer than osteogenic sarcoma and chondrosarcoma and is especially rare in the facial bones and jaws. When it does affect a jaw bone, it is more likely to be the mandible, especially the ramus.

The peak age incidence is in the second decade of

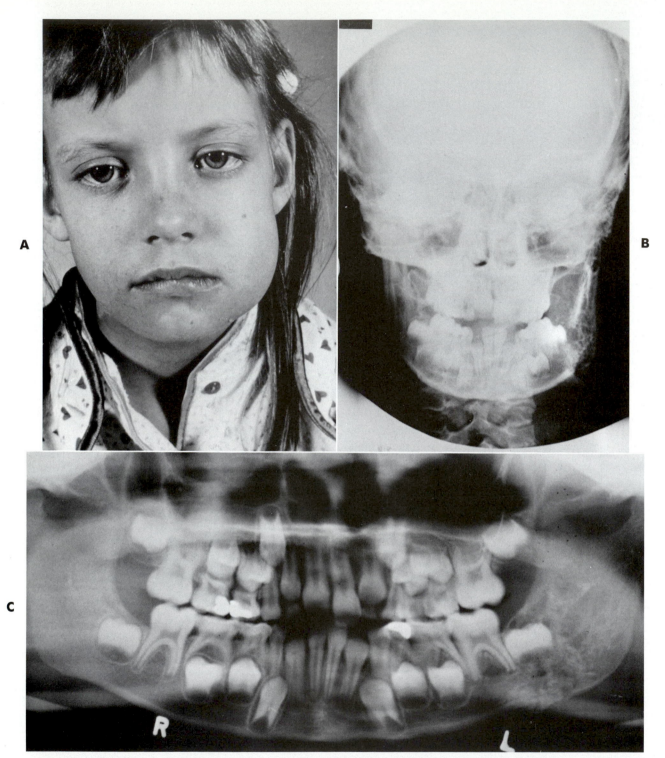

Fig. 9-6 **A,** Note obvious facial asymmetry in this patient with Ewing sarcoma of the left mandible. **B,** Note solitary ill-defined area of bony destruction at left mandibular angle on this posteroanterior projection of patient in **A. C,** Panoramic radiograph demonstrates the periosteal reaction at the lower border of the mandible just anterior to the angle.

life, with 90% of patients between the ages of 5 and 30 years. However, patients as young as 5 months and older than 80 years have also developed the tumor. The mean age of occurrence for primary head and neck tumors is reported to be 10.9 years. The mean age of jaw tumors reported in the literature is 15.9 years, with a range of 2 to 44 years. Ewing sarcoma is twice as prevalent in males as in females and is said to be rare in blacks. Multicentric lesions are well documented, although these may be metastatic in origin.

Signs and symptoms: Clinically the lesions are heralded by local bone pain, fever, a sense of ill health, localized swelling, and deformity. Pain may be referred and of long duration. The area is often tender to palpation. In long bones, pathologic fractures occur. In the jaw, facial neuralgia, swelling, and localized destruction may be present. Loosened teeth and mucosal ulcers may also occur. Cervical lymphadenopathy may be noted.

Laboratory findings: Investigations may reveal anemia, leukocytosis, and an elevated L-lactate dehydrogenase and erythrocyte sedimentation rate.

RADIOLOGIC FEATURES

Cardinal Signs

May be no radiographic changes, especially in the early stages

Solitary, ill-defined area of osseous destruction with infiltrative margins

Expansion of bone with soft tissue mass or masses adjacent to affected bone

Varying degrees of periosteal thickening or cortical erosion

Periosteal reaction of periosteal new bone perpendicular to the original cortex, sunray spicule formation, Codman triangle formation, cortical thickening, and rarely laminar periosteal new bone

Ancillary Signs

Destruction in new periosteal bone

Cystlike areas of destruction

Possible increased vascularity on angiography

Destruction of the lamina dura, contiguous teeth, or adjacent tooth follicles

Differential Diagnosis

Osteomyelitis

Eosinophilic granuloma

Metastatic neuroblastoma

Chondrosarcoma

Osteogenic sarcoma

Non-Hodgkin lymphoma

Metastatic carcinoma

BURKITT LYMPHOMA

Overview

Definition: Burkitt lymphoma is a high-grade, non-Hodgkin lymphoma of B cell lineage. This lesion was first described by Burkitt in 1958 in East Africa. It is grouped with the small noncleaved cell lymphomas in the working formulation for non-Hodgkin lymphoma.

Pathogenesis: The disease is characterized by a translocation of the distal part of chromosomes 8 to 14.

Clinical Features

Demographics: Burkitt lymphoma exists in two forms: endemic African Burkitt lymphoma, affecting children aged 3 to 14 years, and the American form, which affects an older age group. The disease has been reported in an extreme age range of 2 to 60 years.

African Burkitt lymphoma affects boys twice as frequently as girls and involves the mandible, maxilla, retroperitoneum, kidneys, liver, ovaries, and endocrine glands.

Signs and symptoms: In African Burkitt lymphoma extranodal involvement is the norm. It less frequently involves the jaws or viscera.

The tumors grow rapidly when they occur in the jaws, with a potential doubling time of 24 hours. They loosen teeth and destroy alveolar bone. They quickly involve the paranasal sinuses and orbits, producing severe deformities. Pain and paresthesia are frequently present.

RADIOLOGIC FEATURES

Radiologic signs are said to precede clinical signs and symptoms.

Cardinal Signs

Expansive jaw lesion

Multiple well-defined or ill-defined osteolytic regions, starting as small discrete zones and then

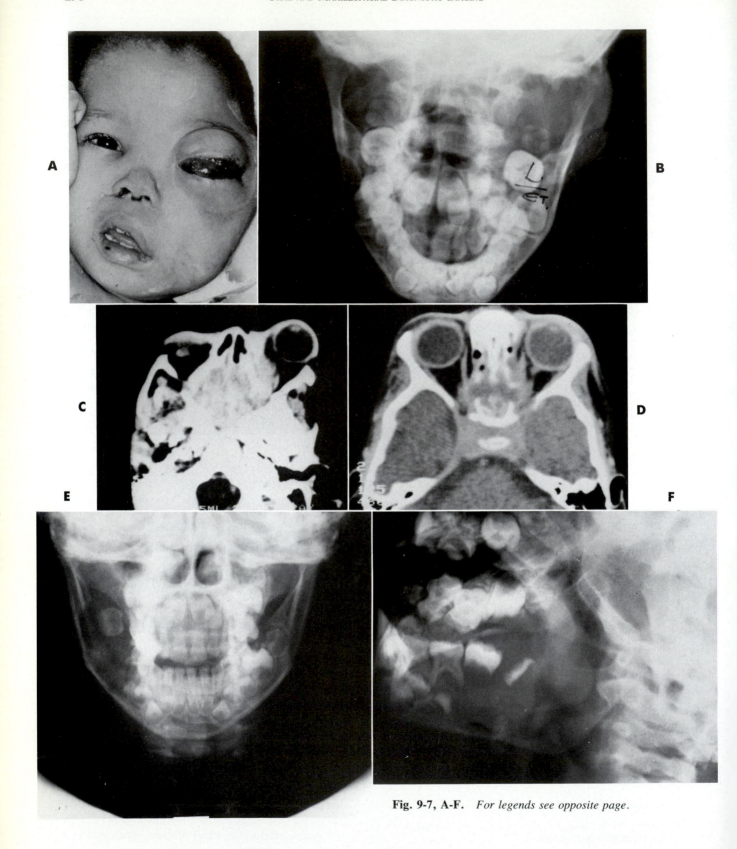

Fig. 9-7, A-F. *For legends see opposite page.*

coalescing to form large radiolucencies

Ballooning, expansion, erosion, or perforation of a bony cortex of the jaw, with associated soft tissue involvement

Destruction of continuous lamina dura, possibly as an initial sign

Displacement of teeth and tooth buds in their crypts and from their crypts

Ancillary Signs

Excessive eruption for the amount of tooth root formation

Effacement of the trabecular bone pattern in the jaw or jaws

Effacement of the cortex of the maxillary sinus or orbit

Sunray spiculation of periosteal bone

Destruction of part or all of the cortex surrounding contiguous unerupted tooth follicles

Destruction of the cortex of the mandibular canal

Evidence of a soft tissue mass in the confines of the maxillary antrum

Proptosis with retro-orbital or paraorbital mass

Thinning of the inferior border of the mandible

Cessation of root development of forming teeth

Destruction of adjacent facial bones by the malignant mass

Differential Diagnosis

Metastatic neuroblastoma

Osteogenic sarcoma

Other Non-Hodgkin lymphomas

Cherubism

HODGKIN DISEASE

Overview

Definition: Hodgkin disease is a form of lymphoma characterized by a pattern of signs and symptoms and specific histologic changes.

Fig. 9-7 **A (opposite page),** Proptosis and left facial swelling in patient with Burkitt lymphoma. **B,** Destruction of the medial pole of the left condyle is evident in this case of Burkitt lymphoma. **C,** Axial CT view shows marked proptosis in case with large retroorbital mass. **D,** Successful chemotherapy of patient in **C** shows shrinkage occurring in only 2 weeks. **E,** Posteroanterior view shows lesion in right mandible. Note complete loss of trabeculation in affected area and displacement of developing molar. **F,** Note destruction of lamina dura around adjacent teeth and tooth displacement in same patient as in **E.**

Clinical Features

Demographics: Hodgkin disease accounts for 0.7% of all new malignancies in the United States, representing 23% of all new cases of malignant lymphomas. Hodgkin and non-Hodgkin lymphomas accounted for 6.8% of all malignant bone tumors in one large series. There is a clinical incidence of osseous involvement in 10% to 20% of cases, with a 34% to 78% incidence at autopsy. Bone involvement is said to be a late manifestation. It occurs in a fairly wide age range, with a clustering of cases in the 15- to 35-year age group. It is rare in children younger than 3 years but does occur in the 9- to 11-year age group. Males are said to be affected more frequently than females. All races are affected.

Signs and symptoms: The clinical features of Hodgkin disease inevitably include enlargement of the regional lymph nodes, with neck nodes being the first group affected in many cases. Fever is often present. Dyspnea, cough, anorexia, weight loss, pruritis, anemia, and fever accompany advanced disease. Extranodal occurrence is less common in Hodgkin disease than in other lymphomas. In the case of osseous lesions pain often precedes radiographic evidence, with pathologic fractures occurring in weight-bearing regions. The mandible is a rare site of involvement.

RADIOLOGIC FEATURES

Cardinal Signs

Large, relatively homogeneous soft tissue proliferations

Ill-defined radiolucency in bone

Productive or destructive sclerotic bony reaction seen in 14% of cases and a mixed blastic/lytic reaction in another 6%

Osseous resorption beneath a malignancy-involved lymph node

Multiple areas of punched-out radiolucency

Ancillary Signs

Possible cortical loss adjacent to the lesion and periosteal reaction in response; periosteal reaction present in 5% of cases

Possible extention into soft tissue from bone

Well-defined mandibular radiolucency related to

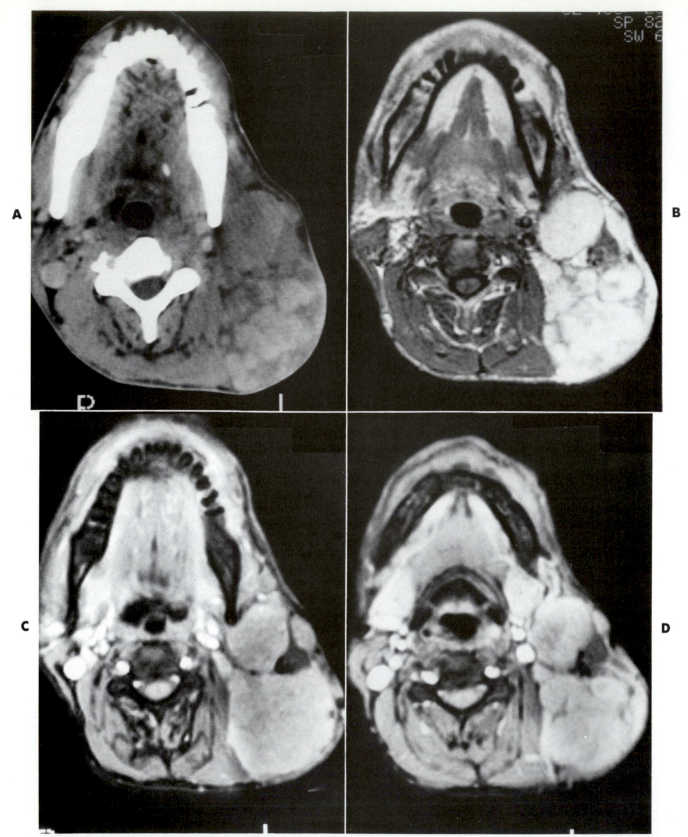

Fig. 9-8, A-D. *For legends see opposite page.*

the apices of teeth with loss of contiguous lamina dura

Differential Diagnosis
Non-Hodgkin lymphoma
Osteomyelitis
Metastatic carcinoma
Multiple myeloma

NON-HODGKIN LYMPHOMA

Overview

Definition: Non-Hodgkin lymphoma is a form of lymphoma not having the characteristic features of Hodgkin lymphoma.

Clinical Features

Demographics: Non-Hodgkin lymphoma (NHL) has its peak incidence in the seventh decade of life, occurring in patients ranging in age from 3 to 95 years. It is rare before the age of 10 years and is more common in males.

Signs and symptoms: Oral sites of involvement include the palate, tonsil, buccal mucosa, floor of the mouth, and retromolar region. Nodal disease is most common, but extranodal involvement is not rare. Extranodal disease occurs in 5% to 25% of cases. Lymphomas in bone account for 5% of all extranodal lymphomas, with the femur, tibia, and humerus being commonly affected bones. The maxillary antrum is frequently affected. It is not certain whether the antrum or the maxilla is the primary site of the lymphoma, and if antral lesions are excluded, the mandible is a more frequent site of involvement than the maxilla. Lymphomas may be primary in bone or metastatic to bone from another primary site.

Gnathic lesions may invade the jawbones or arise in them. Most tumors cause masses. One third of the patients have fever, weight loss, and other constitutional symptoms. Onset may be acute or insidious, with associated lymphadenopathy, abdominal or mediastinal enlargement, fever, night sweats, and weight loss. Lymphoma may spread to other lymph nodes, spleen, liver, and bone marrow, and the cells may spill into the peripheral blood, producing a leukemia. Oral manifestations include pain, fluctuant swellings that tend to ulcerate, tooth mobility, and paresthesia of the mandibular nerve.

Fig. 9-8 A (opposite page), Cervicofacial involvement with late stage Hodgkin lymphoma as shown by axial CT. Note relatively homogeneous soft tissue masses in left cervical region. **B,** Axial MR image of same patient as in **A. C,** Axial MR image of same patient as in **A. D,** Axial MR image of same patient as in **A.**

RADIOLOGIC FEATURES

Cardinal Signs
Ill-defined radiolucent lesion
Generally more destructive than Hodgkin disease
Lesions blending imperceptibly with adjacent normal bone in most cases

Ancillary Signs
If the maxillary sinus is involved, possible opacification with breached cortical walls and associated paraantral or intraantral mass
Multiple areas of destruction separated by normal-appearing bone
Normal sites of bony architecture effaced (e.g., the cortex of the mandibular canal)
Cortices of unerupted tooth buds and lamina dura on adjacent teeth lost
Developing teeth displaced in or out of their follicles
Subperiosteal new bone
Bony cortex possibly widened
Teeth lost prematurely
Expansion of the affected bone
Multiple punched-out radiolucencies
Soft tissue nasopharyngeal mass visible on lateral view or CT of the nasopharynx
Patchy radiopacity
Root resorption of adjacent teeth
Soft tissue mass adjacent to osseous destruction

Differential Diagnosis
Metastatic carcinoma
Ewing sarcoma
Osteogenic sarcoma
Eosinophilic granuloma
Chronic osteomyelitis

METASTATIC DISEASE TO THE JAWS

Overview

Metastatic tumors are the most common malignant tumor affecting the skeleton.

Definition: To qualify as metastatic, a lesion must be localized to bone as distinguished from direct invasion and be microscopically verified as a metastatic lesion. The location of the primary tumor must also be known.

Pathogenesis: The process of metastases occurs by one of three routes: direct seeding of adjacent body

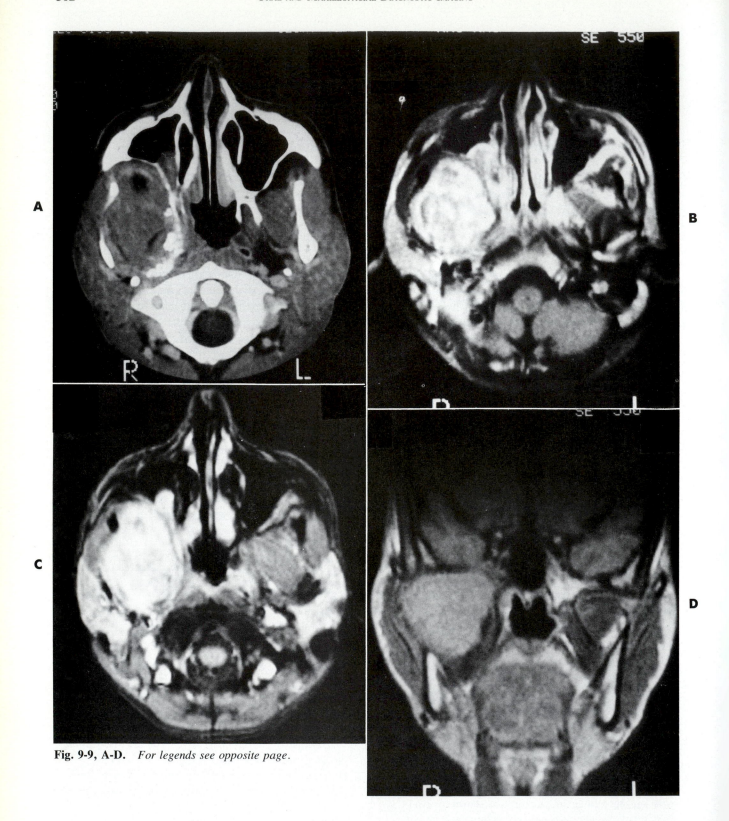

Fig. 9-9, A-D. *For legends see opposite page.*

cavity surfaces, lymphatic spread, and hematogenous dissemination.

Clinical Features

Demographics: Approximately 1% of malignant neoplasms metastasize to the jaws. More aggressive, rapidly growing and large primary tumors favor metastatic spread. Most metastases affect the spine, pelvis, skull, ribs, and humerus. Jaw metastases account for only 1% of all malignant tumors of the oral cavity. Metastases to the jaws are mostly from primary lesions below the clavicle, the most common primary sites being the breast, kidney, lung, colon and rectum, prostate, thyroid, stomach, skin, testes, bladder, ovary, and cervix. In children, in whom metastatic disease to the jaws is rare, neuroblastoma, retinoblastoma, and Wilms tumor may affect the jaws. Jaw metastasis is said to be the initial manifestation of disease in approximately 36% of patients.

Metastatic disease is more common in older age groups, with a mean age in the mid 50s. The mandible is the most likely disease site in the jaws, accounting for approximately 85% of cases. This is because red marrow is present in the posterior part of the jaw. The maxillary sinus is the next most common site, followed by the anterior alveolar processes and the hard palate.

Signs and symptoms: The clinical presentation of metastatic disease to the jaws is nonspecific and includes local pain, swelling, numbness, paresthesia of the lip or chin, and loosening or extrusion of the teeth. Pathologic fractures may also occur, although this is uncommon.

RADIOLOGIC FEATURES

Cardinal Signs

Well circumscribed but uncorticated lytic lesion in

Fig. 9-9 **A (opposite page),** Axial CT of non-Hodgkin lymphoma (B-cell type) affecting right maxilla, maxillary sinus, and adjacent tissues. Note destruction of the ipsilateral pterygoid plates. **B,** Axial MR scan of patient in **A.** The lesion shows a strong signal with patches of inhomogeneity on T2 weighting. **C,** Axial MR image of patient in **A** at level of sphenoid sinus. **D,** Coronal MR image of patient in **A** showing space-occupying lesion in right maxilla encroaching on medial pterygoid and masseter muscle bundles. The outlines of the lesion are smooth.

the posterior mandible is seen.

Metastatic lesions may not appear radiologically until a significant amount of osseous tissue is lost.

Highly irregular lesional shape is typical.

Lytic lesions begin as multiple small areas of bone destruction separated by normal or nearly normal bone, then gradually coalesce to form large ill-defined areas of bone destruction.

Technetium 99methylene diphosphonate bone scans are sensitive markers of metastatic disease.

Ancillary Signs

Possible bone expansion around the metastatic lesion

Possible calcifications in soft tissue accompanying extraosseous or periosteal metastases

Rarely, signs of osteoblastic metastases affecting the jaws (especially from carcinoma of the prostate, less so from metastatic breast tumors, lymphomas, and leukemia); appear as ill-defined zones of increased density with loss of normal architecture and occasionally periosteal osseous reaction

Osteoblastic metastases possibly manifesting as increased girth of individual trabeculae, sclerosing osteitis, and periapical radiopacities

Generalized loss of lamina dura

Periapical radiolucency without evidence of pulpal pathosis

Rarely, external erosion of bone from metastatic disease (more common with primary tumors with direct osseous resorption)

Localized increased density in the calvarium or skull base

Solitary or multiple areas of intracranial density

"Floating" teeth

Failure of an extraction socket to heal or a soft tissue mass extruding from an extraction socket

Differential Diagnosis

Osteomyelitis
Multiple myeloma

Primary malignant tumors cannot be differentiated radiographically from metastatic disease but may be ruled out on the basis of history and physical examination.

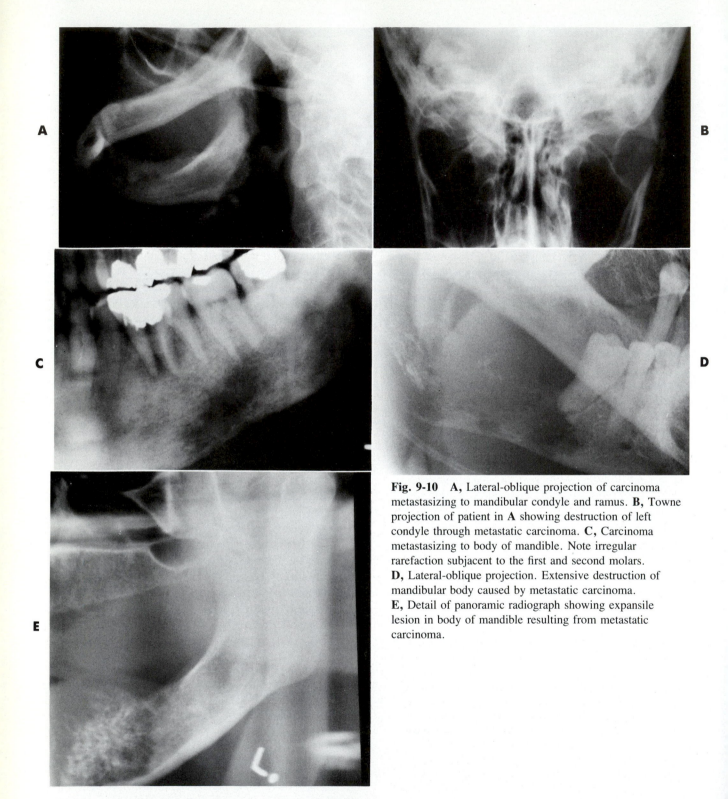

Fig. 9-10 **A,** Lateral-oblique projection of carcinoma metastasizing to mandibular condyle and ramus. **B,** Towne projection of patient in **A** showing destruction of left condyle through metastatic carcinoma. **C,** Carcinoma metastasizing to body of mandible. Note irregular rarefaction subjacent to the first and second molars. **D,** Lateral-oblique projection. Extensive destruction of mandibular body caused by metastatic carcinoma. **E,** Detail of panoramic radiograph showing expansile lesion in body of mandible resulting from metastatic carcinoma.

ANGIOSARCOMAS (HEMANGIOPERICYTOMA, HEMANGIOENDOTHELIOMA, KAPOSI)

Overview

Angiosarcomas comprise less than 1% of malignant bone tumors. The term really refers to hemangiopericytoma and hemangioendothelioma, but Kaposi sarcoma is included here for completeness. Kaposi sarcoma has become much more prevalent because of the spread of human immunodeficiency virus (HIV) infection and the rising incidence of the acquired immunodeficiency syndrome (AIDS).

Hemangioendothelioma

Definition: Hemangioendothelioma is a true neoplasm of vascular origin, characterized primarily by masses of endothelial cells growing in the vicinity of vascular lumina.

Demographics: Hemangioendothelioma occurs in both sexes and in all age groups (mainly in middle life). It can occur anywhere in the body, but skin lesions are the most common. It is rare in the head and neck, occasionally present in the scalp region, and rarely involves the mandible. The most common bones affected are the long tubular ones.

Signs and symptoms: Hemangioendotheliomas grow rapidly but have an insidious clinical onset with minimal symptoms. Occasionally dull local pain, tenderness, and swelling may be present.

Hemangiopericytoma

Definition: Hemangiopericytomas are rare tumors whose cell of origin is the pericytes.

Demographics: Hemangiopericytomas may metastasize to bone but are very rarely primary in bone. When present in children, they tend to behave benignly, occurring in the subcutis. They may arise wherever capillaries are found. Head and neck lesions account for 25% of cases. They have been reported in patients from birth to 92 years of age, with no sex predilection. They rarely involve the jaw bones, although several cases have been reported. In the mouth they most frequently affect the anterior tongue, floor, and buccal mucosa.

Signs and symptoms: The few patients in whom clinical signs and symptoms have been reported had firm, fixed nonpulsatile swellings. Swelling, long duration before presentation, and absence of pain are characteristic. There are no reliable histologic means of differentiating benign from malignant lesions.

Kaposi Sarcoma

Definition: There are four forms of Kaposi sarcoma: The AIDS-related form; the equatorial African AIDS-related form, which occurs in young men; the classic European form, endemic to older men of Mediterranean ancestry; and the immunosuppression form, occurring after organ transplant. Kaposi sarcoma is an unusual multifocal neoplastic disease of the vasculature.

Signs and symptoms: The presentation is overwhelmingly cutaneous, appearing as raised brown to purple blotches. Kaposi sarcoma is frequently found in the mouth and on the tip of the nose in patients with AIDS.

RADIOLOGIC FEATURES

Cardinal Signs

Solitary or multiple areas of destruction with no distinctive radiographic characteristics

Ancillary Signs

Bone formation rarely seen in osteolytic zones

In low-grade tumors persistent scattered trabeculae with somewhat sharper margins; no internal trabeculae in high-grade tumors

Noncharacteristic soft tissue shadow in soft tissue lesions

Expansion and perforation of cortices

Periosteal new bone formation

Tumor permeation well past radiographic margin

Differential Diagnosis

Alveolar bone loss subsequent to Kaposi sarcoma should be differentiated from advanced localized "AIDS periodontitis," with which it shares many features. This may prove difficult if Kaposi lesions about the region of bone loss.

Angiosarcoma is not readily differentiated from malignant central osseous malignancies when it occurs in bone and is not sufficiently different from squamous cell carcinoma involving bone to differentiate it radiologically.

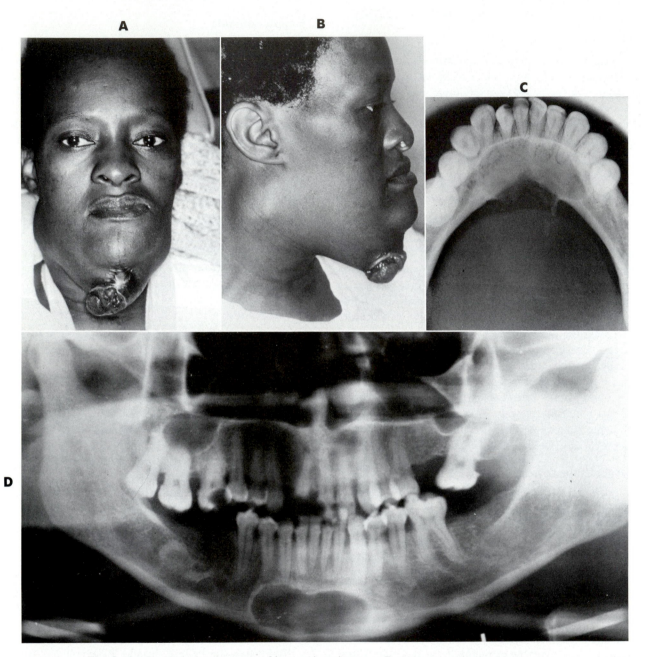

Fig. 9-11 **A,** Clinical appearance of hemangiopericytoma. **B,** Side view of patient in **A.** **C,** True occlusal radiograph of patient in **A.** Hemangiopericytoma showing well-corticated upper margin of lesion with perforation of lingual cortical plate. **D,** Panoramic dental radiograph of patient in **A** showing relatively well-delineated homogeneous radiolucency in midline of mandible. *Continued.*

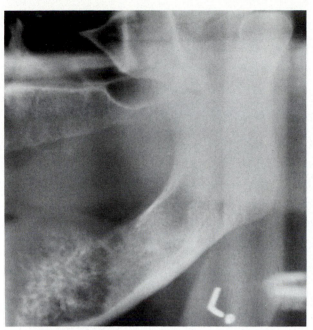

Fig. 9-11, cont'd.   E, Hemangiopericytoma in edentulous mandible. This case shows periosteal new bone formation with "sunray" trabeculations.

PRIMARY CARCINOMA OF THE ORAL CAVITY AND JAWS

Clinical Features

Demographics: Carcinoma is the most common malignancy of the oral cavity. Certain geographic areas of the world have a very high rate of oral cancer. For example, India has a high rate of oral squamous cell carcinoma, and in South China nasopharyngeal carcinoma is prevalent. In the United States, squamous cell carcinoma makes up 4% of all carcinomas in men and 2% in women. Nasopharyngeal carcinoma makes up a scant 0.25% of malignancies among North Americans but accounts for 18% of malignancies in South China. Central carcinomas arising in odontogenic cysts or epithelial cell rests are quite rare compared with oral squamous cell carcinoma invading bone. Central carcinomas may arise in intraosseous glandular tissue, odontogenic cyst lining, embryologically trapped mucous glands, the Tests of Malassez, enamel organ remnants, dentigerous cysts or an ameloblastoma. Primary ameloblastic carcinoma is rarer still.

Eighty-seven percent of oral cancers occur between the ages of 40 and 80 years, although it is not rare in persons younger than 30 years. The mean age at diagnosis for nasopharyngeal carcinoma is 51 years. The use of tobacco is strongly linked to the cause of oral cancer, especially reverse smoking and snuff dipping. Ultraviolet light is also implicated in the development of lip cancer. Paranasal sinus carcinoma has been associated with sinusitis, protracted nasal polyposis, wood dust, and nickel dust. Nasopharyngeal carcinoma is associated with Epstein-Barr virus, chronic rhinosinusitis, poor ventilation, and smoke inhalation.

Signs and symptoms: Primary squamous cell carcinoma is accompanied by erythroplastic lesions with induration and ulceration and eventual spread to regional lymph nodes. Patients with paranasal sinus carcinoma may have pain, paresthesia of involved nerves, swelling, dental pain, loosened maxillary teeth, proptosis, diplopia, trismus, erosion of the palate, and obliteration of the buccal sulcus intraorally. Nasopharyngeal carcinoma may appear as a neck mass or with hearing loss, nasal obstruction, xerophthalmia, facial pain, cranial nerve impingement, or weight loss. Patients may suffer unilateral deafness from eustachian tube involvement.

RADIOLOGIC FEATURES

Cardinal Signs

Ill-defined bone destruction adjacent to intraoral malignant lesion (Invasion of bone may occur in up to 50% of cases.)

Smooth area of bone erosion with a well-defined margin

Combination of the above

Marked alveolar bone loss leading to "floating" teeth

Ancillary Signs

Pathologic fracture with displacement of bone fragments

Increased size of the inferior alveolar nerve canal

Soft tissue mass with underlying bone erosion

Localized increased density beneath a soft tissue mass

Rarely, dental root resorption

If the sinus is involved, sinus cortex possibly not radiographically demonstrable

Possible solitary area of bone destruction with ill-

Text continued on page 311.

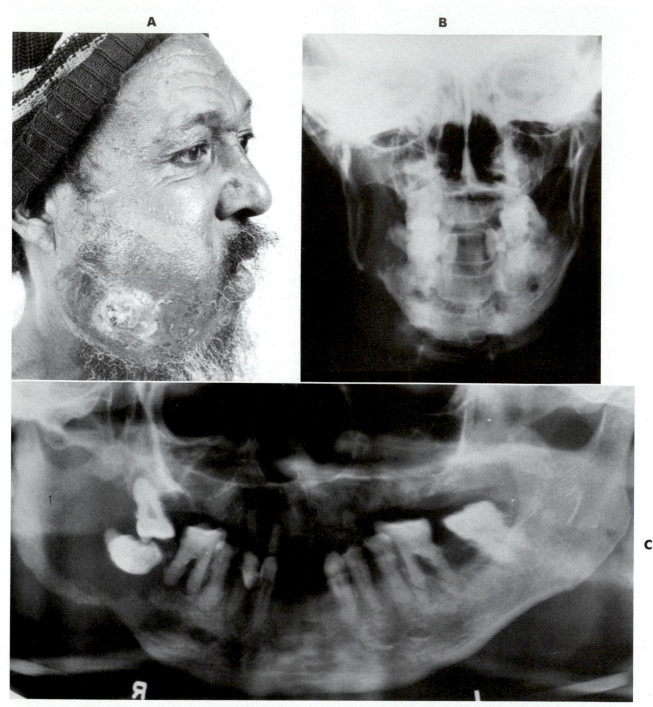

Fig. 9-12 **A,** Squamous carcinoma involving skin of cheek. **B,** Posteroanterior view of patient in **A** showing massive destruction of right mandibular ramus and pathologic fracture. Note "floating" tooth appearance. **C,** Panoramic radiograph of patient in **A** demonstrating "floating" tooth and pathologic fracture in right mandible.   *Continued.*

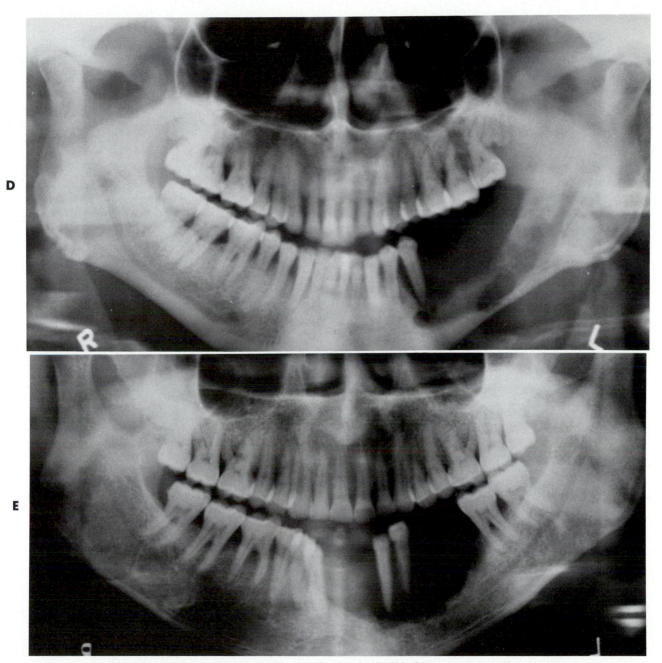

Fig. 9-12, cont'd.   D, Local invasion of left side of mandible from squamous cell carcinoma, with early involvement of ipsilateral maxillary second and third molar region. **E,** Local invasion from squamous cell carcinoma in mandibular anterior and left premolar region.

Continued.

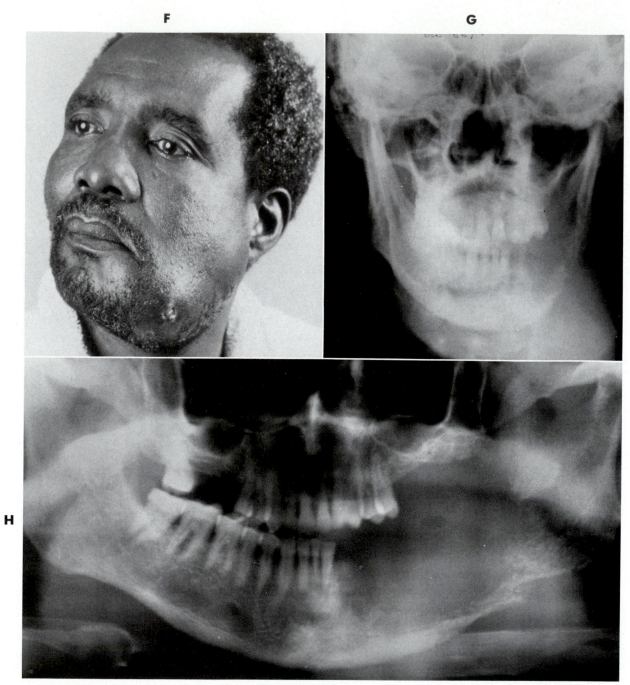

Fig. 9-12, cont'd. **F,** Squamous cell carcinoma. **G,** Posteroanterior view of patient in **F** showing extensive local involvement of left mandible. **H,** Panoramic view of patient in **F.** Note pathologic fracture.   *Continued.*

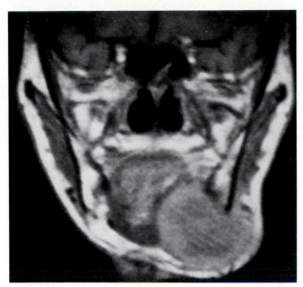

Fig. 9-12, cont'd.   I, T-2 weighted MRI showing carcinoma invading left mandible.

defined border if carcinoma arises intraosseously or if carcinoma affects the buccal or lingual plate

Possible soft tissue shadow appearance of nasopharyngeal carcinoma

Possible bone destruction without remodeling or reshaping with paranasal sinus carcinoma

Periosteal bone production not a feature of oral carcinoma

Paranasal sinus carcinoma possibly affecting the curvature of a sinus wall; destruction of the medial or lateral sinus walls

Sclerosis of the skull base possibly present in nasopharyngeal carcinoma

Differentiation of fluid from tumor possible on MR imaging

Computed tomography and MR imaging possibly useful in demonstrating malignant lymph nodes

Technetium 99methylene diphosphonate possibly useful in demonstrating bone involvement associated with squamous cell carcinoma or metastatic disease

Differential Diagnosis

Carcinomas arising in the bone are not easily differentiated from other central malignancies.

BIBLIOGRAPHY

Osteogenic Sarcoma

Batsakis JG: Osteogenic and chondrogenic sarcomas of the jaws, *Ann Otol Rhinol Laryngol* 96:474, 1987.

Batsakis JG: *Tumors of the head and neck,* ed 2, Baltimore, 1982, Williams & Wilkins, pp 387-390.

Bras JM, et al: Juxta-cortical osteogenic sarcoma of the jaws, *Oral Surg* 50:535, 1980.

Caron AS, Hajdu SI, Strong EW: Osteogenic sarcoma of the facial and cranial bones, *Am J Surg* 122:719, 1971.

Clark JL, et al: Osteosarcoma of the jaw, *Cancer* 51:2311, 1983.

Dahlin DC: *Bone tumors,* ed 3, Springfield, Ill, 1981, Charles C Thomas, pp 226-260.

Forteza G, Colmenero B, Lopez-Barea F: Osteogenic sarcoma of the maxilla and mandible, *Oral Surg* 62:179, 1986.

Gardner DG, Mills DM: The widened periodontal ligament of osteosarcoma of the jaws, *Oral Surg* 41:652, 1976.

Greenfield GB: *Radiology of bone diseases,* ed 3, Philadelphia, 1980, JB Lippincott, pp 530-533.

Greer RO, Mierau GW, Favara BE: *Tumors of the head and neck in children,* New York, 1983, Praeger Scientific, pp 125-133.

Huvos AG: *Bone tumors,* Philadelphia, 1979, WB Saunders, pp 66-74.

Jaffe HL: *Tumors and tumorous conditions of the bone and joints,* Philadelphia, 1958, Lea & Febiger, pp 256-277.

Mendelsohn DB, Hertzanu Y, and Glass RBJ: Computed tomographic findings in primary mandibular osteosarcoma, *Clin Radiol* 34:153, 1983.

Oot RF, Parizel PM, Weber AL: Computed tomography of osteogenic sarcoma of nasal cavity and paranasal sinuses, *J Comput Assist Tomogr* 10:409, 1986.

Present D, Bertoni F, Enneking WF: Osteosarcoma of the mandible arising in fibrous dysplasia, *Clin Orthop* 204:238, 1986.

Rosenmertz SK, Schare HJ: Osteogenic sarcoma arising in Paget's disease of the mandible, *Oral Surg* 28:304, 1969.

Shafer WG, Hine MK, Levy BM: *A textbook of oral pathology,* ed 4, Philadelphia, 1983, WB Saunders.

Som PM, et al: Paget disease of the calvaria and facial bones with an osteosarcoma of the maxilla: CT and MR findings, *J Comput Assist Tomogr* 11:887, 1987.

Spjut HJ, et al: *Tumors of bone and cartilage,* Fascicle 5, Washington, DC, 1983, Armed Forces Institute of Pathology, pp 141-182.

Vener J, Rice DH, Newman AN: Osteosarcoma and chondrosarcoma of the head and neck, *Laryngoscope* 94:240, 1984.

Wood RE, et al: *Handbook of signs in dental and maxillofacial radiology,* Toronto, 1988, Warthog Press.

Worth HM: *Principles and practice of oral radiologic interpretation,* Chicago, 1963, Year Book Medical, pp 563-576.

Yagan R, Radivoyevitch M, Bellon EM: Involvement of the mandibular canal: early sign of osteogenic sarcoma of the mandible, *Oral Surg* 60:56, 1985.

Zarbo RJ, Regezi JA, Baker SR: Periosteal osteogenic sarcoma of the mandible, *Oral Surg* 57:643, 1984.

Chondrosarcoma

Batsakis JG: *Tumors of the head and neck,* ed 2, Baltimore, 1979, Williams & Wilkins, pp 383-387.

Dahlin DC: *Bone tumors,* ed 3, Springfield, Ill, 1981, CC Thomas.

Downey EF, Friedman AC, Finizio J: CT of nasal chondrosarcoma, *AJNR* 3:80, 1982.

Garrington GE, Collett WK: Chondrosarcoma. I. A selected literature review, *J Oral Pathol Med* 17:1, 1988.

Garrington GE, Collett WK: Chondrosarcoma. II. Chondrosarcoma of the jaws: analysis of 37 cases, *J Oral Pathol Med* 17:12, 1988.

Greer RO, Mierau GW, Favara BE: *Tumors of the head and neck in children,* New York, 1983, Praeger, pp 134-142.

Hertzanu Y, et al: Chondrosarcoma of the head and neck: the value of computed tomography, *J Surg Oncol* 28:97, 1985.

Huvos AG: *Bone tumors,* Philadelphia, 1979, WB Saunders, pp 238-241.

Jaffe, HL: *Tumors and tumorous conditions of the bones and joints,* Philadelphia, 1958, Lea & Febiger, pp 317-321.

Shafer WG, Hine MK, Levy BM: *A textbook of oral pathology,* ed 4, Philadelphia, 1983, WB Saunders.

Spjut HJ, et al: *Tumors of bone and cartilage,* Fascicle 5, Washington, DC, 1983, Armed Forces Institute of Pathology, pp 85-116.

Vener J, Rice D, Newman AN: Osteosarcoma and chondrosarcoma of the head and neck, *Laryngoscope* 94:240, 1984.

Wood RE, et al: *Handbook of signs in dental and maxillofacial radiology,* Toronto, 1988, Warthog Press.

Worth HM: *Principles and practice of oral radiologic interpretation,* Chicago, 1963, Year Book Medical, pp 576-578.

Rhabdomyosarcoma

Batsakis JG: *Tumors of the head and neck,* ed 2, Baltimore, 1982, Williams & Wilkins, pp 283-286.

Bras J, Batsakis JG, Luna MA: Rhabdomyosarcoma of the oral soft tissues, *Oral Surg Oral Med Oral Pathol* 64:585, 1987.

Dito WR, Batsakis JG: Rhabdomyosarcoma of the head and neck: an appraisal of the biologic behavior in 170 cases, *Arch Surg* 84:582, 1962.

Greenfield GB: *Radiology of bone diseases,* ed 3, Philadelphia, 1980, JB Lippincott, p 651.

Grieman RB, Katsikeris NK, Symington JM: Rhabdomyosarcoma of the maxillary sinus: review of the literature and report of a case, *J Oral Maxillofac Surg* 46:1090, 1988.

Horn RC, Enterline HT: Rhabdomyosarcoma: a clinicopathological study and classification of 39 cases, *Cancer* 11:181, 1958.

Huvos AG: *Bone tumors,* Philadelphia, 1979, WB Saunders, p 335.

Kurita S, et al: Sarcoma of the maxilla and the maxillary sinus, *Kurume Med J* 29(suppl):S165-S173, 1982.

Lattes R: *Tumors of the soft tissues,* Washington, DC, 1982, Armed Forces Institute of Pathology, pp 169-181.

Masson JK, Soule EH: Embryonal rhabdomyosarcoma of the head and neck: report of 88 cases, *Am J Surg* 110:585, 1965.

O'Day RA, Soule EH, Goresg RJ: Soft tissue sarcomas of the oral cavity, *Mayo Clin Proc* 39:169, 1964.

Shafer WG, Hine MK, Levy B: *A textbook of oral pathology,* ed 4, Philadelphia, 1983, WB Saunders, pp 199-202.

Stobbe GD, Dargeon HW: Embryonal rhabdomyosarcoma of the head and neck in children and adolescents, *Cancer* 3:826, 1950.

Weinblatt ME, Miller JH: Radionuclide scanning in children with rhabdomyosarcoma, *Med Pediatr Oncol* 9:293, 1981.

Wood RE, et al: *Handbook of signs in dental and maxillofacial radiology,* Toronto, 1988, Warthog Press.

Multiple Myeloma

Cotran RS, Kumar V, Robbins S: *Pathologic basis of disease,* ed 4, Philadelphia, 1989, WB Saunders, pp 739-743.

Dahlin DC: *Bone tumors,* ed 3, Springfield, Ill, 1981, Charles C Thomas, pp 159-172.

Epstein JB, Voss NJS, Stevenson-Moore P: Maxillofacial manifestations of multiple myeloma, *Oral Surg* 57:267, 1984.

Greenfield GB: *Radiology of bone diseases,* ed 3, Philadelphia, 1980, JB Lippincott, pp 421-430.

Huvos AG: *Bone tumors,* Philadelphia, 1979, WB Saunders, pp 413-431.

Regezi JA, Sciubba JJ: *Oral pathology clinical-pathologic correlations,* Philadelphia, 1989, WB Saunders, pp 421-424.

Shafer WG, Hine MK, Levy BM: *A textbook of oral pathology,* ed 3, Philadelphia, 1983, WB Saunders, pp 191-194.

Spjut HJ, et al: *Tumors of bone and cartilage,* Fascicle 5, Washington, DC, 1983, Armed Forces Institute of Pathology, pp 201-216.

Worth HM: *Principles and practice of oral radiologic interpretation,* Chicago, 1963, Year Book Medical, pp 582-587.

Leukemia

Cotran RS, Kumar V, Robbins S: *Robbins pathologic basis of disease,* ed 4, Philadelphia, 1989, WB Saunders, pp 722-739.

Ficarra G, et al: Granulocytic sarcoma (chloroma) of the oral cavity: a case with aleukemic presentation, *Oral Surg Oral Med Oral Pathol* 63:709, 1987.

Greenfield, GB: *Radiology of bone diseases,* ed 3, Philadelphia, 1980, JB Lippincott, pp 454-464.

Greer RO, Mierau GW, Favara BE: *Tumors of the head and neck in children,* New York, 1983, Praeger Scientific, pp 294-298.

Huvos AG: *Bone tumors,* Philadelphia, 1979, WB Saunders, pp 403-406.

Spjut HJ, et al: *Tumors of bone and cartilage,* Washington, DC, 1983, Armed Forces Institute of Pathology, pp 381-387.

Wood RE, et al: *Handbook of signs in dental and maxillofacial radiology,* Toronto, 1988, Warthog Press.

Worth HM: *Principles and practice of oral radiologic interpretation,* Chicago, 1963, Year Book Medical, pp 370-372, 587.

Ewing Sarcoma

Batsakis JG: *Tumors of the head and neck,* ed 2, Baltimore, 1982, Williams & Wilkins, pp 454-460.

Cotran RS, Kumar V, and Robbins SL: *Robbins pathologic basis of disease,* ed 4, Philadelphia, 1989, WB Saunders, pp 248-249.

Dahlin DC: *Bone tumors,* ed 3, Springfield, Ill, 1981, Charles C Thomas, pp 274-284.

Greenfield GB: *Radiology of bone disease,* ed 3, Philadelphia, 1980, JB Lippincott, pp 548-554.

Greer RO, Mierau GW, Favara BE: *Tumors of the head and neck in children,* New York, 1983, Praeger, pp 157-161.

Huvos AG: *Bone tumors,* Philadelphia, 1979, WB Saunders, pp 322-344.

Jaffe HL: *Tumors and tumorous conditions of the bones and joints,* Philadelphia, 1958, Lea & Febiger, pp 350-368.

Regezi, JA, Sciubba JJ: *Oral pathology,* Philadelphia, 1989, WB Saunders, pp 417-419.

Shafer WG, Hine MK, Levy B: *A textbook of oral pathology,* ed 4, Philadelphia, 1983, WB Saunders, pp 188-189.

Spjut HJ, et al: *Tumors of bone and cartilage,* Washington, DC, 1983, Armed Forces Institute of Pathology, pp 216-229.

Wood RE, et al: Ewing's sarcoma, *Oral Surg Oral Med Oral Pathol* 69:120, 1990.

Wood RE, et al: *Handbook of signs in dental and maxillofacial radiology,* Toronto, 1988, Warthog.

Worth HM: *Principles and practice of oral radiologic interpretation,* Chicago, 1963, Year Book Medical, pp 580-581.

Burkitt Lymphoma

Adatia AK: Radiology of Burkitt's tumor in the jaws, *East Afr Med J* 43:290, 1966.

Adatia AK: Significance of jaw lesions in Burkitt's lymphoma, *Br Dent J* 145:263, 1978.

Batsakis JG: *Tumors of the head and neck,* ed 2, Baltimore, 1982, Williams & Wilkins, pp 452-453.

Burkitt D: A sarcoma involving the jaws in African children, *Br J Surg* 46:218, 1958.

Cotran RS, Kumar V, Robbins SL: *Robbins pathologic basis of disease,* ed 4, Philadelphia, 1989, WB Saunders, pp 715-722.

Greenfield GB: *Radiology of bone disease,* ed 3, Philadelphia, 1980, JB Lippincott, pp 464-466.

Huvos AG: *Bone tumors,* Philadelphia, 1979, WB Saunders, pp 399-400.

Levine PH, et al: The American Burkitt's lymphoma registry: eight years experience, *Cancer* 49:1016, 1982.

Regezi JA, Sciubba JJ: *Oral pathology,* Philadelphia, 1989, WB Saunders, pp 419-421.

Sariban E, Donahue A, Magrath IT: Jaw involvement in American Burkitt's lymphoma, *Cancer* 53:1777, 1984.

Shafer WG, Hine MK, Levy B: *A textbook of oral pathology,* ed 4, Philadelphia, 1983, WB Saunders, pp 188-189.

Wood RE, et al: *Handbook of signs in dental and maxillofacial radiology,* Toronto, 1988, Warthog.

Hodgkin Disease

Batsakis JG: *Tumors of the head and neck,* ed 2, Baltimore, 1982, Williams & Wilkins, pp 454-460.

Cotran RS, Kumar V, and Robbins SL: *Robbins pathologic basis of disease,* ed 4, Philadelphia, 1989, WB Saunders, pp 248-249.

Dahlin DC: *Bone tumors,* ed 3, Springfield, Ill, 1981, Charles C Thomas, pp 174-176.

Greenfield GB: *Radiology of bone diseases,* ed 3, Philadelphia, 1980, JB Lippincott, pp 610-611.

Greer RO, Mierau GW, Favara BE: *Tumors of the head and neck in children,* New York, 1983, Praeger, pp 302-303.

Huvos AG: *Bone tumors,* ed 3, Philadelphia, 1979, WB Saunders, pp 406-410.

Jaffe HL: *Tumors and tumorous conditions of the bones and joints,* Philadelphia, 1958, Lea & Febiger, pp 407-410.

Regezi JA, Sciubba JJ: *Oral pathology,* Philadelphia, 1989, WB Saunders, pp 287-290.

Shafer WG, Hine MK, Levy B: *A textbook of oral pathology,* ed 4, Philadelphia, 1983, WB Saunders, pp 189-191.

Spjut HJ, et al: *Tumors of bone and cartilage,* Fascicle 5, Washington, DC, 1983, Armed Forces Institute of Pathology, p 385.

Wood RE, et al: *Handbook of signs in dental and maxillofacial radiology,* Toronto, 1988, Warthog Press.

Worth HM: *Principles and practice of oral radiologic interpretation,* Chicago, 1963, Year Book Medical, pp 587-590.

Non-Hodgkin Lymphoma

Baker CG, Tichler JM: Malignant disease in the jaws, *Can Assoc Radiol J* 28:129, 1977.

Batsakis JG: *Tumors of the head and neck,* ed 2, Baltimore, 1982, Williams & Wilkins, pp 414-416.

Cotran RS, Kumar V, Robbins SL: *Robbins pathologic basis of disease,* ed 4, Philadelphia, 1989, WB Saunders, pp 708-722.

Dahlin DC: *Bone tumors,* ed 3, Springfield, Ill, 1981, Charles C Thomas, pp 173-189.

Greenfield GB: *Radiology of bone disease,* ed 3, Philadelphia, 1980, JB Lippincott, pp 390, 414.

Greer RO, Mierau GW, Favara BE: Tumors of the head and neck in children, New York, 1983, Praeger, pp 302-304.

Huvos AG: *Bone tumors,* Philadelphia, 1979, WB Saunders, pp 392-402.

Jaffe JL: *Tumors and tumorous conditions of the bones and joints,* Philadelphia, 1958, Lea & Febiger, pp 415-424.

Regezi JA, Sciubba JJ: *Oral pathology,* Philadelphia, 1989, WB Saunders. pp 290-297.

Shafer WG, Hine MK, Levy BM: *A textbook of oral pathology,* ed 4, Philadelphia, 1983, WB Saunders, pp 184-188.

Spjut HJ, et al: *Tumors of bone and cartilage,* Washington, DC, 1983, Armed Forces Institute of Pathology, pp 381-387.

Wong DS, et al: Extranodal non-Hodgkin's lymphoma of the head and neck, *AJR* 123:471, 1975.

Wood RE, et al: *Handbook of signs in dental and maxillofacial radiology,* Toronto, 1988, Warthog.

Worth HM: *Principles and practice of oral radiologic interpretation,* Chicago, 1963, Year Book Medical, pp 591-592.

Metastatic Disease to the Jaws

Appenzeller J, Weitzner S, Long GW: Hepatocellular carcinoma metastatic to the mandible: report of a case and review of literature, *J Oral Maxillofac Surg* 29:668, 1971.

Batsakis JG: *Tumors of the head and neck,* ed 2, Baltimore, 1982, Williams & Wilkins, pp 240-250.

Buchner A, Ramon Y: Distant metastases to the jaws: report of four cases, *J Oral Maxillofac Surg* 25:246, 1967.

Carl W: Metastatic cancers in the mouth, *Compend Contin Educ Dent VII,* 1986.

Ciola B: Oral radiographic manifestations of a metastatic prostatic carcinoma, *Oral Surg* 52:105, 1981.

Cohen D, et al: Maxillary metastases of a transitional cell carcinoma: report of a case, *Oral Surg Oral Med Oral Pathol* 67:185, 1989.

Cotran RS, Kumar V, Robbins SL: *Robbins pathologic basis of disease,* ed 4, Philadelphia, 1989, WB Saunders, pp 248-249.

Curtin J: Mandibular metastases from a primary adenocarcinoma of the fallopian tube, *J Oral Maxillofac Surg* 43:636, 1985.

Dahlin DC: *Bone tumors,* ed 3, Springfield, Ill, 1981, Charles C Thomas, pp 356-357.

Draper BW, et al: Follicular thyroid carcinoma metastatic to the mandible, *J Oral Maxillofac Surg* 37:736, 1979.

Greenfield GB: *Radiology of bone diseases,* ed 3, Philadelphia, 1980, JB Lippincott, pp 380, 390, 402, 410.

Hashimoto N, et al: Pathological characteristics of metastatic carcinoma in the human mandible, *J Oral Pathol Med* 16:362, 1987.

Jaffe HL: *Tumors and tumorous conditions of the bones and joints,* Philadelphia, 1958, Lea & Febiger, pp 407-410.

Mast HL, Nissenblatt MJ: Metastatic colon carcinoma to the jaw: a case report and review of the literature, *J Surg Oncol* 34:202, 1987.

Mucitelli Dr, Zuna RE, Archard HO: Hepatocellular carcinoma presenting as an oral cavity lesion, *Oral Surg Oral Med Oral Pathol* 66:701, 1988.

Nevins A, et al: Metastatic carcinoma of the mandible mimicking periapical lesion of endodontic origin, *Endod Dent Traumatol* 4:238, 1988.

Nishimura Y, et al: Metastatic thyroid carcinoma of the mandible, *J Oral Maxillofac Surg* 40:221, 1982.

Redman RS, Behrens AS, Calhoun NR: Carcinoma of the lung presenting as a mandibular metastasis, *J Oral Maxillofac Surg* 40:745, 1982.

Regezi JA, Sciubba JJ: *Oral pathology,* Philadelphia, 1989, WB Saunders, pp 424-425.

Shafer WG, Hine MK, Levy BM: *A textbook of oral pathology,* ed 4, Philadelphia, 1983, WB Saunders, pp 213-215.

Spjut HJ, et al: *Tumors of bone and cartilage,* Fascicle 5, Washington, DC, 1983, Armed Forces Institute of Pathology, pp 367-378.

Vigneul JC, et al: Metastatic hepatocellular carcinoma of the mandible, *J Oral Maxillofac Surg* 40:745, 1982.

Wood RE, et al: *Handbook of signs in dental and maxillofacial radiology,* Toronto, 1988, Warthog.

Yagan R, Bellon EM, Radivoyevitch M: Breast carcinoma metastatic to the mandible mimicking ameloblastoma, *Oral Surg* 57:189, 1984.

Angiosarcomas

Austermann KH, et al: Klinishce, rontegenologisch un histomorphologische aspekte des haemangioperizytoms in Kopf-Hals-Bereich, *Dtsch Zahn* 31:257, 1976.

Batsakis JG: *Tumors of the head and neck,* Baltimore, 1982, Williams & Wilkins, pp 473-475.

Cotran RS, Kumar V, Robbins S: *Robbins pathologic basis of disease,* ed 4, Philadelphia, 1989, WB Saunders, pp 590-592, 1291-1292.

Dahlin DC: *Bone tumors,* ed 3, Springfield, Ill, 1981, Charles C Thomas, pp 344-355.

Greenfield GB: *Radiology of bone diseases,* ed 3, Philadelphia, 1980, JB Lippincott, p 609.

Greer RO, Mierau GW, Favara BE: *Tumors of the head and neck in children,* New York, 1983, Praeger, pp 382-385.

Gupta OP, Jain RK, Gupta S: Hemangiopericytoma of the head and neck, *Ear Nose Throat J* 64:76, 1985.

Huvos AG: *Bone tumors,* Philadelphia, 1979, WB Saunders, pp 358-372.

Kwon HJ, et al: Haemangiopericytoma of the tongue: report of a case, *J Am Dent Assoc* 109:583, 1984.

Powell DB, SLE OW: Unusual sinus tumors, *Tex Med J* 59:690, 1963.

Sage HH, Salman I: Malignant hemangiopericytome in the area of a previous ameloblastoma of the mandible, *J Oral Maxillofac Surg* 26:275, 1968.

Unni KK, et al: Hemangioma, hemangiopericytoma and hemangioendothelialoma (angiosarcoma) of bone, *Cancer* 27:1403, 1971.

Vilasco J, et al: Un cas d'hémangiopéricitome mandibulaire, *Rev Stomat* (Paris) 71:50, 1970.

Wood RE, et al: Haemangiopericytoma of the mandible: review of the literature and report of an intra-osseous case, *Dentomaxillofac Radiol* 17:133, 1988.

Wood RE, et al: *Handbook of signs in dental and maxillofacial radiology,* Toronto, 1988, Warthog.

Primary Carcinoma of the Oral Cavity and Jaws

Baker CG, Tishler JM: Malignant disease in the jaws, *Can Assoc Radiol J* 26:129, 1977.

Batsakis JG: *Tumors of the head and neck,* Baltimore, 1982, Williams & Wilkins, pp 144-199, 416, 560.

Myers EN: *Cancer of the head and neck,* ed 2, New York, 1989, Churchill Livingstone, pp 311-508.

Noyek AM, et al: The radiologic diagnosis of malignant tumors of the paranasal sinuses and related structures, *J Otolaryngol* 6:399, 1977.

Regezi JA, Sciubba JJ: *Oral pathology,* Philadelphia, 1989, WB Saunders, pp 70-83, 346.

Schaefer SD, et al: Magnetic resonance imaging vs computed tomography, *Arch Otolaryngol Head Neck Surg* 111:730, 1985.

Shafer WG, Hine MK, Levy BM: *A textbook of oral pathology,* ed 4, Philadelphia, 1983, WB Saunders, pp 112-127.

Valvassori GE, et al: *Radiology of the ear, nose, and throat,* Philadelphia, 1982, WB Saunders, pp 193-209, 260-266.

Virapongse C, Mancuso A, Fitzsimmons J: Value of magnetic resonance imaging in assessing bone destruction in head and neck lesions, *Laryngoscope* 96:284, 1986.

Watkinson JC, Maisey MN: Imaging head and neck cancer using radioisotopes: a review, *J R Soc Med* 81:653, 1988.

Whitehouse GH: Radiological bone changes produced by intraoral squamous carcinomata involving the lower alveolus, *Clin Otolaryngol* 1:45, 1976.

Wood RE, et al: *Handbook of signs in dental and maxillofacial radiology,* Toronto, 1988, Warthog.

Worth HM: *Principles and practice of oral radiologic interpretation,* Chicago, 1963, Year Book Medical, pp 549-558.

10

FIBRO-OSSEOUS LESIONS

FIBROUS DYSPLASIA

Overview

Definition: In fibrous dysplasia, normal medullary bone is replaced by fibrous tissue. It can affect just one bone (monostotic) or multiple bones (polyostotic). When multiple bones in the head and neck region only are affected, it is termed *craniofacial*. Occasionally, fibrous dysplasia is found in association with a variety of endocrine conditions, including precocious puberty in females (Albright syndrome).

Pathogenesis: The condition is idiopathic; it may represent a nonneoplastic, hamartomatous growth of mesenchymal elements. No hereditary basis for fibrous dysplasia has been found.

Clinical Features

Demographics: Monostotic fibrous dysplasia accounts for about 80% of all cases, and jaw involvement is common, especially the maxilla. The long bones and ribs are also commonly affected. The sexes are equally affected.

Symptoms and signs: Patients with fibrous dysplasia have painless, slow, and progressive enlargement of the affected bone during childhood or adolescence. When the jaws are affected, there is gradually increasing facial asymmetry. Buccal swelling is more common than lingual expansion. There may be consequential spacing of the teeth and malocclusion. Growth tends to cease in the late teens. Skin pigmentation (cafe au lait macules) is found in Albright syndrome.

Laboratory tests: Serum calcium, phosphorus, and alkaline phosphatase levels are within the normal range.

RADIOLOGIC FEATURES

Cardinal Signs

Initially radiolucent, either unilocular or multilocular

Mottled radiopacity in intermediate stage

Densely radiopaque with time

"Ground glass" (frosted glass) appearance on extraoral radiographs.

"Orange peel" *(peau d'orange)* appearance with the higher resolution of intraoral radiographs

Imperceptible merging with surrounding normal bone during radiopaque phase (cf. ossifying fibroma, which has a well-demarcated/"encapsulated" margin)

Ancillary Signs

Fusiform rather than spheroidal outline

Differential Diagnosis

Ossifying fibroma

Paget disease of bone

Florid osseous dysplasia

Osteopetrosis

Pyknodysostosis

Oculodentoosseous dysplasia

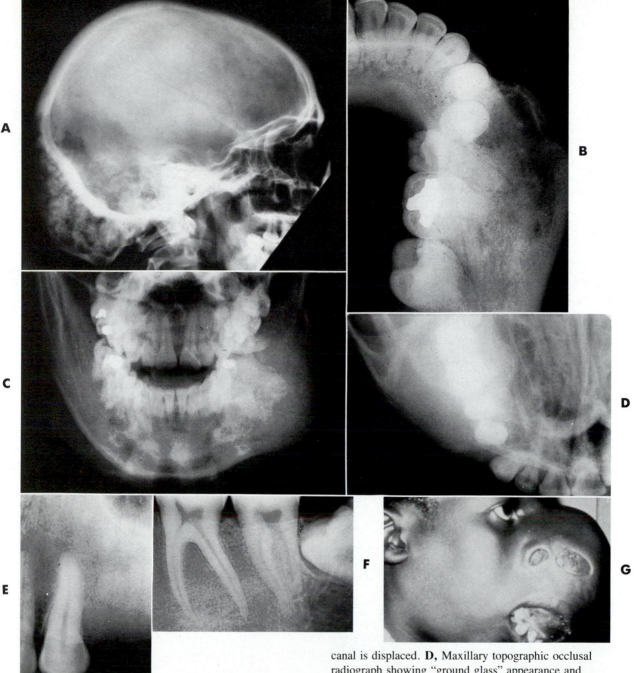

Fig. 10-1 **A,** Lateral skull radiograph showing fibrous dysplasia in occipital region. Note enlargement of affected area and presence of granular opacities and radiolucent components of the lesion. **B,** Buccal expansion of mandible seen on occlusal radiograph. The lesion merges imperceptibly with the surrounding normal bone. **C,** Posteroanterior view of same patient as in **B.** This lesion has a typical "ground glass" appearance and merges imperceptibly with the surrounding bone. The expansion is fusiform and exclusively buccally directed. The mandibular canal is displaced. **D,** Maxillary topographic occlusal radiograph showing "ground glass" appearance and predominantly buccal expansion from late-stage fibrous dysplasia. **E,** Intraoral periapical radiograph showing "orange peel" appearance of fibrous dysplasia in the left maxillary canine/premolar region. **F,** Intraoral periapical radiograph of mandibular molar region showing "orange peel" trabeculation in patient with fibrous dysplasia. Note the change to a normal trabecular pattern anterior to the unerupted third molar. The lesion merges imperceptibly with surrounding bone rather than having a discrete margin. **G,** Facial asymmetry can be marked in fibrous dysplasia.
Continued.

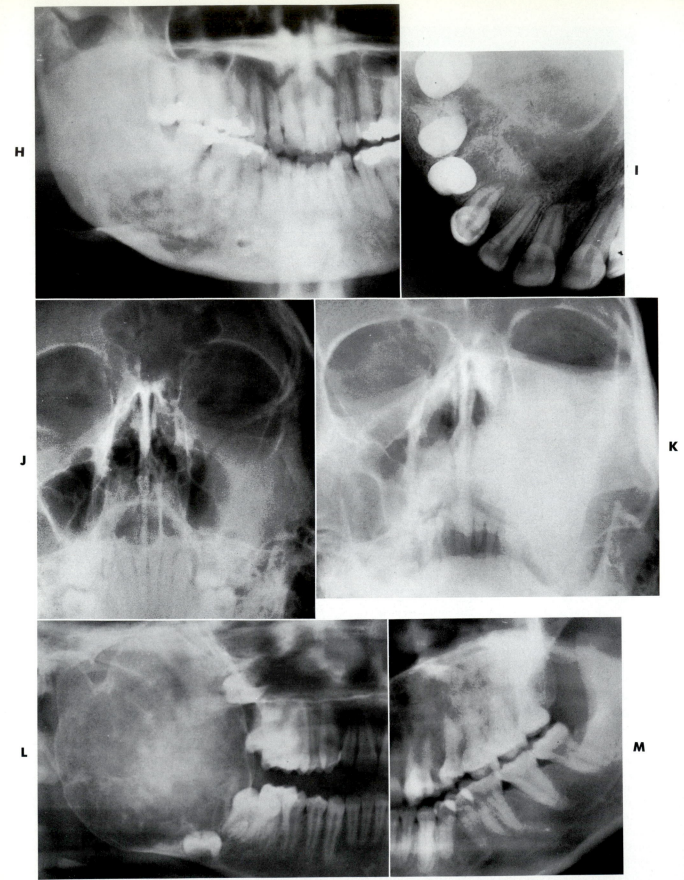

For legend see opposite page.

FLORID OSSEOUS DYSPLASIA (GIGANTIFORM CEMENTOMA)

Overview

Definition: Florid osseous dysplasia is an idiopathic progressive patchy sclerosis of the jaws found predominantly in black women aged 25 years and older.

Pathogenesis: The disease is idiopathic in most cases, though a familial pattern is sometimes present.

Clinical Features

Demographics: Women, particularly black women, are more frequently affected than men. Close to 90% of cases involve the mandible, and nearly 60% involve all four jaw quadrants. The premolar region is the most commonly affected.

Symptoms and signs: Florid osseous dysplasia is usually asymptomatic unless secondary osteomyelitis or chronic diffuse sclerosing osteomyelitis is superimposed. The condition is generally found incidentally during radiographic examination of the jaws.

Laboratory tests: Serologic levels are within the normal range. Histologic examination shows solid calcified masses with few cellular inclusions.

Opposite page. Fig. 10-1, cont'd.　H, Cropped panoramic radiograph showing fibrous dysplasia of right mandible. Note patchy increased mineralization and enlargement of the affected segment. The outlines of the teeth are less clearly seen through the dysplastic mass. **I,** Topographic occlusal radiograph showing mild fibrous dysplasia in right maxilla. **J,** Waters view demonstrating fibrous dysplasia of left maxilla, which causes smoothly outlined radiopacity of maxilla to be superimposed over maxillary sinus on affected side. **K,** Fibrous dysplasia of left maxilla. The lesion is restricted to one bone and does not cross the midline. This lesion has displaced the floor of the orbit and left lateral wall of the nasal passage. **L,** Panoramic radiograph showing fibrous dysplasia of right mandibular ramus at the intermediate stage of maturation (mixed radiolucency/radiopacity). The mandibular condyle is spared but the coronoid process is greatly expanded. The ipsilateral third molar is displaced towards the lower border of the mandible. **M,** Cropped panoramic radiograph showing fibrous dysplasia of left maxilla. The lesion is radiopaque with some radiolucent mottling.

RADIOLOGIC FEATURES

Cardinal Signs

Multiple sclerotic masses

Pagetoid cotton wool appearance

Occasionally, a thin radiolucent band at the periphery of sclerotic masses

Eventual coalescence of masses to form a single lobulated diffuse mass

"Ground glass" appearance of alveolar bone with loss of detail of periodontal ligament spaces.

Ancillary Signs

Generally, zone of normal bone between lesions and cortex of mandibular lower border

Extension of lesions to surface of mandibular edentulous ridge

Slight jaw expansion in some cases

Mixed radiolucency/radiopacity similar to a benign tumor in patients with concurrent traumatic bone cyst. (Such cysts are much more common in patients with florid osseous dysplasia than in the general population.)

Sequestration of sclerotic masses in some edentulous patients, particularly those with complicating chronic osteomyelitis

Uncommonly, tooth displacement

Differential Diagnosis

Paget disease of bone

Fibrous dysplasia

Enostosis/osteoma

Gardner syndrome

Osteopetrosis

Pyknodysostosis

Oculodentoosseous dysplasia

Ossifying/cementifying fibroma

Condensing osteitis

Chronic diffuse sclerosing osteomyelitis

PERIAPICAL CEMENTAL DYSPLASIA (CEMENTOMA, PERIAPICAL OSSEOUS DYSPLASIA)

Overview

Definition: Periapical cemental dysplasia consists of multiple reactive lesions in the periapical bone, most frequently associated with mandibular permanent incisor teeth.

Pathogenesis: The condition is idiopathic.

Text continued on page 324.

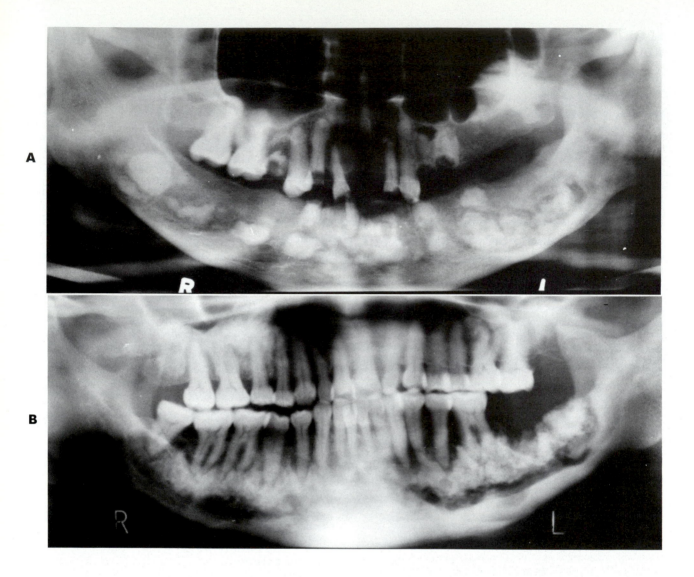

Fig. 10-2, above. **A,** Panoramic radiograph showing "cotton wool" radiopacities throughout the body of the mandible, largely above the mandibular canal. Some of the lesions are surrounded by a thin radiolucent margin. Sclerotic masses are also seen in the left maxilla; however, these are associated with retained dental roots. The mental foramina are unaffected. **B,** Panoramic radiograph showing fused sclerotic masses in all four quadrants. The periodontal ligament spaces are clearly demonstrated. In the mandible, the lesions are primarily positioned above the mandibular canal.

Opposite page. **C,** Panoramic radiograph showing sclerotic masses in all four quadrants. The mass in the anterior mandible has resulted in enlargement of the jaw. This mass is confluent with more typical lesions of florid osseous dysplasia in the posterior segments of the body of the mandible. **D,** Lateral radiograph of lesion shown in **C.** Note expansion of jawbone in anterior mandible. **E,** Intraoral photograph of florid osseous dysplasia in maxilla showing expansion of jaw. Serologic findings were within normal limits. **F,** Panoramic radiograph showing diffuse sclerotic mass in left maxilla (same case as **E**).

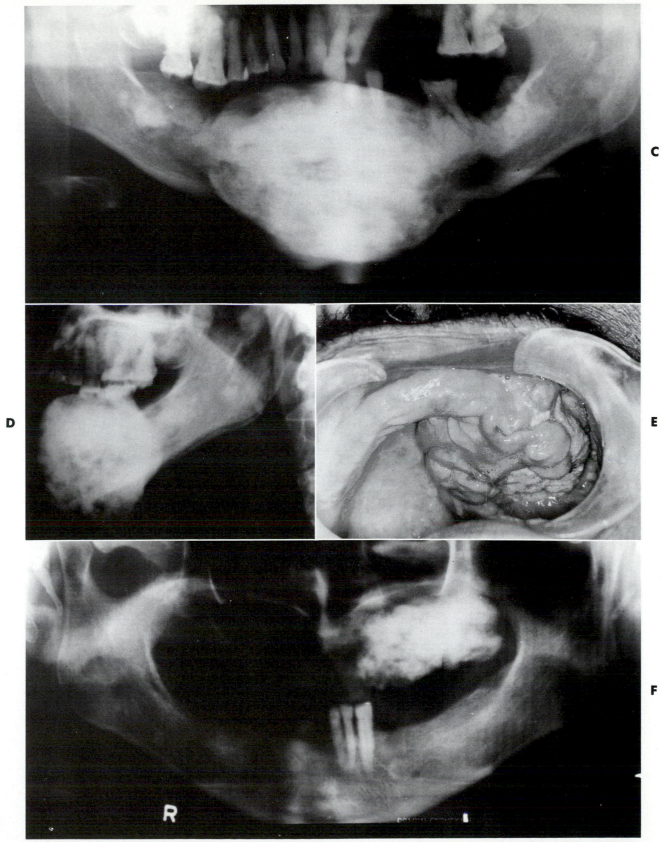

C

D

E

F

Continued.

G

H

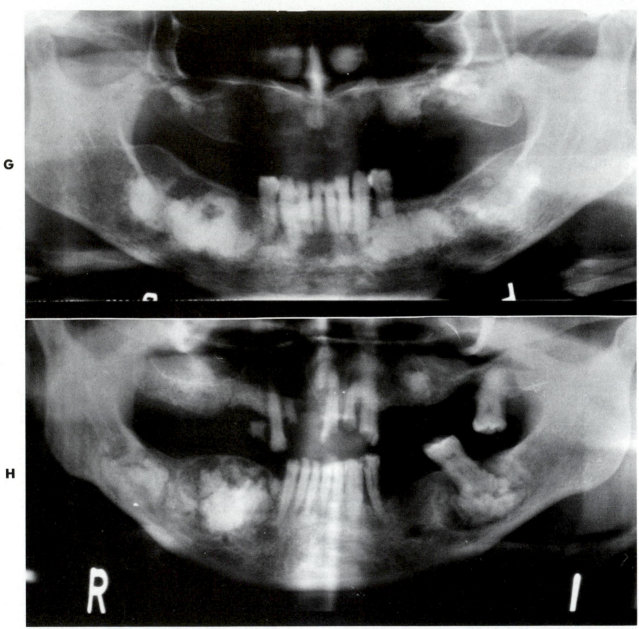

For legend see opposite page.
Continued.

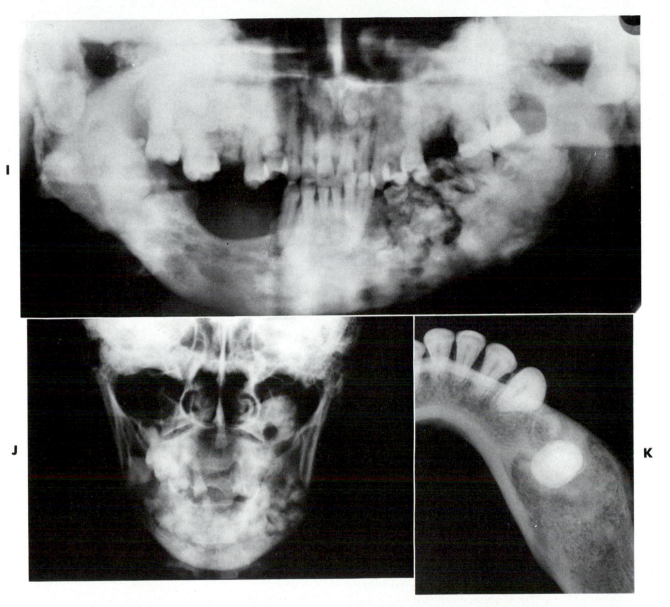

Fig. 10-2, cont'd. Opposite page.   G, Panoramic radiograph showing diffuse sclerotic lesions in all four quadrants of the jaws. **H,** Panoramic radiograph showing sclerotic masses surrounded by radiolucent margins in mandible. Note expansion of the premolar region of the right side of the mandible.

Above.   I, Panoramic radiograph showing extensive florid osseous dysplasia in both jaws. Secondary osteomyelitis in the left mandible results in a mixed radiolucency/ radiopacity. **J,** Posteroanterior radiograph showing sclerotic masses in all four jaw quadrants. **K,** Mandibular occlusal radiograph showing patchy sclerosis in premolar region. The jaw is somewhat expanded; however, the sclerotic masses do not reach the mandibular cortex.

A   **B**   **C**

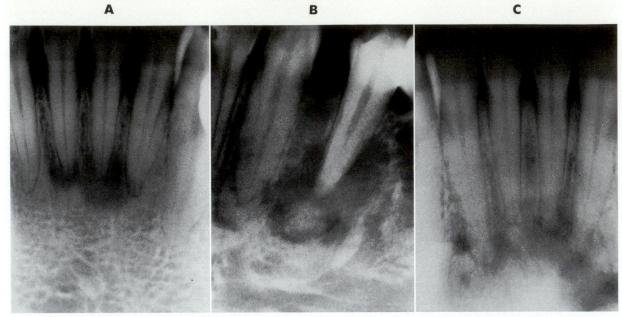

Fig. 10-3   A, Stage I periapical cemental dysplasia. The teeth are intact, as are the periodontal ligament spaces. Periapical radiolucencies have smooth outlines without a sclerotic rim. **B,** Target lesion (stage II) below premolar tooth. This lesion has a sclerotic rim at its deep margin, but no such margin more superficially. The lesion beneath the canine tooth is stage III, i.e., homogeneously radiopaque except for a radiolucent outline. Note that the periodontal ligament space is intact. **C,** Periapical radiolucencies of adjacent teeth are fused and there are patchy "cotton wool" calcifications.

Clinical Features

Demographics: Periapical cemental dysplasia is most common in Black women around middle age (40 years). It is rarely seen before age 20 years.

Symptoms and signs: The condition is usually found incidentally during radiography of the teeth and jaws. Stage I lesions are radiolucent. The periodontal ligament space is intact and the teeth are vital to pulp testing. No treatment is necessary, so it is important to differentiate between stage I lesions and apical radiolucencies of inflammatory origin. In time the lesions calcify, first being mixed radiolucent/radiopaque (stage II), and then radiopaque (stage III).

Laboratory tests: Serologic testing is within the normal range. Histologic examination shows active fibrous tissue with calcifications resembling the active stages of fibrous dysplasia. (N.B.: Histologic evaluation is not required to diagnose this condition; radiology and vitality testing of the teeth are sufficient.

RADIOLOGIC FEATURES

Cardinal Signs

Stage I: Radiolucencies associated with apices of teeth (usually anterior mandibular teeth)

Intact periodontal ligament space

Noncorticated, smooth outline

Stage II: "Cotton wool" radiopacity within the apical radiolucencies with a "targetlike" appearance.

Stage III: Radiopaque lesion; Fusion of lesions from adjacent teeth gives superficial appearance of florid osseous dysplasia

Ancillary Signs

Sclerotic rim around lesions in some cases, particularly at lower borders

Differential Diagnosis

Multiple periapical cysts, granulomas, or abscesses

Condensing osteitis

Florid osseous dysplasia

PAGET DISEASE OF BONE (OSTEITIS DEFORMANS)

Overview

Definition: Paget disease is a chronic, slowly progressive disease of bone in which there is abnormal resorption and deposition, leading eventually to sclerosis and expansion of affected bones. The disease can be divided into three stages: (1) initial bone resorptive phase, (2) vascular phase with osteoblastic repair, and (3) appositional/sclerosing phase.

Pathogenesis: The condition is idiopathic. Postulated causes have included autoimmunity, hyperthyroidism, inborn error of connective tissue metabolism, autonomic-mediated vascular defect, paramyxovirus infection, and slow virus infection.

Clinical Features

Demographics: The condition is common in the elderly and has been estimated to occur in about 1% of the population. The jaws are involved in approximately one in five cases, with the maxilla being affected about twice as frequently as the mandible.

Signs and symptoms: During the initial phase of bone resorption, the affected bones may be deformed or painful, particularly the weight-bearing structures such as the long bones of the legs. Later the affected bones expand; this is common in the maxilla, mandible, or skull. At this stage the dental patient who wears full dentures may complain that the fit of the dentures is becoming progressively worse; hat sizes may also become progressively larger. When the maxilla is affected, the alveolar ridge widens and the palatal vault can flatten. When teeth are present, they may become increasingly spaced. With extensive jaw enlargement it may become impossible to close the mouth fully.

Neurologic complaints can result from increased deposition of bone in the areas of the foramina of the skull, namely headaches, auditory disorders progressing to deafness, visual disorders progressing to blindness, facial paresis, and vertigo.

In the latter stages the bone, which is increased in density, is like unreinforced concrete, the marrow in normal bone being like the steel in reinforced concrete. The bones are relatively brittle; hence, fractures are likely.

Osteogenic sarcoma is well documented as a complication of Paget disease, occurring in 1% to 15% of cases in reported series.

Laboratory tests: Serum alkaline phosphatase level is markedly elevated. Urinary calcium and hydroxyproline levels are also increased. Histopathologic examination shows haphazard resorption and deposition of bone, with osteoblastic and osteoclastic activity often noted side by side. Eventually, bone deposition exceeds resorption and "marble bone," with sparse marrow and multiple reversal lines, results. Biopsy of lesions can be risky, with abnormal vascular patterns carrying the potential for hemorrhage and reduced marrow predisposing to infection.

RADIOLOGIC FEATURES

Cardinal Signs

Patchy osteoporosis in early stages (osteoporosis circumscripta)

Generalized radiolucency/osteoporosis

Intermediate stage with mixed radiolucency/radiopacity

"Driven snow" coarse trabeculation

"Cotton wool" radiopacities in final stage

Enlarged bones

Affects the whole of an involved bone

Ancillary Signs

Fractures of weight-bearing bones

Hypercementosis

Loss of lamina dura and obliteration of periodontal ligament spaces

External root resorption

Positive radionuclide scans for affected bones (technetium 99 methylene diphosphonate)

Differential Diagnosis

Acromegaly

Florid osseous dysplasia

Sclerosing osteomyelitis

Fibrous dysplasia

Osteopetrosis

Pyknodysostosis

Oculodentoosseous dysplasia

Periostitis ossificans

Osteogenic sarcoma

Hyperparathyroidism

Hypoparathyroidism

Thalassemia

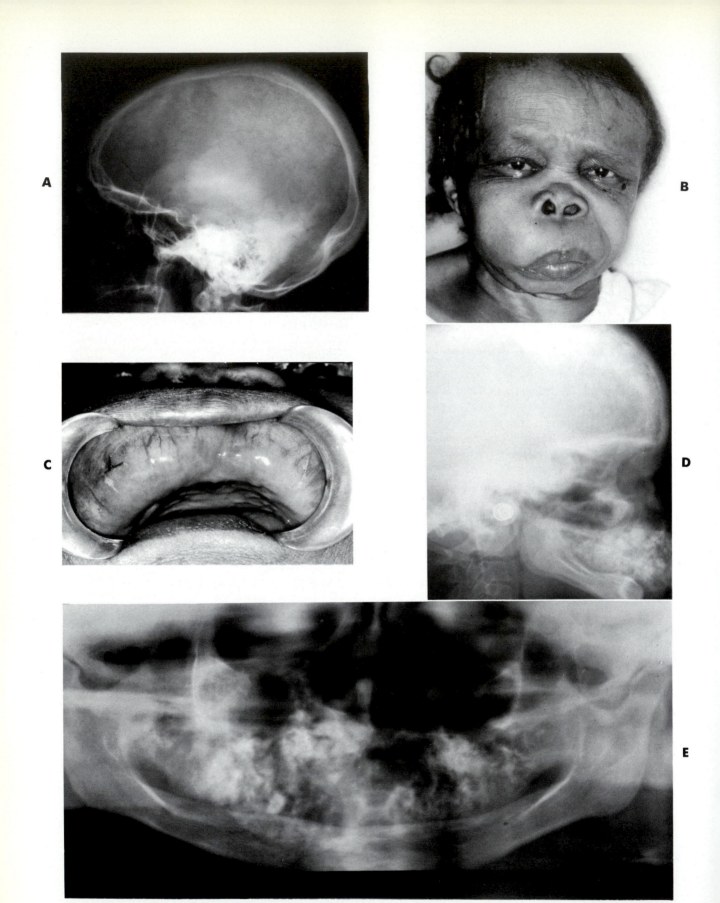

Continued.

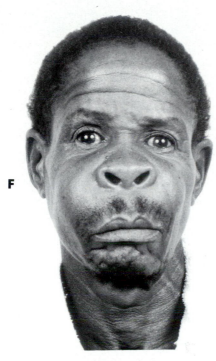

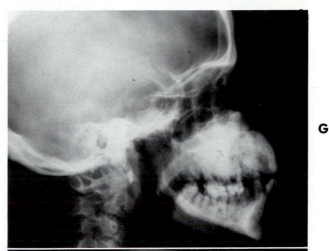

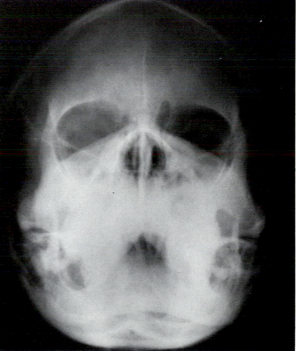

G

H

Fig. 10-4, opposite page. **A,** Lateral skull radiograph showing osteoporosis imperfecta in anterior and posterior parts of skull, along with thickening of calvarium in cranial vault. **B,** Clinical features of Paget disease affecting the maxilla. Unlike fibrous dysplasia, Paget disease crosses the midline when the maxilla is involved. **C,** Same patient as in **B.** Intraoral examination reveals a widened alveolar ridge and flattening of the palate. **D,** Same patient as in **B.** "Cotton wool" radiopacities are seen in the expanded maxilla and in the frontal region of the skull. **E,** Panoramic radiograph showing mixed radiopacity/radiolucency of maxilla in an edentulous patient. The lesion involves all of the illustrated walls of the right maxillary sinus. Right, **F,** Facial appearance of patient with Paget disease affecting the maxilla. **G,** Lateral radiograph of patient in **F.** Note dense sclerosis of maxilla. **H,** Waters projection showing obliteration of maxillary sinuses in patient in **F.**

Continued.

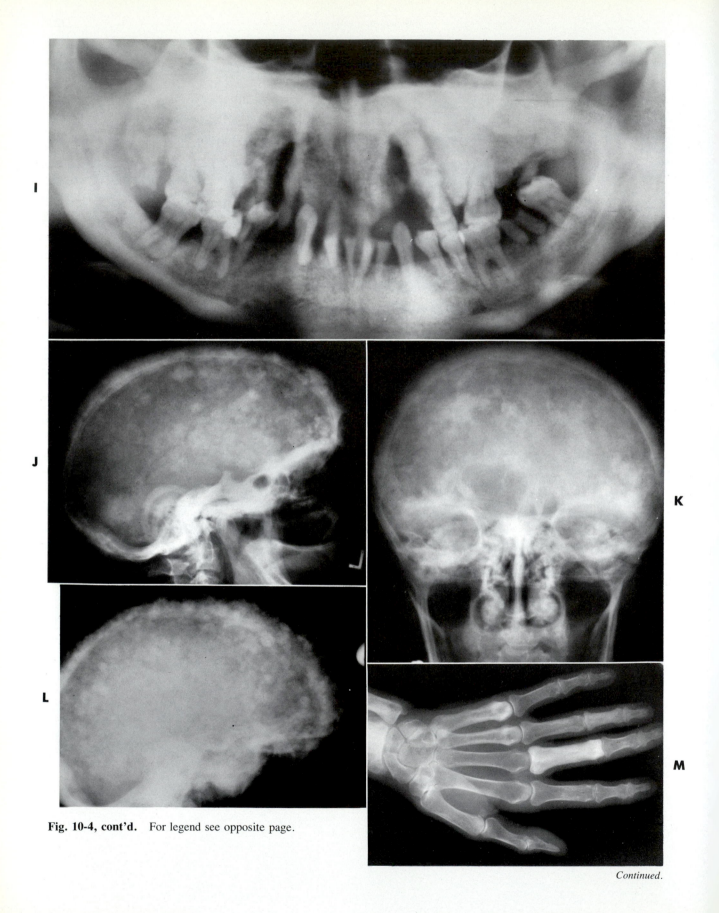

Fig. 10-4, cont'd. For legend see opposite page.

Continued.

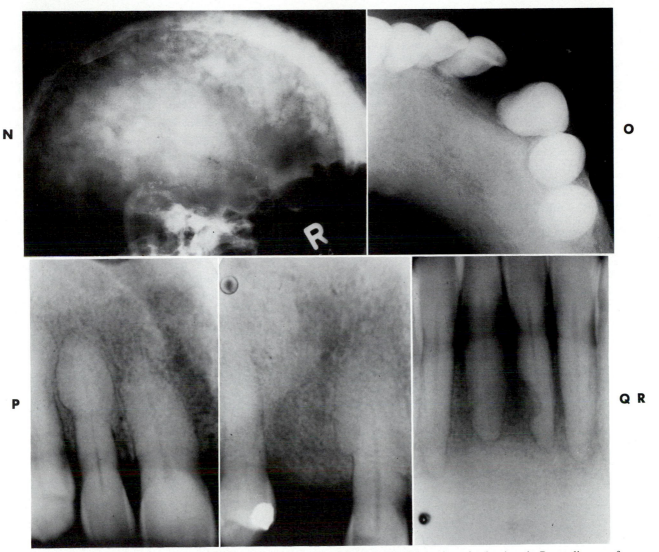

Fig. 10-4, cont'd. Opposite page,   I, Panoramic radiograph showing marked sclerosis of maxilla and "cotton wool" lesion in mandibular left canine region. **J,** Lateral radiograph showing "cotton wool" radiopacities in skull. The base of the skull shows dense sclerosis. **K,** Posteroanterior radiograph of patient in **J. L,** Lateral skull radiograph showing "cotton wool" sclerosis in skull. **M,** Hand-wrist radiograph of patient in **L** showing Paget disease in phalanx of third digit. The affected bone is enlarged and sclerotic.

Above.   N, Thickening of calvarium in Paget disease of bone (lateral skull projection). **O,** Mandibular occlusal radiograph showing generalized radiopacity and jaw enlargement. **P,** Periapical radiograph showing hypercementosis of lateral incisor and canine with loss of definition of periodontal ligament space, most noticeable on central incisor, in patient with Paget disease of bone. **Q,** Hypercementosis and bone sclerosis in patient with Paget disease of bone. The periodontal ligament space is obliterated apically (periapical radiograph). **R,** Periapical radiograph of mandibular incisor region. There is external resorption of the mesial root surface of the left central incisor. The surrounding bone is densely sclerotic.

BIBLIOGRAPHY

Fibrous Dysplasia

Eversole LR, Sabes, WR, Rovin S: Fibrous dysplasia: a nosologic problem in the diagnosis of fibro-osseous lesions, *J Oral Pathol* 1:189, 1972.

Stewart JCB: *Benign non-odontogenic tumors.* In Regezi JA, Sciubba JJ, editors: *Oral pathology,* Philadelphia, 1989, WB Saunders, pp 372-375.

Waldron CA, Giansanti JS: Benign fibro-osseous lesions of the jaws: a clinical-radiologic-histologic review of sixty-five cases. I. Fibrous dysplasia of the jaws, *Oral Med Oral Pathol* 35:190, 1973.

Florid Osseous Dysplasia

Bhaskar SN, Cutright DE: Multiple enostosis: report of 16 cases, *J Oral Surg* 26:321, 1968.

Langlais RP: *Radiology of the jaws.* In DelBalso AM, editor: *Maxillofacial Imaging,* Philadelphia, 1990, WB Saunders, pp 361-3.

Melrose FJ, Abrams AM, Mills BG: Florid osseous dysplasia: a clinical pathological study of 34 cases, *Oral Med Oral Pathol* 41:62, 1976.

Waldron CA: Fibro-osseous lesions of the jaws, *J Oral Maxillofac Surg* 43:249, 1985.

Waldron CA, Giansanti JS: Benign fibro-osseous lesions of jaws: a clinico-radiologic-histologic review of sixty-five cases. II. Benign fibro-osseous lesions of periodontal ligament origin, *Oral Surg Oral Med Oral Pathol* 35:340, 1973.

Periapical Cemental Dysplasia

Hamner JE, Scofield HH, Cornyn J: Benign fibro-osseous jaw lesions of periodontal membrane origin, *Cancer* 22:861, 1968.

Langlais RB: *Radiology of the jaws.* In *Maxillofacial imaging,* Philadelphia, 1990, WB Saunders, pp 344-346.

Zegarelli EV, et al: The cementoma, *Oral Med Oral Pathol* 18:219, 1964.

Paget Disease of Bone

Basle MF, et al: On the trail of paramyxoviruses in Paget's disease of bone, *Clin Orthop* 217:9, 1987.

Crespi P: *Metabolic and genetic jaw disease.* In Regezi JA, Sciubba JJ, editors: *Oral pathology,* Philadelphia, 1989, WB Saunders, pp 427-430.

Ellis G, Connole P: Diffuse mandibular enlargement caused by osteitis deformans, *Ear Nose Throat J* 64:466, 1985.

Otis LL, Terezhalmy GT, Glass BJ: Paget's disease of bone: etiological theories and report of a case, *J Oral Med* 41:214, 1986.

CHAPTER

11

METABOLIC AND SYSTEMIC DISEASES

ACROMEGALY (HYPERPITUITARISM)

Overview

Definition and pathogenesis: Hyperpituitarism is generally idiopathic in children and caused by an acidophilic adenoma of the anterior lobe of the pituitary gland in adults. In childhood hyperpituitarism leads to gigantism; in adulthood it causes acromegaly.

Clinical Features

Symptoms and signs: When hyperpituitarism occurs after epiphyseal closure, acromegaly results. The terminal phalanges of the hands and feet are enlarged, and ribs are increased in size. Growth of the mandibular condyles and rami results in marked prognathism, and this, together with macroglossia, leads to dental malocclusion. Temporomandibular joint dysfunction can occur. The enlarged tongue shows indentations on the sides because of pressure against the teeth. The skin is coarse, and the lips become thickened. Headaches, photophobia, and reduced vision may also be present.

If the condition occurs in individuals in whom the epiphyses of the long bones have not closed, gigantism results. This is characterized by a symmetric overgrowth of the body. Some persons reach more than 8 feet in height. Such individuals have been found to have underdeveloped genitals. Relative nonspecific complaints later in life include joint pain, headaches, lassitude, fatigue, and excessive perspiration. The dentition in gigantism has normal crown size but relatively long roots through hypercementosis. This leads to spacing between the teeth, as the dental arch is relatively wide. There is an enlarged cranium with a large sella turcica and prominent frontal sinus.

RADIOLOGIC FEATURES

Cardinal Signs

Enlarged sella turcica
Large skull
Prominent frontal sinus
Prognathic mandible with class III dental malocclusion

Ancillary Signs

Increased length of long bones (gigantism only)
Increased length of dental arch causing dental spacing (gigantism only)
Hypercementosis
Occasional accelerated dental eruption

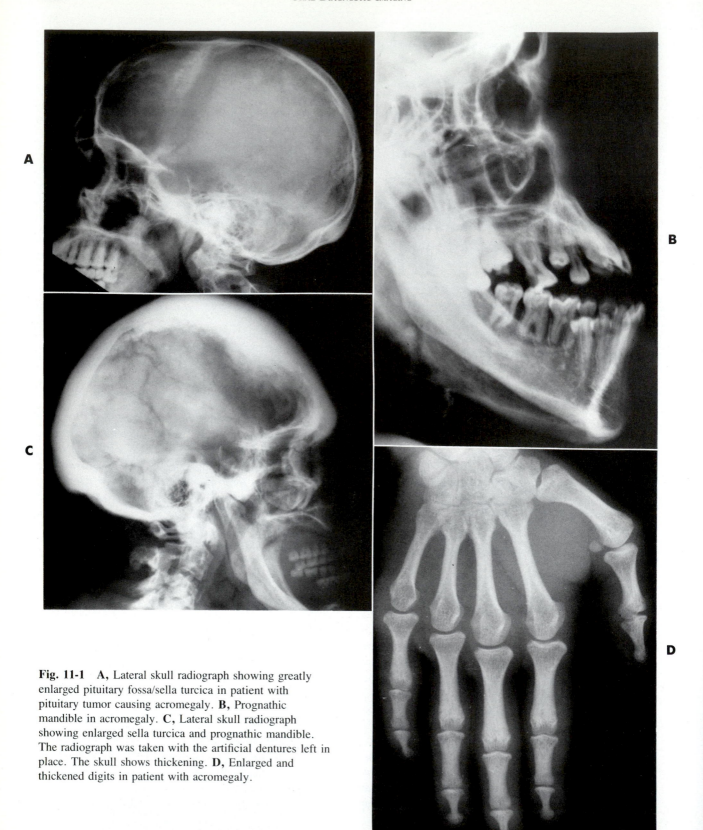

Fig. 11-1 **A,** Lateral skull radiograph showing greatly enlarged pituitary fossa/sella turcica in patient with pituitary tumor causing acromegaly. **B,** Prognathic mandible in acromegaly. **C,** Lateral skull radiograph showing enlarged sella turcica and prognathic mandible. The radiograph was taken with the artificial dentures left in place. The skull shows thickening. **D,** Enlarged and thickened digits in patient with acromegaly.

PRIMARY HYPERPARATHYROIDISM

Overview

Definition: Primary hyperparathyroidism results from excessive secretion of parathyroid hormone caused by functional benign or malignant tumors of the parathyroid glands. It is relatively rare.

Clinical Features

Demographics: Although it can be found in any age group, primary hyperparathyroidism is most frequent in middle age. The condition is three times more common in females than in males.

Signs and symptoms: Urinary tract stones are common early findings, but occasionally the first sign is a giant cell tumor (brown tumor) seen radiographically as a cystic radiolucency.

There is a generalized osteoporosis from loss of phosphorus and calcium. Malocclusion caused by sudden drifting and spacing of the teeth has been reported as an early feature of the condition.

RADIOLOGIC FEATURES

Cardinal Signs

Generalized osteoporosis
Unilocular or multilocular cystic radiolucency (Brown tumor) consistent with that of giant cell tumor or granuloma
Absence of lamina dura
Calcification in muscles and subcutaneous tissues

Ancillary Signs

Absence of radiopaque outline of maxillary sinuses
Thinning of inferior mandibular cortex
Saucer-shaped erosion of bone
Dental malocclusion
Crestal radiolucency leading to loss of alveolar bone
Ballooning or blisterlike expansion of mandibular cortex
Single or multiple separate well-defined radiolucencies
Generalized increased calvarial density
Granular-appearing bone in skull
Enlargement of sella turcica
Multiple intracranial opacities
Return to normal after treatment

Differential Diagnosis

Hypercorticosteroidism
Osteopetrosis
Benign odontogenic cyst or tumor
Central giant cell granuloma
Osteoclastoma
Aneurysmal bone cyst
Paget disease of bone

SECONDARY HYPERPARATHYROIDISM

Overview

Definition: Secondary hyperparathyroidism is the excessive secretion of parathyroid hormone caused by parathyroid hyperplasia. This occurs to compensate for another metabolic disorder that has resulted in retention of phosphate or depletion of serum calcium levels.

Pathogenesis: Secondary hyperparathyroidism most commonly occurs as a complication of end-stage renal disease. The likelihood of its occurrence increases with time on dialysis. The bone changes are identical to those found in primary hyperparathyroidism.

RADIOLOGIC FEATURES

Cardinal Signs

Generalized osteoporosis
Unilocular or multilocular cystic radiolucency (brown tumor)
Absence of lamina dura

Ancillary Signs

Absence of radiopaque outline of maxillary sinuses
Occasionally increased radiopacity (surrounding tooth roots)
Diffuse periradicular granular opacity
Mandibular enostoses

Differential Diagnosis

Hypercorticosteroidism
Osteopetrosis
Benign odontogenic cyst or tumor
Central giant cell granuloma
Osteoclastoma
Aneurysmal bone cyst

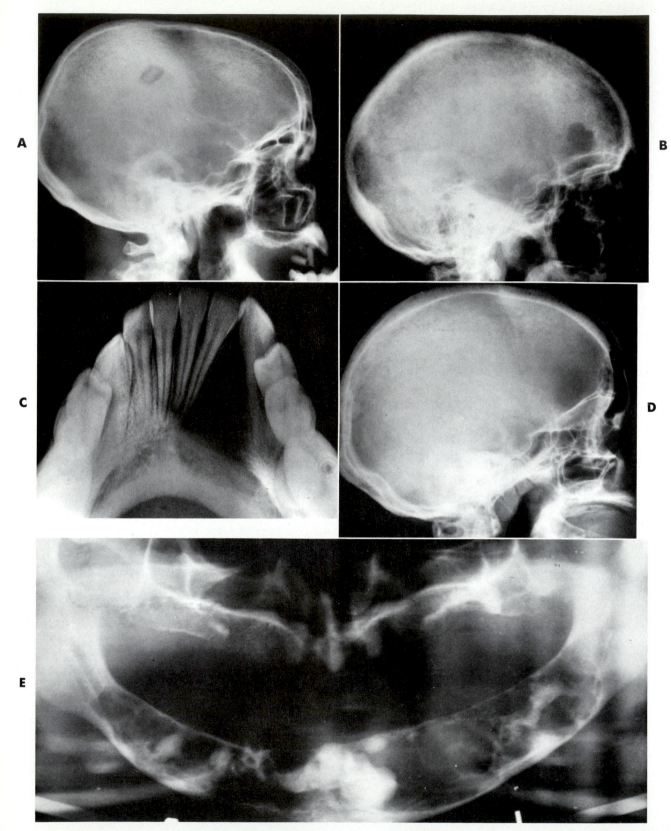

Continued.

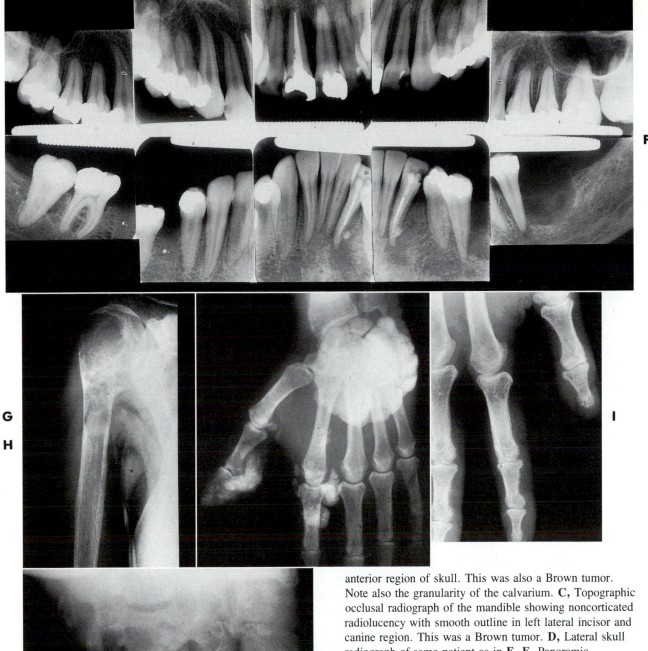

Fig. 11-2 **A,** Lateral skull radiograph showing solitary "punched-out" radiolucency in parietal region. This was a Brown tumor. **B,** Lateral skull radiograph showing crenated radiolucency with well-defined noncorticated margins in anterior region of skull. This was also a Brown tumor. Note also the granularity of the calvarium. **C,** Topographic occlusal radiograph of the mandible showing noncorticated radiolucency with smooth outline in left lateral incisor and canine region. This was a Brown tumor. **D,** Lateral skull radiograph of same patient as in **E. E,** Panoramic radiograph showing generalized radiolucency of jaws with multilocular radiolucent lesions in mandible. The latter proved to be Brown tumors. Note granularity of skull. **F,** Periapical radiographs from same patient as in **G.** A Brown tumor is seen distal to the left mandibular premolar. The lamina dura in that site has been resorbed. The right maxillary incisor and canine regions also show a relative radiolucency of the alveolar bone. **G,** Right humerus. Note radiolucency with coarse internal trabeculation and blister lesion of periosteum on medial surface. **H,** Metastatic calcifications in hand and wrist of patient with primary hyperparathyroidism. **I,** Digits of patient in **D.** Note patchy demineralization and periosteal new bone formation. **J,** Metastatic calcifications in soft tissues adjacent to spine and brown tumor demineralization of vertebrae.

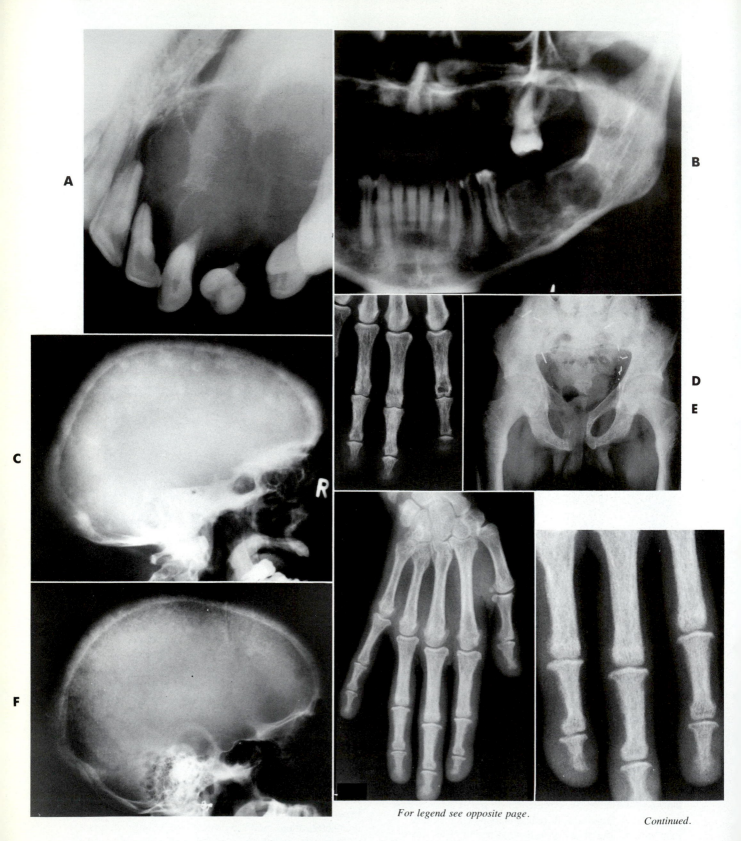

For legend see opposite page.

Continued.

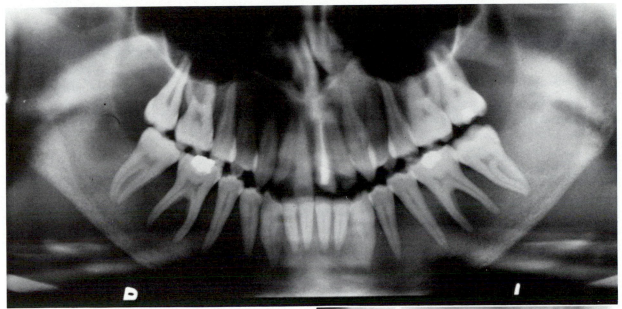

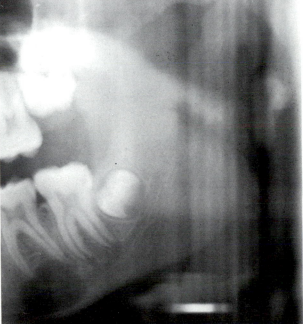

Fig. 11-3, opposite page. **A,** Lateral maxillary occlusal projection in patient with chronic renal failure. There is a multilocular radiolucency with loss of lamina dura around left first premolar and lateral incisor teeth. **B,** Cropped panoramic radiograph demonstrating Brown tumor in left mandibular edentulous molar segment. **C,** Patchy increased mineralization in skull of patient with chronic renal failure and secondary hyperparathyroidism. **D,** Patchy demineralization of digit in patient in **C.** A periosteal response is also noted. **E,** Lysis of bone in right pelvis through brown tumor in same patient as in **D. F,** Lateral skull radiograph of patient with secondary hyperparathyroidism caused by renal osteodystrophy. Note granular appearance of skull. The radiopaque outlines of the maxillary sinuses are not evident. **G,** Note granularity of trabecular pattern in bones of the hand and wrist in same patient as in **F. H,** Detail of **G. This page, I,** Panoramic radiograph of patient in **F.** There is a generalized relative rarefaction of the jawbones and absence of lamina dura around the teeth. Brown tumors are present in the regions distal to the molars in all four segments. **J,** Cropped panoramic radiograph of patient with secondary hyperparathyroidism with Brown tumor subjacent to mandibular first permanent molar.

HYPOPARATHYROIDISM

Overview

Definition and pathogenesis: Hypoparathyroidism is insufficient parathyroid hormone production because of surgical removal of parathyroid glands, destruction of parathyroid gland from thrombosis, or rare congenital absence.

Clinical Features

Symptoms and signs: Hypoparathyroidism results in decreased excretion of calcium. Increased neuromuscular excitability occurs if serum calcium falls below 8 mg/dl. Characteristic carpopedal spasm can occur with tetany when serum calcium drops below 6 mg/dl.

If hypoparathyroidism develops before the teeth are fully formed, the teeth can be hypoplastic. Chronic candidiasis is often seen as an early feature of hypoparathyroidism.

Laboratory tests: Serum calcium is low, and serum phosphorus is high.

RADIOLOGIC FEATURES

Cardinal Signs

Aplasia and hypoplasia of teeth
Increased bone density

Ancillary Signs

Osteoporosis
Delayed dental eruption
Dilaceration of tooth roots
Multiple external resorption of teeth
Radiopacity in region of basal ganglion
Subcutaneous soft tissue mineralization

HYPOVITAMINOSIS D (SIMPLE RICKETS)

Overview

Vitamin D (1,25-dihydroxycholecalciferol), D_2 (ergocalciferol) derived from the action of sunlight on dietary ergosterol, and D_3 (cholecalciferol) derived from the action of sunlight on endogenous 7-dehydrocholesterol are hydroxylated cholecalciferol compounds that are antirachitic. The origins and actions of this group of compounds are between that of a vitamin and a hormone. Vitamin D itself can be produced by the action

of hepatic 25-hydroxylase and renal 1-α-hydroxylase on either of the other two compounds. Vitamin D acts to increase intestinal calcium uptake, bone calcium mobilization, and renal calcium reabsorption. Hypovitaminosis D leads to nondeposition of calcium salt in bone matrix.

Clinical Features

Symptoms and signs: Hypovitaminosis D causes simple rickets, with malformed limbs and thorax, enlargement of the wrists and ankles, craniotabes, and an increased incidence of bone fractures. Osteoporosis may be seen in the oral region.

RADIOLOGIC FEATURES

Cardinal Signs

Osteoporosis with thinning and decrease in number of trabeculae
Radiolucency of jaws and skull
Bulging of frontal, parietal, and occipital regions of skull

Ancillary Signs

Attenuation of lamina dura
Attenuation of crypt outlines of unerupted teeth
Enamel hypoplasia
Delayed eruption of teeth
Unusual sequencing of eruption of teeth
Thinning of mandibular inferior cortex

Differential Diagnosis

Vitamin D–resistant rickets
Osteoporosis

VITAMIN D–RESISTANT RICKETS (HYPOPHOSPHATEMIA)

Overview

Definition: Vitamin D–resistant rickets is an isolated renal tubular defect inhibiting reabsorption of inorganic phosphates, resulting in hyperphosphaturia.

Pathogenesis: Vitamin D–resistant rickets is inherited as an X-linked dominant trait.

Clinical Features

Symptoms and signs: The full manifestation of vitamin D–resistant rickets is rickets or osteomalacia

Text continued on page 342.

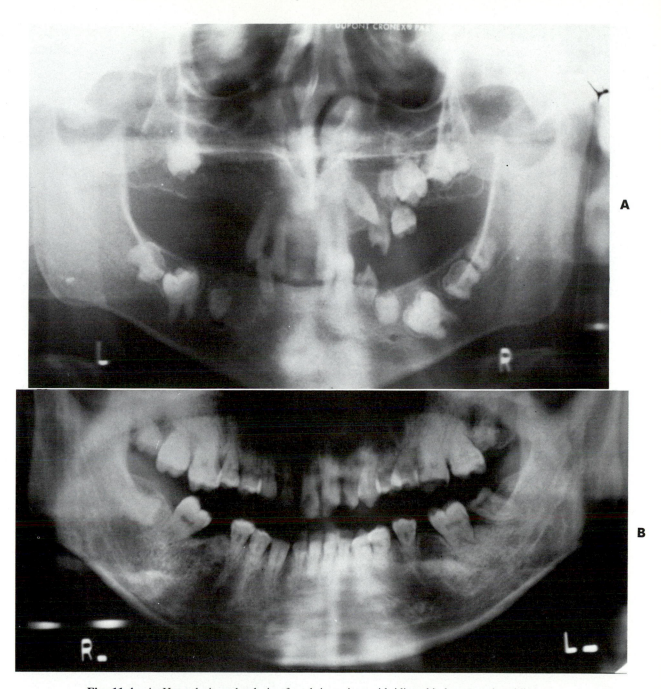

Fig. 11-4 A, Hypoplasia and aplasia of teeth in patient with idiopathic hypoparathyroidism (panoramic radiograph). **B,** Panoramic radiograph showing aberrant short tooth root formation in patient with idiopathic hypoparathyroidism. There is also enamel hypoplasia.

Continued.

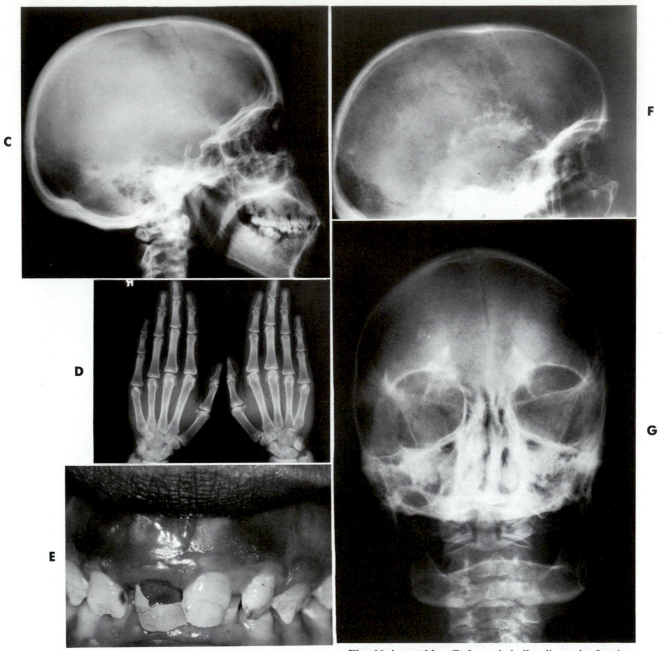

Fig. 11-4, cont'd.   C, Lateral skull radiograph of patient in **B. D,** Hand and wrist radiographs of patient in **B.** Note multiple extra sesamoid bones associated with metacarpals. **E,** Clinical appearance of enamel hyperplasia in patient in **B. F,** Soft tissue calcification of the brain in patient with hypoparathyroidism. **G,** Posteroanterior radiograph showing increased mineralization of orofacial structures.

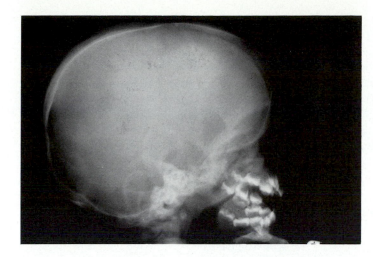

Fig. 11-5 Lateral skull radiograph from child with vitamin D deficiency (rickets). Note the bulging of the frontal region of the skull and attenuation of the outlines of the dental crypts.

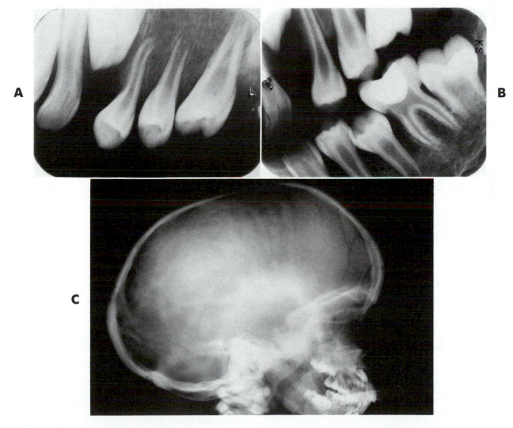

Fig. 11-6 **A,** Periapical radiograph of left maxillary premolar region. Note the large pulp cavities and the attenuation of the lamina dura and dental crypts. **B,** Bitewing radiograph from same patient as in **A.** Note relative lack of mineralization of alveolar crestal bone in this child. The pulp chambers are relatively large. There is cervical caries on the mesial aspect of the left mandibular first permanent molar tooth. **C,** Lateral skull radiograph showing radiolucency of jaws and skull.

nonrespondent to vitamin D therapy, as vitamin D metabolism is normal. However, there is diminished intestinal calcium and phosphate absorption. Patients with the milder form may be slightly shorter than normal siblings, with no other manifestations. Females tend to show fewer signs than their brothers. Dental features have been reported on several occasions. These include elongated and high pulp horns and marked hypocalcification of the dentin, with globular dentin formation and clefting. Cementum is also abnormal, and the lamina dura is poorly defined or absent.

Laboratory tests: Serum calcium is in the normal range, and parathyroid hormone levels are in the high-normal range.

RADIOLOGIC FEATURES

Cardinal Signs:

  Elongated pulp horns and generalized enlargement of pulp

  Attenuation of lamina dura and follicular cortices of teeth

  Osteoporosis with thinning and decrease in number of trabeculae

  Radiolucency of jaws and skull

Ancillary Signs

  Rapid progression of dental caries

HYPOPHOSPHATASIA (HYPOPHOSPHATESEMIA)

Overview

Definition and pathogenesis: Hypophosphatasia is a hereditary disease transmitted as an autosomal recessive trait. Patients have a deficiency of serum and tissue levels of alkaline phosphatase. The onset of hypophosphatasia may occur in infancy, childhood, or adulthood.

Clinical Features

Symptoms and signs: The infantile form of hypophosphatasia is characterized by hypercalcemia and severe ricketslike lesions. In most cases it is rapidly lethal. When it originates in childhood, there is severe growth retardation with marked ricketslike deformities. There is costochondral junction enlargement,

producing the classic rachitic rosary appearance; calcification of the calvarium is inhibited; and the propensity for infection is increased. Hypocalcified teeth with large pulp chambers and premature shedding of deciduous teeth have been reported. The adult onset form is associated with a high propensity for fractures, osseous radiolucencies, and a history of rickets.

Laboratory tests: Excretion of phosphoethanolamine in urine is a common laboratory finding.

RADIOLOGIC FEATURES

Cardinal Signs

  Irregular metaphyseal ossification
  Costochondral junction rachitic rosary
  Relative radiolucency of calvarium
  Hypocalcified teeth with large pulp chambers and root canals
  Premature exfoliation of primary dentition
  Alveolar bone loss (never properly calcified)
  Generalized osseous rarefaction

Ancillary Signs

  Craniostenosis
  Localized thinning of calvarium
  Multiple calvarial wormian bones
  Defective cranial ossification

Differential Diagnosis

  Rickets (hypovitaminosis D)
  Vitamin D–resistant rickets (hypophosphatemia)
  Pseudohypophosphatasia
  Pink disease

OSTEOPOROSIS

Overview

Definition: Osteoporosis is abnormal porosity of bone, most prevalent in postmenopausal women, in sedentary or immobilized individuals, and in patients on long-term steroid therapy. It is the most common type of metabolic bone disease.

Clinical Features

Symptoms and signs: Osteoporosis can cause pain, especially in the lower back; pathologic fracture; loss of physical stature; and various deformities, including severe kyphosis. It may be idiopathic or sub-

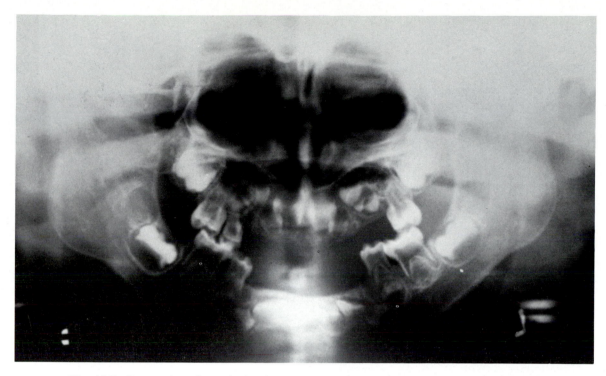

Fig. 11-7 Panoramic radiograph showing enlarged pulp chambers in primary teeth and alveolar bone loss (particularly in anterior segments of both jaws). There is also evidence of enamel hypoplasia.

sequent to thyrotoxicosis or hyperparathyroidism. As skeletal mass in old age is proportional to skeletal mass at maturity, childhood calcium intake may play a major role in the occurrence and severity of the disease in later years.

RADIOLOGIC FEATURES

Cardinal Signs:

  Generalized osteopenia (most prominent in spine)
  Thinning and accentuation of cortices
  Accentuation of primary and loss of secondary trabeculation
  Change in structure of vertebral body

Ancillary Signs

  Spontaneous, atraumatic fracture (especially of the spine, wrist, hip, or ribs)
  Basilar invagination of skull base
  Granular-appearing bone in skull

Differential Diagnosis

  Juvenile rickets
  Osteomalacia
  Scurvy
  Hyperparathyroidism
  Early Paget disease of bone

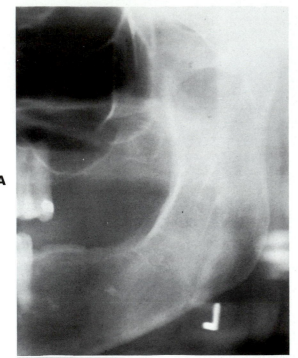

A

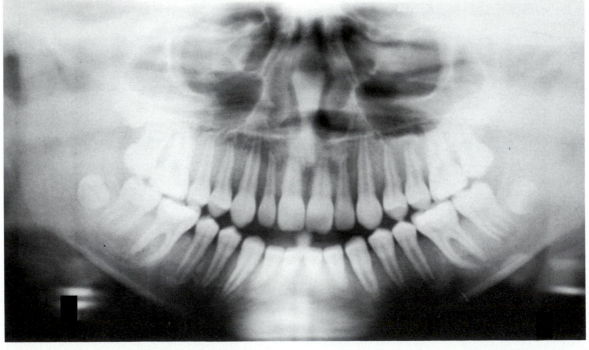

B

Fig. 11-8 **A,** Cropped panoramic radiograph showing relative radiolucency of both jaws with reduced definition of cortices. **B,** Panoramic radiograph showing generalized osteoporosis in nephrotic syndrome.

BIBLIOGRAPHY

Acromegaly (Hyperpituitarism)

Gibilisco JA, editor: *Stafne's oral radiographic diagnosis,* ed 5, Philadelphia, 1985, WB Saunders.

Hampton RE: Acromegaly and resulting myofascial pain and temporomandibular joint dysfunction, *J Am Dent Assoc* 114:625, 1987.

Jadresic A, et al: The acromegaly syndrome: relation between clinical features, growth, hormone values, and radiological characteristics of pituitary tumors, *Q J Med* 51:189, 1982.

Primary Hyperparathyroidism

Bramley P. Dwyer D: Primary hyperparathyroidism: its effects on a mother and her children, *Oral Surg Oral Med Oral Pathol* 30:464, 1970.

Kennett S, Pollick H: Jaw lesions in familial hyperparathyroidism, *Oral Surg Oral Med Oral Pathol* 31:502, 1971.

Rosenberg EH, Guralnick WC: Hyperparathyroidism: a review of 220 proved cases, with special emphasis on findings in the jaws, *Oral Surg Oral Med Oral Pathol* 15(suppl 2):84, 1962.

Schour I, Massler M: Endocrines and dentistry, *J Am Dent Assoc* 30:597, 763, 943, 1943.

Silverman S, et al: The dental structures in hyperparathyroidism, *Oral Surg Oral Med Oral Pathol* 15:426, 1962.

Silverman S, Jr Ware WH, Gillooly C Jr: Dental aspects of hyperparathyroidism, *Oral Surg Oral Med Oral Pathol* 26:184, 1968.

Teng CT, Nathan NH: Primary hyperparathyroidism, *Am J Roentgenol Radium Ther Nucl Med* 83:716, 1960.

Secondary Hyperparathyroidism

Massry SG, et al: Secondary hyperparathyroidism in chronic renal failure, *Arch Intern Med* 124:431, 1969.

Shear M, Copelyn M: Metastatic calcification of the oral mucosa in renal hyperparathyroidism, *Br J Oral Maxillofac Surg* 42:81, 1966.

Spolnik KJ, et al: Dental radiographic features of end-stage renal disease, *Dent Radiog Photog* 54:21, 1981.

Hypoparathyroidism

Keller EE, Stafne EC, Gibilisco JA: *Oral manifestations of systemic disease.* In Gibilisco JA, editor: *Stafne's oral radiographic diagnosis,* ed 2, Philadelphia, 1985, WB Saunders, pp 263-264.

Poyton HG, Pharoah MJ: *Oral radiology,* ed 2, Philadelphia, 1989, BC Decker, p 246.

Hypovitaminosis D (Simple Rickets)

Haussler MR, McCain TA: Basic and clinical concepts related to vitamin D metabolism and action I, *New Engl J Med* 297:974, 1977.

Haussler MR, McCain TA: Basic and clinical concepts related to vitamin D metabolism and action II, *New Engl J Med* 297:1041, 1977.

Poyton HG: *Oral radiology,* Baltimore, 1982, Williams & Wilkins, p 256.

Shafer WG, Hine MK, Levy BM: *A textbook of oral pathology,* ed 4, Philadelphia, 1983, WB Saunders, p 640.

Vitamin D–Resistant Rickets (Hypophosphatemia)

Ainley JE: Manifestations of familial hypophosphatemia, *J Endocrinol* 4:26, 1978.

Archard HO, Witkop CJ Jr: Hereditary hypophosphatemia (vitamin D–resistant rickets) presenting primary dental manifestations, *Oral Surg Oral Med Oral Pathol* 22:184, 1966.

Marks SC, Lindahl RL, Bawden JW: Dental and cephalometric findings in vitamin D–resistant rickets, *ASDC J Dent Child* 32:259, 1965.

Tracy WE, et al: Analysis of dentine pathogenesis in vitamin D–resistant rickets, *Oral Surg Oral Med Oral Pathol* 32:38, 1971.

Vasilakis GJ, Nygaard VK, DiPalma DM: Vitamin D–resistant rickets: a review and case report of an adolescent boy with a history of dental problems, *J Oral Pathol Med* 35:19, 1980.

Hypophosphatasia (Hypophosphatesemia)

Beumer J, et al: Childhood hypophosphatasia and the premature loss of teeth, *Oral Surg Oral Med Oral Pathol* 35:631, 1973.

Brittain JM, Oldenberg TR, Burkes EJ: Odontohypophosphatasia: a report of two cases, *ASDC J Dent Child* 43:38, 1976.

Houpt MI, Kenny FM, Listgarten M: Hypophosphatasia: case reports, *ASDC J Dent Child* 37:126, 1970.

Kjellman M, et al: Five cases of hypophosphatasia with dental findings, *Int J Oral Maxillofac Surg* 2:152, 1973.

Witkop CJ, Rao S: Inherited defects in tooth structure, *Birth Defects* 7:153, 1971.

Osteoporosis

Genant HK, Vogler JB, Block JE: *Radiology of osteoporosis.* In Riggs BL, Melon LJ III, editors: *Osteoporosis: etiology, diagnosis and management,* New York, 1988, Raven Press, p 181.

CHAPTER

12

ARTICULAR DISORDERS

HYPERPLASIA OF THE MANDIBLE OR MANDIBULAR CONDYLE

Overview

Definition: Enlargement of one mandibular condylar process may occur in isolation or in association with enlargement of part of the mandibular ramus and body.

Pathogenesis: Most cases of mandibular hyperplasia, especially hemihyperplasia, are developmental and thus may be genetic in origin. Postulated causes include neoplasia, excessive repair proliferation following trauma, exuberant response to infection, or abnormal function.

Clinical Features

Demographics: Unilateral hyperplasia of the condyle, either as an isolated finding or as part of hemihyperplasia of the mandible, is usually a coincidental finding on radiographs made for another purpose. With the widespread use of pantomography in dentistry, and to a slightly lesser degree in medicine, it has become easy to compare the morphology of the left and right sides of the mandible. Although minor asymmetries are common, from time to time more striking asymmetries are found. There is no apparent sex predilection.

Signs and symptoms: The extent of hyperplasia determines whether it is clinically apparent. There are usually no associated symptoms and the patient is unaware of the situation; sometimes, however, the pa-

tient presents with temporomandibular joint (TMJ) dysfunction.

Special tests: Before hyperplasia of the condyle or mandible is diagnosed, care should be taken to rule out asymmetric placement of the patient into the radiographic unit, which could result in a greater magnification of one side relative to the other. It is often useful to compare the apparent size of the teeth and other surrounding structures, although teeth may also be involved in unilateral size differences.

Technetium 99m bone scintigraphy may be useful to determine if active growth is still occurring.

RADIOLOGIC FEATURES

Cardinal Signs

Increased size of the condylar neck and head compared to the normal population or, in unilateral cases, compared to the contralateral side.

Ancillary Signs

Malocclusion of teeth
Shift in midline of mandible

Differential Diagnosis

Acromegaly
Osteochondroma
Congenital hemifacial hyperplasia

346

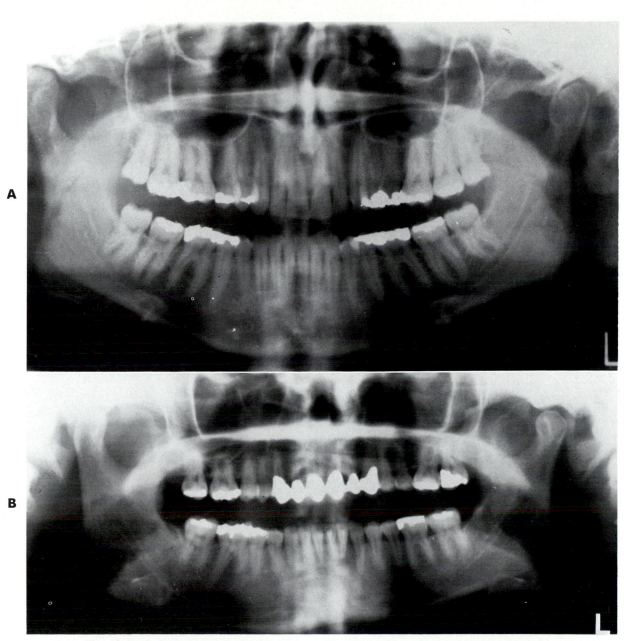

Fig. 12-1 A, Pantomograph of a 24-year-old white woman who was seen for routine dental care. Note the elongated right condylar neck. Comparison with other bilateral structures shows that the patient was symmetrically placed into the x-ray unit. She was unaware of any problem in the area, and no relevant history could be elicited. Clinically, although the right side did appear slightly larger, it was no more so than would be expected in the population at large, and the difference would not have been noted except for the radiographic finding. **B,** Pantomograph of a 46-year-old white man shows a similar condylar enlargement to that in **A,** except that there is also a noticeable alteration in the morphology of the condylar neck and head compared to the opposite side. Also, in this case it is the left side that is enlarged. Again, the patient seems to have been symmetrically placed into the unit. There is some suggestion that the entire left side of the mandible is slightly enlarged. The history and clinical examination were noncontributory.

Continued.

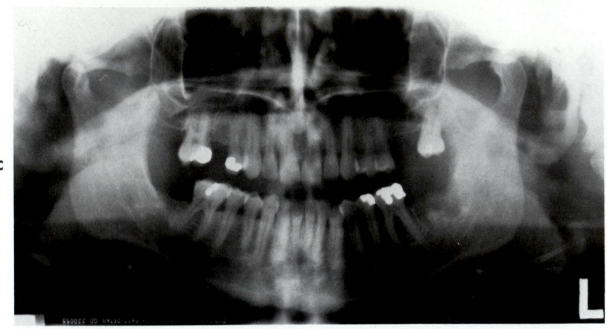

Fig. 12-1, cont'd   C, Patient with enlargement of the right condyle and obvious enlargement of the entire left side of the mandible. The teeth and the entire left and right arch of the maxilla are symmetric, again confirming that the patient was symmetrically placed into the unit. This case is more correctly called hemihyperplasia of the mandible than unilateral condylar hyperplasia. Clinical examination revealed slight enlargement of the right side compared with the left, but the soft tissue masked the bulk of the enlargement such that it would have been only slightly apparent to the casual examiner.

CORONOID PROCESS HYPERPLASIA

Overview

Definition: Coronoid process hyperplasia is said to exist if the tip of the process extends 1 cm above lower edge of the zygomatic arch.

Pathogenesis: Elongation of coronoid processes may result from ankylosis or restriction of movement in the TMJ. It may also occur as a primary phenomenon. In this situation it becomes a TMJ problem, in that the hyperplastic processes impinge on the zygomatic process of the maxilla and the zygomatic bone, thus preventing the condyles from moving in and out of the glenoid fossa. Although some authors have suggested trauma as a cause, the cause of coronoid process hyperplasia is still unknown.

Clinical Features

Demographics: Coronoid hyperplasia is rare and has no particular demographic distribution. Hall, Orbach, & Landberg[3] have stated that unilateral hyperplasia may occur in either gender but bilateral involvement is predominantly found in males.

Signs and symptoms: Affected patients are to open the mouth fully.

Special tests: No special tests are required.

RADIOLOGIC FEATURES

Cardinal Signs

Location of the tip of the coronoid process more than 1 cm above lower edge of the zygomatic arch; shape of the process should be pointed.

Ancillary Signs

Inability to move the condyle to the crest of the articular eminence on open-mouth TMJ views; larger than usual coronoid process.

Differential Diagnosis

Ankylosis of the TMJ
Osteochondroma of the coronoid process

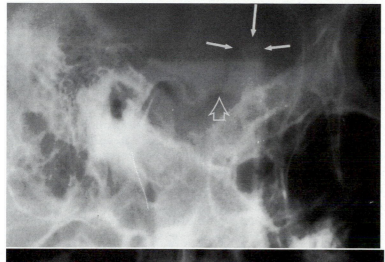

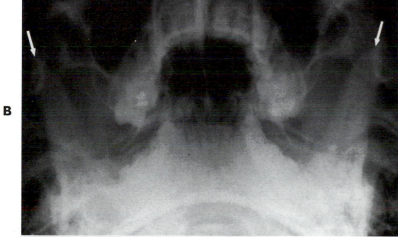

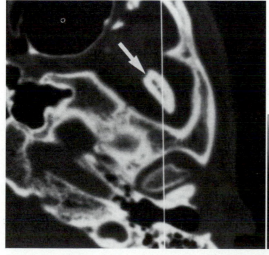

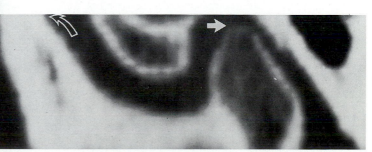

Fig. 12-2 A 19-year-old white man who presented with moderate limitation of opening. *A,* The plain-film lateral skull view shows major elongation of the coronoid process *(closed arrows),* well beyond the criterion for elongated coronoid process: 1 cm superior to the inferior border of the zygomatic arch *(open arrow).* **B,** The occipitomental view also shows major elongation of the coronoid processes *(arrows)* beyond the inferior border of the zygomatic arch. *C,* The axial CT view also shows the coronoid process *(arrow)* plainly above the level at which it is normally found. **D,** The parasagittal CT view, reformatted along the line in **C,** confirms that the coronoid process *(open arrow)* is plainly visible above the level of the mandibular condyle *(closed arrow).* There is no evidence of a neoplastic process. Rather, there is bilateral symmetry of both coronoid processes, more in keeping with a developmental anomaly.

HYPOPLASIA OF THE MANDIBULAR CONDYLE

Overview

Definition: In hypoplasia of the mandibular condyle, the condyle fails to develop to its full size.

Pathogenesis: Hypoplasia of the condyle refers to a smaller than normal condyle resulting from lack of full development, as opposed to loss of condylar mass resulting from an acquired disease. Some cases of hypoplasia seem to result from trauma or infection. Juvenile rheumatoid arthritis has also been implicated. Another specific cause is Hurler syndrome, one of the mucopolysaccharidoses (MPS). This condition, designated as MPS I, is inherited as an autosomal recessive disease.

Clinical Features

Demographics: Hypoplasia is often a coincidental finding on radiographs made for unrelated reasons; thus its prevalence or distribution in the population is not known. It does not appear to be a common finding. It may, however, be related to a specific disease, such as Hurler syndrome, Morquio syndrome, or Weill-Marchesani syndrome.

Signs and symptoms: The patient may have no signs or symptoms. Deviation of the mandibular midline to the affected side may be noted in unilateral cases, or retrognathia may be present. In Hurler syndrome there may be hernia before age 6; mental retardation; small stature; and multiple skeletal anomalies, including kyphosis, flattened vertebrae, genu valgum, coxa valga, pes planus, and talipes equinovarus.

Special tests: For Hurler syndrome, the urine should be checked for elevated mucopolysaccharide levels, especially chondroitin sulfate B and heparin sulfate.

RADIOLOGIC FEATURES

Cardinal Signs

Smaller than usual condyle and condylar neck; glenoid fossa is also smaller than normal. Bone in the area is well corticated, smooth, and of normal radiopacity.

Ancillary Signs

In Hurler syndrome: J-shaped sella turcica, in addition to the other anomalies described previously.

Differential Diagnosis

Fracture of the condylar neck with displacement of the proximal fragment

Dislocation of the condyle

MANDIBULAR CONDYLE DISLOCATION

Overview

Definition: Mandibular condyle dislocation exists when the mandibular condyle is displaced from the glenoid fossa—usually anterior to the anterior articular eminence—and the patient is not able to return it to the glenoid fossa by normal masticatory muscle action.

Pathogenesis: Dislocation, also called luxation, of the TMJ may result from a variety of causes, ranging from a yawn to a blow to the jaws, especially while the mouth is open. Extensive dental procedures, such as third molar extraction, have also been implicated.

In dislocation of the TMJ, the head of the condyle moves to a position anterior to the anterior articular eminence. This results from laxity of the capsule and ligaments or from sudden force applied to the jaw that forces it to rotate, stretching or tearing the capsule and forcing the condylar head anteriorly. If this is followed by muscle contraction and spasm, the patient is unable to move the condyle back into the glenoid fossa. The dislocation may be unilateral or bilateral.

Clinical Features

Demographics: Condylar dislocation may be more likely in individuals with shallow anterior articular eminences and those with lax capsules and ligaments. Certainly people who have had a previous dislocation

Fig. 12-4, opposite page,   **A,** Lateral view of a patient injured in a motor vehicle accident, who was being investigated to rule out a vertebral column injury, shows that the mandibular condyle *(A)* is anterior to the crest of the articular eminence *(B).* Also apparent is the anterior open bite *(C),* which extends along one side of the dental arch. **B,** The AP view of the cervical skull confirms the unilateral open bite *C* by showing that the teeth of the opposite side are in occlusion *(D).* There is no apparent midline shift in the mandible. The patient was not, however, able to open fully to show the vertebral column properly, presumably because of muscle spasm.

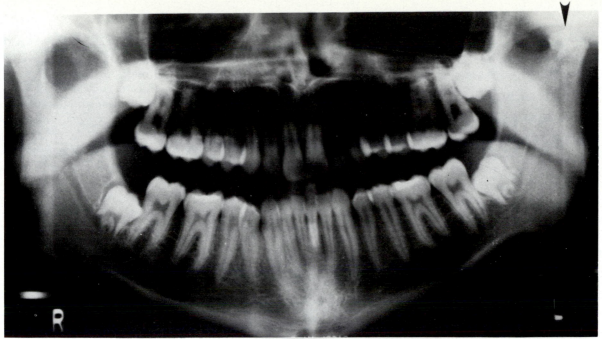

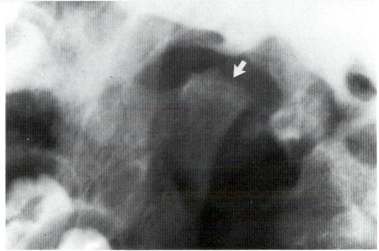

Fig. 12-3 A, The left condyle *(arrow)* is smaller and altered in morphology compared with the right condyle. No cause was suggested by the patient's history. *B,* The left condyle *(arrow)* is smaller than expected and altered in morphology. Although the appearance is similar to that in **A,** this patient was diagnosed as having Hurler syndrome (mucopolysaccharidosis I).

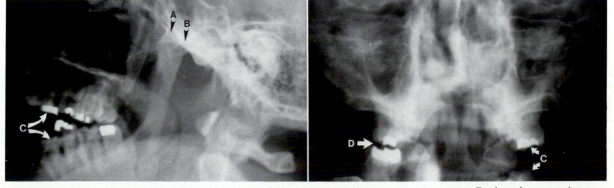

For legend see opposite page.

of the TMJ are more likely to have a dislocation in the future. However, because the dislocation may result from trauma, it may happen to almost anyone in the population.

Signs and symptoms: The most likely clinical finding is anterior apertognathia, with only the most posterior teeth in some form of occlusion, or unilateral anterolateral apertognathia, with only the posterior teeth on one side in occlusion. In the latter case, the mandibular midline is displaced to the unaffected side. The patient is unable to close the mouth or move the mandible from side to side.

There may be pain due to muscle spasm and inability to speak, eat, or drink properly.

Special tests: There are no special tests, other than asking the patient to attempt to close the mouth properly.

RADIOLOGIC FEATURES

Cardinal Signs

Absence of the condyle from the glenoid fossa. It is often displaced to a position anterosuperior to the anterior articular eminence on both open- and closed-mouth views.

Ancillary Signs

Only the most posterior teeth in the arches, if included on the radiographs, are seen to occlude. In unilateral dislocation, only the teeth on the opposite side occlude. In the latter case the midlines of the two dental arches may also be non-aligned.

Differential Diagnosis

Lack of patient cooperation in closing the mouth and biting
Fracture of the mandibular condylar neck or body with displacement of the proximal fragment
Aplasia/hypoplasia of the condyle
Resorption of the condyle caused by inflammatory or malignant disease

MANDIBULAR CONDYLE NECK FRACTURES

Overview

Definition: Mandibular condylar neck fractures are unilateral or bilateral traumatic discontinuities of the mandible above the body of the ramus and inferior to

the head of the condyle. These fractures may be extracapsular or intracapsular.

Pathogenesis: Fractures of the mandibular condyle are not rare, especially since the advent of high-speed motor vehicle transportation. A blow to the chin in an anteroposterior direction transmits the force horizontally along the mandibular body. To dissipate the force, the mandible must either give way as a unit or collapse in some fashion. The latter is more likely, resulting in a fracture of the weakest part of the bone, the condylar neck. The same is true of a more posterolaterally directed blow, except that only one condylar neck may be fractured.

Clinical Features

Demographics: Condylar neck fractures are commonly seen in patients involved in contact sports, motor vehicle accidents, or physical altercations.

Signs and symptoms

Inability to open and/or move the mandible in a normal fashion
Pain
Preauricular swelling
Possible anterior open bite

Special tests: No special tests are required.

RADIOLOGIC FEATURES

Cardinal Signs

The usual radiographic finding is anteromedial displacement of the proximal fragment of the head and part of the neck of the condyle. The glenoid fossa is empty on the closed view. On pantomographs or lateral skull views there may be increased radiopacity of the neck of the condyle where the proximal and distal fragments overlap. On lateral skull views the fragment is usually found lying horizontally anterior to the normal position. Towne views usually reveal the medial position of the head.

Ancillary Signs

An area of increased radiopacity in the neck of the condyle may result from superimposition of parts of the two fragments.

Differential Diagnosis

Dislocation of the TMJ
Condylar hypoplasia

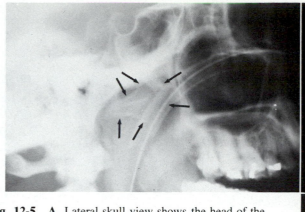
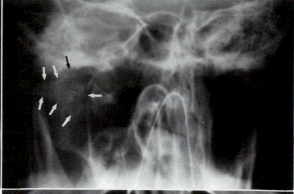
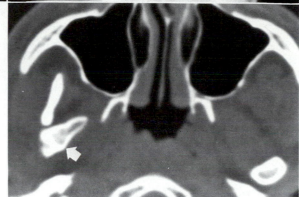

Fig. 12-5   A, Lateral skull view shows the head of the condyle lying horizontally, with its articulating surface directed anteriorly *(arrows)*. Note the anterior open bite and occlusion on only one side. **B,** Towne view reveals the medial position of the head *(arrows)* and articular surface. The coronoid process is higher on the fracture side than on the unaffected side because of muscle pull elevating the affected side. **C,** Axial CT section at the level of the condylar neck shows medial displacement of the condylar fragment *(arrow)*. Note also that part of the ramus of the affected side is visible because of the upward shift of that side due to muscle pull. There is no evidence of the ramus, other than the condyle, on the unaffected side.

SAGITTAL FRACTURE OF THE MANDIBULAR CONDYLE

Overview

Definition: Sagittal fracture occurs through the head of the mandibular condyle in an anteroposterior direction, splitting the head into two almost equally large medial and lateral segments.

Pathogenesis: The fracture results from a high-force blow, such as in a car accident, that causes the bone to break at its weakest point or in a plane in the direction of the force.

Clinical Features

Demographics: Although sagittal fractures of the condyle were thought to be uncommon, the use of computerized tomography (CT) imaging of the TMJ area after motor vehicle accidents is changing that opinion. Such fractures may be seen fairly regularly in a busy trauma center on CT images made for neurologic investigation. They may even be seen as unsuspected findings, at least with respect to the actual morphology of the fracture.

Signs and symptoms
    Pain no moving the mandible or inability to move the mandible on the affected side
    Preauricular swelling

Special tests: No special tests are required.

RADIOLOGIC FINDINGS

Cardinal Signs

    Separation of the medial from the lateral side of the condyle in an axial view, especially on CT.

Ancillary Signs

    Scissorlike separation of the medial and lateral poles of the condyle on lateral projections such as plain transcranial views, pantomographs, and lateral tomographs.

Differential Diagnosis

    Bifid condyle

A   **B**

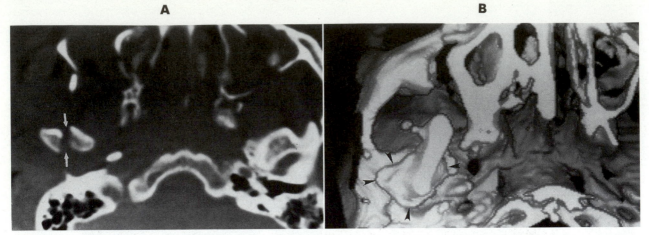

Fig. 12-6   A, Axial bone mode CT clearly shows the separation of the medial and lateral fragments *(arrows)*. Also visible is the interruption of various osseous structures of the midface region. **B,** Three dimensionally reformatted CT view shows abnormal morphology of the head of the condyle. However, it does not reveal the fracture line, which is so clearly seen on the axial unreformatted view, because of the algorithm "smoothing" techniques used to produce this image.

ANKYLOSIS OF THE MANDIBLE AND SURROUNDING BONES

Definition: Ankylosis is the bony or fibrous union of part of the mandible with one of the surrounding bones, resulting in immobility of the TMJ. This union may be within the capsule of the joint (intracapsular) or away from the joint proper (extracapsular).

OSSEOUS ANKYLOSIS OF THE TMJ

Overview

Definition: Osseous ankylosis of the TMJ is the bony union of the mandibular condyle with part of the temporal bone, resulting in immobility of the joint.

Pathogenesis: Osseous ankylosis of the TMJ most commonly results from inflammatory destruction of the synovial lining of the joint, resulting in contact between the underlying osseous structures. The inflammation may result from primary infection of the joint; extension from a neighboring infection such as otitis media, mastoiditis, or osteomyelitis of the mandible; blood-borne infections from several sources; trauma to the joint; or one of the rheumatoid diseases such as rheumatoid arthritis, ankylosing spondylitis, psoriatic arthritis, and Reiter syndrome. It may also result from hemarthrosis, such as may occur in hemophiliacs.

Clinical Features

Demographics: Because of the large number of possible causes, there are no clear demographic features associated with ankylosis of the TMJ.

Signs and symptoms: True ankylosis, or osseous union between the condyle and temporal bone, manifests as a painless inability to open the mouth properly. The degree of this inability is variable, because the bone of the mandible is somewhat flexible; thus even with bilateral ankylosis there is not complete lack of movement of bone.

If the ankylosis is bilateral and has been present since before the end of somatic growth, retrognathia and downward growth of the mandible may be present. In unilateral cases there is usually a fullness of the face on the affected side and flattening of the face on the unaffected side. Deviation of the midline toward the affected side may also be present, a result of unilateral normal growth.

Special tests: There are no special tests, other than asking the patient to open the mouth as widely as possible. If necessary, local anesthesia may be used to overcome possible muscle spasms, the results of which could mimic ankylosis.

If a specific disease such as rheumatoid arthritis is suspected, specific tests must be carried out.

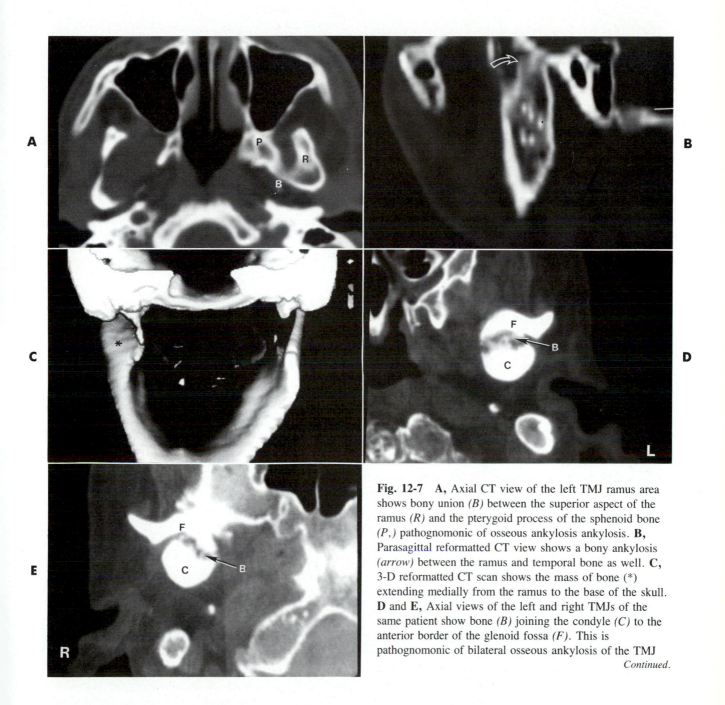

Fig. 12-7 **A,** Axial CT view of the left TMJ ramus area shows bony union *(B)* between the superior aspect of the ramus *(R)* and the pterygoid process of the sphenoid bone *(P,)* pathognomonic of osseous ankylosis ankylosis. **B,** Parasagittal reformatted CT view shows a bony ankylosis *(arrow)* between the ramus and temporal bone as well. **C,** 3-D reformatted CT scan shows the mass of bone (*) extending medially from the ramus to the base of the skull. **D** and **E,** Axial views of the left and right TMJs of the same patient show bone *(B)* joining the condyle *(C)* to the anterior border of the glenoid fossa *(F)*. This is pathognomonic of bilateral osseous ankylosis of the TMJ

Continued.

RADIOLOGIC FEATURES

Cardinal Signs

Lack of a demonstrable joint space on plain and tomographic views, usually accompanied by increased radiopacity of the joint area, which results from increased bone across the former joint space.

Ancillary Signs

Lack of movement of the osseous components between open- and closed-mouth views.

Differential Diagnosis

Osseous ankylosis of the TMJ
Extracapsular ankylosis between the mandible and temporal or zygomatic bone
Muscle spasm
Fracture of the mandible

OSSEOUS ANKYLOSIS OF BONES OTHER THAN THE TMJ

Overview

Definition: Osseous ankylosis of the coronoid process of the mandible is the bony union of the coronoid process of the mandible with part of the temporal bone, zygomatic bone, or maxilla, resulting in immobility of the joint.

Pathogenesis: Ankylosis of the coronoid process often results from direct trauma to the area, which causes bleeding with osseous organization.

Clinical Features

Demographics: Because of the traumatic origin of the lesion, it may be found in anyone who has received sufficient trauma to the area of the mandibular coronoid process.

Signs and symptoms: The patient is unable to move the mandible freely and may have deviation to the affected side on opening. If the injury occurs before the completion of growth of the mandible, midline is deviated to the affected side, giving the face a flattened appearance on the affected side and a fuller appearance on the unaffected side. The ankylosis itself is usually asymptomatic.

Special tests: There are no special tests, other than asking the patient to attempt to open and move the mandible anteriorly and toward the unaffected side.

RADIOLOGIC FEATURES

Cardinal Signs

Loss of the osseous architecture in the coronoid process area, often combined with a mass of bone where the coronoid process would be

Ancillary Signs

Possible hypoplasia of the ramus of the mandible on the same side; signs of degenerative joint disease resulting from altered function
Deviation of the midline may to the affected side

Differential Diagnosis

Ankylosis of the TMJ
Osteochondroma of the coronoid process

FIBROUS ANKYLOSIS OF THE TMJ

Overview

Definition: Fibrous ankylosis of the TMJ is the fibrous union of the condyle of the mandible with part of the temporal bone, resulting in immobility of the joint.

Pathogenesis: In fibrous ankylosis of the TMJ, which is probably a variant of osseous ankylosis, the osseous components are united by fibrous tissue that has not undergone ossification. The causes are therefore the same as those of osseous ankylosis, namely inflammation resulting from localized infection; trauma to the joint; one of the rheumatoid diseases such as rheumatoid arthritis, ankylosing spondylitis, psoriatic arthritis, and Reiter syndrome; or hemarthrosis, such as may occur in hemophiliacs.

Clinical Features

Demographics: Because of the large number of possible causes, there are no clear demographic features associated with fibrous ankylosis of the TMJ.

Signs and symptoms: Fibrous ankylosis between the condyle and temporal bone manifests with the gradual onset of a painless inability to open the mouth properly. The degree to which this occurs is variable, as the fibrous tissue may allow some movement between the two bony components of the mandible. This, added to the innate ability of the mandible to flex somewhat, means that varying amounts of movement will be possible.

Special tests: There are no special tests, other than asking the patient to open as widely as possible. If

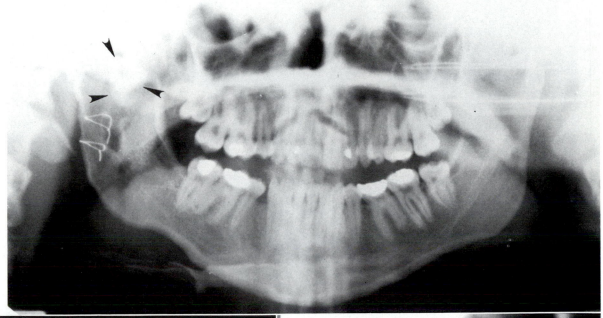

F

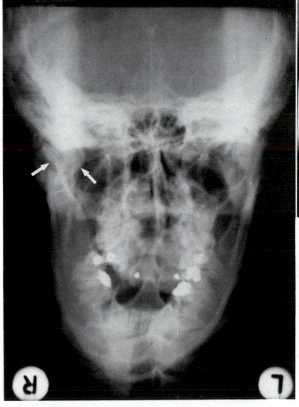

G

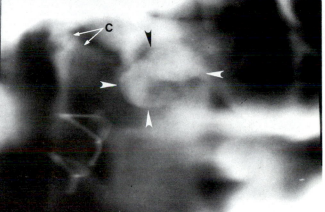

H

Fig. 12-7, cont'd. **F,** The region of the right coronoid process reveals a large osseous mass *(arrowheads),* which may be continuous with both the coronoid process and from the zygomatic arch. The metallic sutures are from a previous trauma-related operation. **G,** Modified Towne view shows a mass of bone in the same mediolateral position as the right coronoid process *(arrows).* The midline of the jaw has deviated toward the right. **H,** Lateral tomogram of the right mandibular ramus area shows a large osseous mass extending from the coronoid process (which no longer actually exists) to the zygomatic arch *(arrowheads).* The altered morphology of the condyle *(C),* with flattening and erosion, and the shortening of the neck are consistent with degenerative joint disease.

Continued.

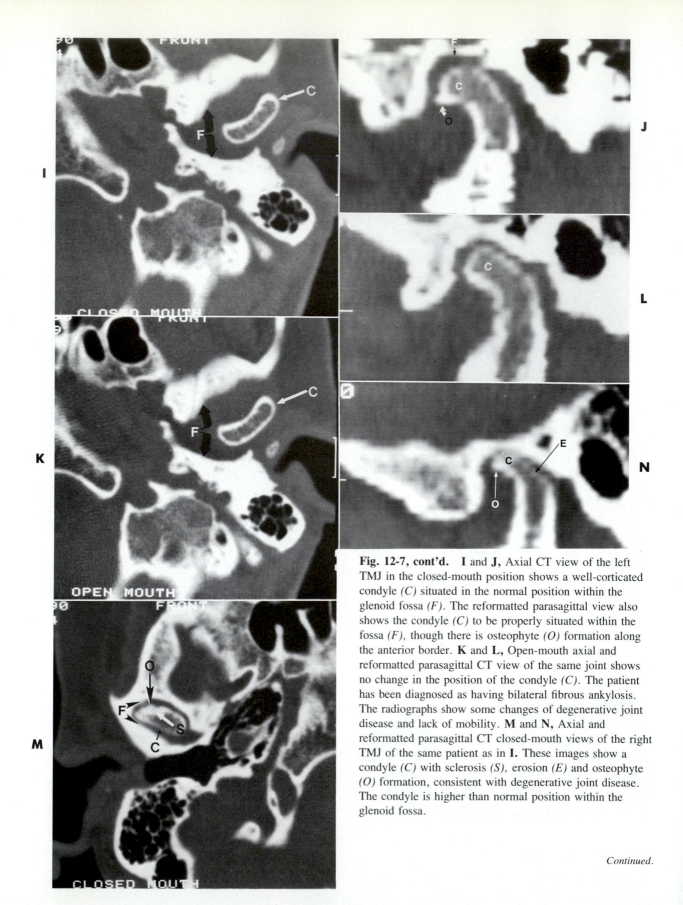

Fig. 12-7, cont'd.   **I** and **J,** Axial CT view of the left TMJ in the closed-mouth position shows a well-corticated condyle *(C)* situated in the normal position within the glenoid fossa *(F)*. The reformatted parasagittal view also shows the condyle *(C)* to be properly situated within the fossa *(F)*, though there is osteophyte *(O)* formation along the anterior border. **K** and **L,** Open-mouth axial and reformatted parasagittal CT view of the same joint shows no change in the position of the condyle *(C)*. The patient has been diagnosed as having bilateral fibrous ankylosis. The radiographs show some changes of degenerative joint disease and lack of mobility. **M** and **N,** Axial and reformatted parasagittal CT closed-mouth views of the right TMJ of the same patient as in **I.** These images show a condyle *(C)* with sclerosis *(S)*, erosion *(E)* and osteophyte *(O)* formation, consistent with degenerative joint disease. The condyle is higher than normal position within the glenoid fossa.

Continued.

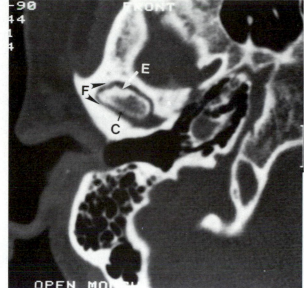

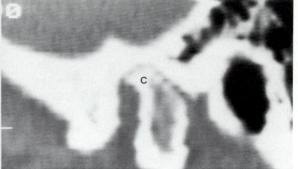

Fig. 12-7, cont'd. **O** and **P,** No movement of the condyle is seen between the closed-mouth views of **M** and **N,** and these open-mouth views. This finding is consistent with fibrous ankylosis.

necessary, local anesthesia may be used to overcome possible muscle spasms, the results of which could mimic ankylosis.

RADIOLOGIC FEATURES

Cardinal Signs

The appearance of fibrous union is not as well defined as that of osseous union. There may be some loss of the smooth cortication of the bony components of the joint, although the appearance may be similar to that of fibrous union of fracture, in which a clear cortex is visible. There may be some destructive or proliferative bone changes, and the size of the joint space may be decreased.

Ancillary Signs

Limited movement of the bony components of the joint between open- and closed-mouth radiographs

Differential Diagnosis

Osseous ankylosis of the TMJ
Extracapsular ankylosis between the mandible and temporal or zygomatic bone
Muscle spasm
Fracture of the mandible

INTERNAL DERANGEMENTS OF THE TMJ

Overview

Definition: Internal derangement of the TMJ is an abnormal relationship of the disk relative to the condyle, anterior articular eminence, or glenoid fossa.

Pathogenesis: The underlying abnormality is subluxation or dislocation of the articular disk. An understanding of the normal meniscal-condylar movements is necessary to interpret the imaging studies.

Normally the biconcave articular disk is interposed between the condyle and the articular surface of the temporal bone. The thinner central portion, known as the intermediate zone, occupies the narrowest part of the joint between the eminence and the condyle. The thicker anterior and posterior bands lie, respectively, in front of and behind this region. On opening of the mouth, the condyle glides forward over the eminence and carries the disk with it. However, to maintain the congruity of the joint, the disk also rotates posteriorly with respect to the condyle. Even with the mouth fully open, the intermediate zone still occupies the narrowest point between the eminence and the condyle. The normal position of the disk is partly maintained by its biconcave shape. Also contributing to its stability is a balance between the forward pull of the superior head of the lateral pterygoid and the backward pull of the elastic bilaminar zone, which connects the posterior disk band to the tympanic plate and condylar neck.

With internal derangements, the disk is usually displaced anteriorly or anteromedially. Two major forms are described: anterior displacement with and without reduction.

Anterior displacement with reduction: Anterior displacement with reduction is the less advanced form, its mildest variant being anterior displacement with early reduction to the normal position on opening of the mouth. With the mouth closed, the posterior band comes to lie anterior to the condyle. In this case the anterior part of the bilaminar zone occupies the narrowest part of the joint. On opening of the mouth, the condyle passes over the posterior band so as to articulate normally with the intermediate zone. More advanced stages are associated with reduction of the disk at progressively later stages of opening. On closing of the mouth, the disk returns to its abnormal anterior position.

Anterior displacement without reduction: When the bilaminar zone becomes overstretched because of anterior dislocation of the disk, it can lose its elasticity. When this happens it will no longer hold the disk back sufficiently to allow the condyle to pass over the posterior band and reduce the dislocation. The disk therefore remains dislocated anteriorly, with the posterior band in front of instead of behind the condyle. It can then cause a mechanical obstruction to the normal anterior translation of the condyle on opening of the mouth. With further overstretching, the bilaminar zone may become perforated or detached from the posterior band and degenerative changes may eventually ensue.

Clinical Features

Demographics: Internal derangement of the TMJ occurs in up to 28% of adults and can be a major cause of pain and dysfunction. It is particularly common in relatively young women, although post mortem studies suggest that the prevalence of disk dislocation actually increases with age. Women are affected more frequently than men, with some series reporting a ratio of greater than 10:1. The condition is particularly common in people with benign hypermobile joint syndrome, another condition that is much more common among women.

Signs and symptoms

Anterior displacement with reduction: The classic sign of anterior displacement with reduction is the "reciprocal click." When the condyle moves forward over the anteriorly dislocated posterior band, the disk suddenly "snaps" posteriorly to regain its normal position. In so doing it can create a click, which is often audible to both the patient and other people nearby. The click may be palpated by the examining clinician. When the mouth is closed again and the disk returns to the dislocated position, a second click may occur, although this is usually far less noticeable than the opening click. Early reduction of the disk is associated with an early opening click; more advanced cases are associated with later opening clicks.

Anterior displacement without reduction: The classic sign of anterior displacement without reduction is the "closed lock." There is typically a history of a previous reciprocal click. This click will have ceased at the same time that limitation of opening of the mouth began. The limitation of motion results from mechanical obstruction of anterior translation caused by the anteriorly situated disk.

Special tests: When a closed lock is unilateral, the jaw moves towards the affected side on opening.

RADIOLOGIC FEATURES

Because the vast majority of internal derangements are caused by soft tissue abnormalities, plain films and conventional tomography are of limited value. Computer tomography has been used with varying success, but its delineation of soft tissue structures is not as good as that of either arthrography or magnetic resonance (MR) imaging. We feel that CT is better reserved for conditions that primarily affect bony structures.

Cardinal Signs

Anterior displacement with reduction

Fluoroscopy during arthrography—The disk appears as a filling defect in the contrast. The disk is observed to be displaced anteriorly while the mouth is closed. As the mouth opens, the disk is initially compressed by the forward movement of the condyle. At some stage during the opening phase, the disk moves suddenly in a posterior direction so that the posterior band lies posterior to the condyle. On closing of the mouth, the disk initially moves posteriorly with the condyle. Before closing is complete, the disk moves forward again to an abnormal position, with the posterior band anterior to the condyle.

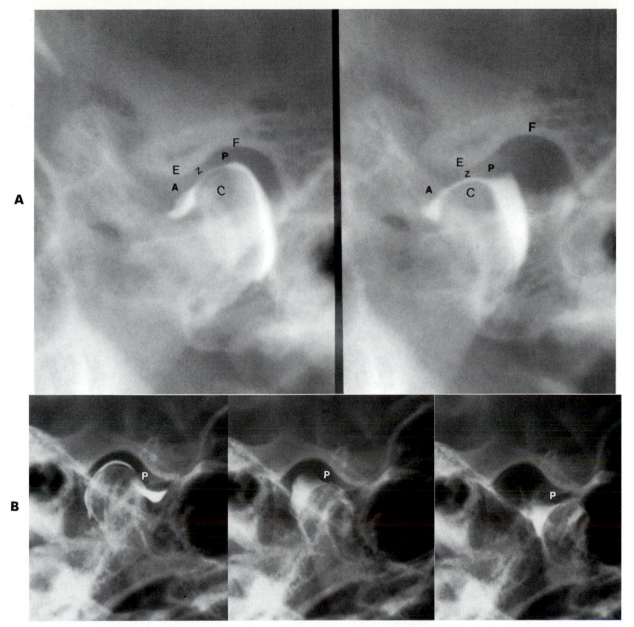

Fig. 12-8 **A,** *Left,* Normal TMJ arthrogram; closed mouth. Contrast in the inferior compartment outlines the inferior surface of the disk. The intermediate zone *(Z)* lies in the narrowest part of the joint between the condyle *(C)* and the anterior articular eminence *(E).* The anterior *(A)* and posterior *(P)* bands occupy the wider parts of the joint that lie in front of and behind the condyle, respectively. *F* indicates the glenoid fossa. *Right,* Open mouth. The condyle has translated anteriorly and the disk has moved forwards with it. It has also rotated posteriorly relative to the condyle, thus maintaining congruous articular surfaces between the condyle and the eminence. Note that the intermediate zone continues to occupy the narrowest point between the condyle and the eminence. **B,** *Left,* Arthrogram showing anterior displacement with early reduction; closed mouth. Anterior impression on the contrast represents the anteriorly displaced disk. The posterior band *(P)* is difficult to identify clearly in this static image. *Center,* Partially open mouth. The posterior band has reduced to the normal position and now lies behind the condyle. The reduction was easily detected on fluoroscopy, and the sudden posterior movement of the posterior band coincided with an audible click. *Right,* Open mouth. Appearances remain normal, with the disk rotating posteriorly with respect to the condyle. *Continued.*

Spot films during arthrography—Closed-mouth views show a filling defect anterior to the condyle; this represents the displaced disk. Open-mouth views appear normal, with the condyle forward on the eminence and the disk interposed between the condyle and the eminence.

Magnetic resonance imaging—Closed- and open-mouthed sagittal T1-weighted images show the disk as a low-signal structure that is displaced anterior to the condyle with the mouth closed but is in normal position with the mouth open. Coronal images may demonstrate associated medial, or occasionally lateral, disk displacement.

Anterior Displacement without Reduction

Arthrography—The disk appears as a filling defect in the contrast and is observed to be displaced anteriorly. During attempts to open the mouth, the condyle shows limited anterior translation. The disk either moves forward with the condyle or almost completely obstructs any forward translation. An advanced closed lock may look almost identical with the mouth open or closed.

Magnetic resonance imaging—Closed- and open-mouth views show the disk to be displaced anteriorly and often buckled, particularly in the open-mouth images. Coronal images may demonstrate associated medial, and occasionally lateral, disk displacement.

Disk Detachment and Perforation

Arthrography—Contrast injected into the posterior aspect of the inferior compartment immediately fills both the inferior and superior compartments. This may be result from a small perforation in the intermediate zone or from a free communication behind the posterior band, the result of detachment from the bilaminar zone.

Magnetic resonance imaging—Perforations and detachments cannot be reliably diagnosed with MR; however, they may be suspected when the disk appears fragmented or shows markedly increased signal.

Ancillary Signs

Changes of degenerative joint disease are often associated with internal derangement. Degenerative changes are more easily detected with MR imaging or conventional radiography than with arthrography.

Perforations and detachments are nearly always associated with anterior displacement of the disk, usually without reduction.

Differential Diagnosis

Degenerative joint disease may cause crepitus, which can be confused with the clicks of a dislocating disk.

In both arthrography and MR imaging, anterior displacement with reduction can be confused with anterior displacement without reduction if the patient does not open the mouth sufficiently to cause relocation of the dislocated disk.

Text continued on page 366.

Fig. 12-8, cont'd. C, *Left,* Arthrogram showing anterior displacement without reduction in a patient with only a minor restriction of opening; closed mouth. Anterior filling defect in the contrast represents the anteriorly displaced disk *(D)*. Typically, it is not possible to identify the different parts of the disk. *Right,* Open mouth. As the condyle has moved forward so has disk, with anterior translation sufficient to restrict mouth opening only minimally. **D,** *Left,* Arthrogram showing anterior displacement without reduction in a patient with a closed lock; closed mouth. The disk *(D)* is displaced anteriorly. *Right,* Open mouth. Although the condyle can be seen to have rotated slightly, consistent with the earliest movement of mouth opening, the anteriorly displaced disk has remained in the same position, effectively blocking any anterior translation of the condyle. **E,** *Left,* Arthrogram showing anterior displacement with detachment of the posterior band from the bilaminar zone; closed mouth. Contrast has filled a common superior and inferior compartment that is no longer separated by disk or bilaminar zone. The condyle *(C)* and the anteriorly displaced disk are outlined by the contrast. **E,** *Right,* Open mouth. The condyle has moved forward, carrying the disk with it. There is some obstruction to anterior translation by the persistently displaced disk.

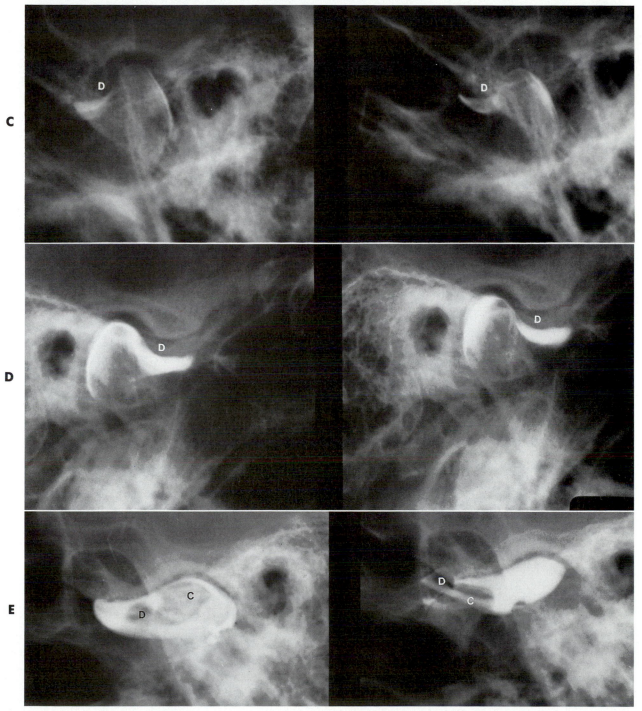

Continued.

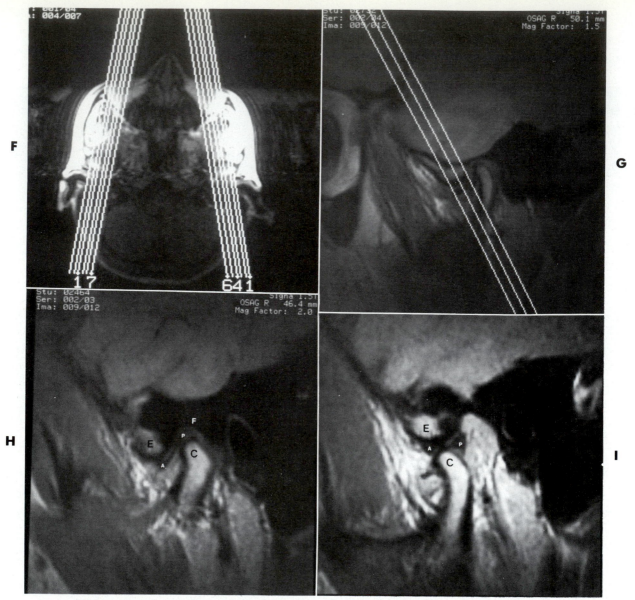

Fig. 12-8, cont'd. **F,** Corrected sagittal planes for MR of the TMJ. Axial scout for planning sagittal views: Oblique sagittal images in the plane of the mandible, as shown here, generally demonstrate anatomic structures in a manner that is more readily appreciated than the straight sagittal views. **G,** Sagittal scout for planning coronal views: Coronal images performed with a forwards tilt, as shown in this scout, facilitate interpretation of mediolateral disk displacement, as the anatomic landmarks of the anterior articular eminence and condyle can usually be seen in the same images as the displaced disk. **H,** Normal MR image of TMJ (T1-weighted image; TR450, TE20); closed mouth. The condyle *(C)* and anterior articular eminence *(E)* both contain normal fatty bone marrow and are therefore high signal (light). The overlying cortex is low signal (black), as is the adjacent dense temporal bone of the glenoid fossa *(F)*. Note the normal positions of the anterior *(A)* and posterior *(P)* bands of the disk. The articular disk in this patient is quite thin but within normal limits. Its low signal intensity results from its fibrocartilaginous composition. **I,** Open mouth. The condyle *(C)* and the disk have moved forward, and the disk has also rotated posteriorly over the condyle. The anterior *(A)* and posterior *(P)* bands continue to lie in front of and behind the condyle, respectively. As is often the case, the disk is more easily identified in the open-mouthed view as moves away from other low signal intensity structures. Also, as its contour changes to accommodate the articular surfaces, it assumes more of the classical "bowtie" shape.

Continued.

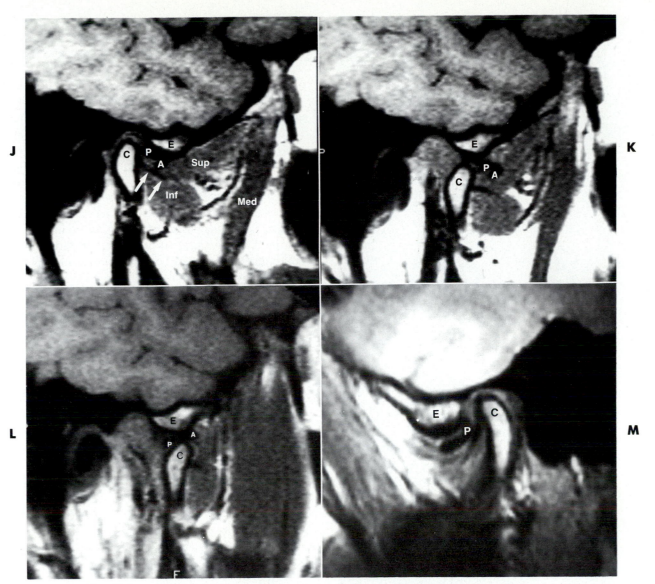

Fig. 12-8, cont'd. **J,** MR image shows anterior displacement with late opening reduction (T1-weighted image; TR450, TE20); closed mouth. The disk is displaced anterior to the condyle *(C)* and below the eminence *(E)*. The disk is also buckled so that the anterior band *(A)* lies below and slightly in front of the posterior band *(P)*. Note also the medial pterygoid muscle *Med)* and the superior *(Sup)* and inferior *(Inf)* heads of the lateral pterygoid muscle. The linear low signal intensity structure extending from the neck of the mandible is the tendon of the inferior head of lateral pterygoid *(arrows)*. This can sometimes be mistaken for an anteriorly displaced disk. **K,** Partially open mouth. The condyle *(C)* has moved forward but the disk remains displaced, with the posterior band *(P)* trapped anterior to the narrow region between the condyle and the anterior articular eminence *(E)*. **L,** Open mouth. The condyle *(C)* has moved forward to just beyond the anterior articular eminence *(E)* and the disk has reduced, with the posterior band *(P)* moving back to its normal position behind the condyle. The anterior band *(A)* remains in front of the condyle, and the disk has regained its normal "bowtie" configuration. **M,** MR image showing anterior displacement without reduction (T1-weighted images; TR450, TE20); closed-mouth sagittal view. The disk is displaced, with the posterior band *(P)* lying anterior to the condyle *(C)*. *E* indicates the anterior articular eminence.

Continued.

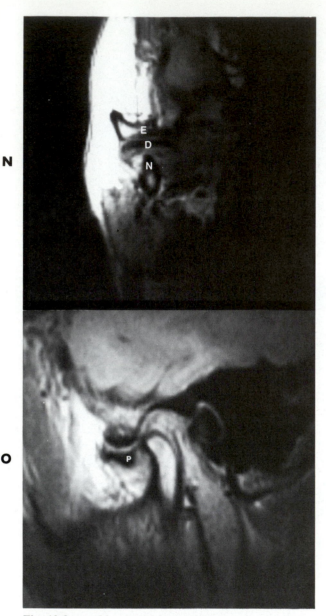

Fig. 12-8, cont'd. **N,** Closed-mouth oblique coronal view. The disk *(D)* lies midway between the anterior articular eminence *(E)* above and the neck of the mandible *(N)* below. There is no evidence of medial or lateral displacement. **O,** Open-mouthed sagittal view. The disk has deformed slightly as it obstructs the forward movement of the condyle. The posterior band *(P)* continues to lie anterior to the condyle.

OSTEOARTHROSIS OF THE TMJ

Overview

Definition: In osteoarthrosis of the TMJ, the primary abnormality is degeneration of articular cartilage.

Pathogenesis: Osteoarthrosis results from the failure of intraarticular structures to resist the forces that are applied to the joint. Primary and secondary forms of osteoarthrosis have been described. In primary disease, there are no initiating factors besides age and use; this is probably uncommon in the TMJ. Secondary osteoarthrosis occurs when the joint is damaged either by an initiating event, such as trauma or infection, or by a more continuous or repetitive process, such as internal derangement. As discussed in the section on TMJ implants, secondary osteoarthrosis may be a sequela of foreign body reaction to implants or other introduced material.

Clinical Features

Demographics: Osteoarthrosis is the most common disease of the TMJ. It becomes progressively more common with advancing age, but it can be seen as early as the second decade of life in patients with internal derangements. It is more common in women.

Signs and symptoms: Audible and palpable crepitus

Pain and limitation of movement

Special tests: No special tests are required.

RADIOLOGIC FEATURES

Cardinal Signs

Narrowing of the "joint space," flattening of the condyle and anterior articular eminence, formation of subcortical cysts and erosion, osteophytosis, and eburnation

Ancillary Signs

Increased tracer uptake on bone scintigraphy

Differential Diagnosis

Clinically the crepitus of osteoarthrosis may be confused with the clicks of internal derangement

Increased tracer uptake is nonspecific; it is seen in any condition associated with increased osteoblastic activity

Destruction of cartilage and erosion are also seen in inflammatory arthritides, such as rheumatoid arthritis

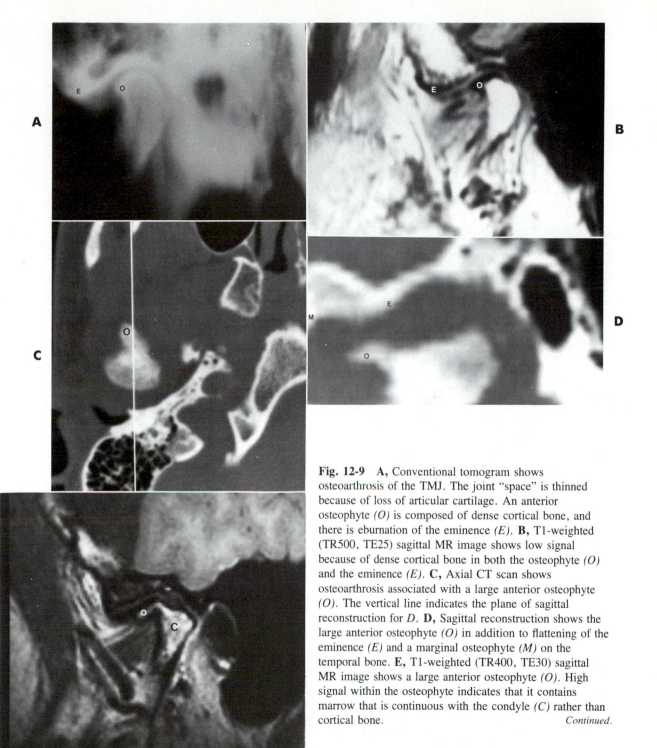

Fig. 12-9 A, Conventional tomogram shows osteoarthrosis of the TMJ. The joint "space" is thinned because of loss of articular cartilage. An anterior osteophyte *(O)* is composed of dense cortical bone, and there is eburnation of the eminence *(E)*. **B,** T1-weighted (TR500, TE25) sagittal MR image shows low signal because of dense cortical bone in both the osteophyte *(O)* and the eminence *(E)*. **C,** Axial CT scan shows osteoarthrosis associated with a large anterior osteophyte *(O)*. The vertical line indicates the plane of sagittal reconstruction for *D*. **D,** Sagittal reconstruction shows the large anterior osteophyte *(O)* in addition to flattening of the eminence *(E)* and a marginal osteophyte *(M)* on the temporal bone. **E,** T1-weighted (TR400, TE30) sagittal MR image shows a large anterior osteophyte *(O)*. High signal within the osteophyte indicates that it contains marrow that is continuous with the condyle *(C)* rather than cortical bone.   *Continued.*

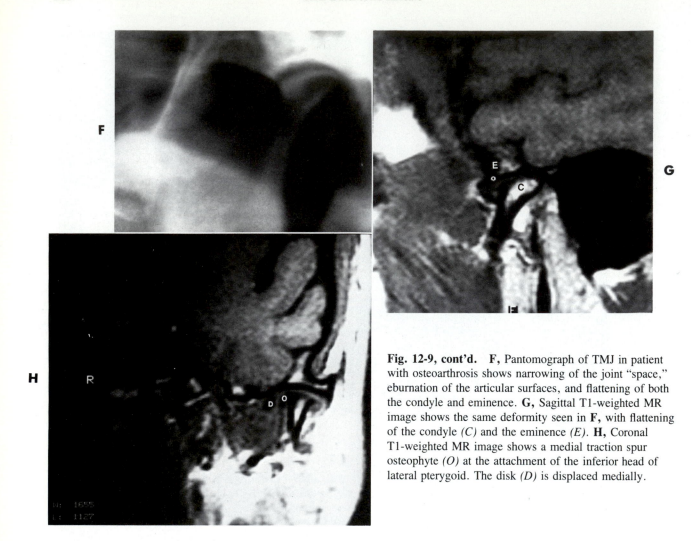

Fig. 12-9, cont'd.   F, Pantomograph of TMJ in patient with osteoarthrosis shows narrowing of the joint "space," eburnation of the articular surfaces, and flattening of both the condyle and eminence. **G,** Sagittal T1-weighted MR image shows the same deformity seen in **F,** with flattening of the condyle *(C)* and the eminence *(E)*. **H,** Coronal T1-weighted MR image shows a medial traction spur osteophyte *(O)* at the attachment of the inferior head of lateral pterygoid. The disk *(D)* is displaced medially.

RHEUMATOID CHANGES IN THE TMJ

Overview

Only some of the features of the various diseases causing rheumatoid changes in the TMJ will be considered here. The complexity and variability of each of these disease processes is such that the reader is encouraged to consult references in standard textbooks for each individually.

Definition: Rheumatoid arthritis and many related arthritides are assumed to be autoimmune diseases involving several joints, including the TMJ.

Pathogenesis: Involvement of the TMJ in rheumatoid arthritis is highly likely. Rheumatoid changes in the TMJ may also occur in association with one of the other spondyloarthropathies (ankylosing spondylitis, psoriatic arthritis, and Reiter syndrome), as well as with gout or Lyme disease. These diseases, which are generally considered to have an autoimmune component, may result from a genetic predisposition. Environmental factors such as trauma or an infectious or toxic agent may also be involved.

Clinical Features

Demographics
Rheumatoid arthritis
    20 to 60 years
    More common under 40 years in women; equal gender incidence over 40

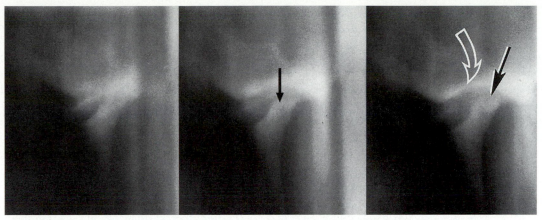

Fig. 12-10   Three corrected lateral linear tomograms of the TMJ show advanced erosion of the head of the condyle *(white arrow),* possible subarticular cyst formation *(black arrow),* and loss of anterior articular eminence height. There is sclerosis of the border of the glenoid fossa *(open arrow),* posterior positioning of the condyle within the fossa, and no evidence of loss of joint space.

Reiter syndrome
    20 to 40 years
    50:1 male predilection
Psoriatic arthritis
    20 to 50 years
    No sex predilection
Ankylosing spondylitis
    15 to 35 years
    10:1 male predilection
Gouty arthritis
    30 to 50 years
    20:1 male predilection

Signs and symptoms: The presenting features of ankylosing spondylitis may be inability to flex the spine freely and, in jaw involvement, may range from minimal pain and inflammation to inability to move the mandible because of ankylosis. Soft tissue swelling may also be present, although among the early signs of rheumatoid diseases, this may be difficult to evaluate in the TMJ. Psoriatic skin lesions may be seen in psoriatic arthritis.

Special tests: In rheumatoid arthritis, erythrocyte sedimentation rate, C-reactive protein, and rheumatoid factor, especially the immunoglobulin G type, are usually elevated. Human leukocyte antigen DR4 is also found in rheumatoid arthritis. Serum uric acid is usually elevated in gouty arthritis.

RADIOLOGIC FEATURES

Cardinal Signs

The major radiographic findings are resorption of the articulating surface of the head of the condyle and articular eminence; sclerosis of the osseous components; a possible decrease in the size of the "joint space"; and, in advanced cases, ankylosis.

Ancillary Signs

Anterior disk location or structure or disk destruction
Posterior positioning of the condyle within the glenoid fossa
Osteophyte formation
Subcortical cyst formation
Some of these result from secondary osteoarthrosis

Differential Diagnosis

Each of these rheumatoid diseases is included in the differential diagnosis for the others:
Ankylosing spondylitis
Rheumatoid arthritis
Psoriatic arthritis
Reiter syndrome
Gouty arthritis
Degenerative joint disease

COSTOCHONDRAL GRAFT IN THE TMJ

Overview

Definition: A costochondral graft is a cartilaginous autograft from the costochondral region of a rib. It is commonly used for replacement of the mandibular condylar head.

Pathogenesis: Such surgical replacement of a damaged component of the TMJ may be done after trauma, infection/inflammation, or neoplasm.

Clinical Features

Demographics: Placement of autogenous implants for a variety of TMJ diseases has increased; as such, there is no particular segment of the population that is more likely to have such an implant.

Signs and symptoms: There are no signs or symptoms unless secondary problems arise.

Special tests: No special tests are required, other than to elicit a history of previous autograft surgery.

RADIOLOGIC FEATURES

Cardinal Signs

An altered shape of the mandibular condyle with radiolucent areas scattered throughout, or a radiolucent condyle with ossification scattered throughout; either of these may represent cartilage with ossification

Ancillary Signs

Metallic sutures or other fixation devices that attach the graft to the rest of the mandible

Differential Diagnosis

Osteoarthrosis
Metastasis to the condyle

TEMPOROMANDIBULAR JOINT IMPLANT AND OTHER FOREIGN BODY REACTIONS

Overview

Definition: Any of a number of foreign materials may be injected or surgically placed into the TMJ, or used to replace part or all of the joint.

Pathogenesis: Implants have long been used to replace part or all of the TMJ structure. Joint compo-nents may be destroyed by arthritis, trauma, or infection; implants may be made of metal, polymers, or combinations of the two. One of the more widely used implants in recent years was Proplast Teflon for disk replacement. This material was not as stable and resistant as originally thought; it broke down, resulting in noticeable damage to the joints. Another popular material is Delrin, which is used as a condylar replacement. Unrelated, except that they too are foreign materials, are injections of various medications into the joint.

Clinical Features

Demographics: Implants are placed for a variety of causes, such as replacement for joint components damaged by degenerative joint disease, ankylosis, or surgery for neoplasm. As such, there is no specific population or age group in which implants might be expected, although in general the patients will be older.

Signs and symptoms: There may be no signs or symptoms if the implants are functioning properly. Pain and obvious asymmetry may result from secondary degenerative disease, inflammation, and implant malpositioning. In the case of infected foreign materials, severe degenerative joint disease may occur with attendant pain and dysfunction.

RADIOLOGIC FEATURES

Cardinal Signs

The Proplast Teflon disk replacement appears as a slightly radiopaque thick line, either in the area where the disk should be or, if displaced, in a paracondylar or parafossa position. The osseous structures associated with the implant often exhibit the changes of degenerative joint disease (osteoarthrosis), which range from erosion to osteophyte formation and sclerosis.

In the case of Delrin implants, the condyle may have normal external morphology but lack the radiopacity, cortex, or trabecular pattern associated with normal bone. Delrin appears homogeneous and much more radiolucent.

Injections such as sclerosing solutions into the joint may cause foreign body reactions. These may result in erosive changes, often associated with areas of bone sclerosis. In some cases there may

Text continued on page 374.

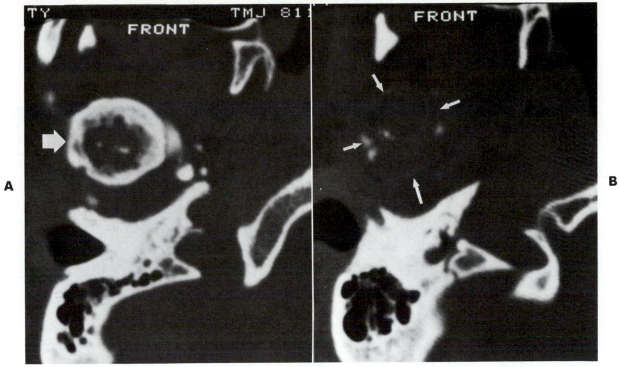

Fig. 12-11 Axial CT views, at different levels, of costochondral implants show a mixed radiolucent/radiopaque irregular osseous structure in place of the normal osseous pattern and altered morphology of the heads of the condyle *(arrows)*. This pattern is consistent with the radiographic appearance of cartilage.

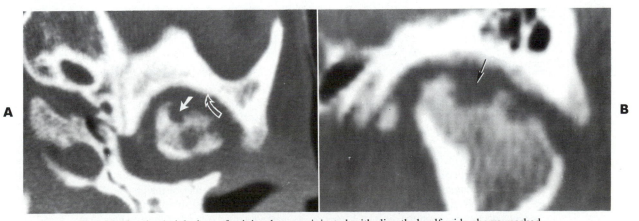

Fig. 12-12 **A,** Axial view of a joint that was injected with dimethyl sulfoxide shows marked erosion *(closed arrows)* and altered morphology of the condyle and sclerosis of the bone of the glenoid fossa *(open arrow)*. **B,** 2D parasagittal reconstruction shows loss of cortical bone on the superior surface and large radiolucent areas of erosion or cartilage formation *(arrows)*.

Continued.

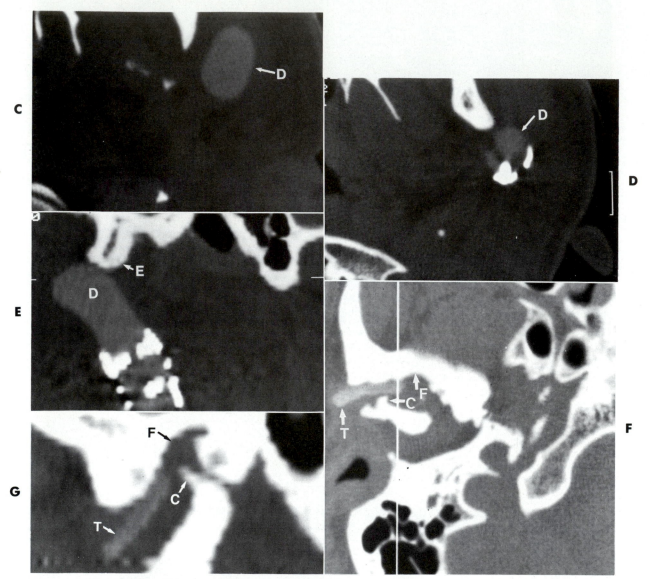

Fig. 12-12, cont'd.   **C** and **D,** Axial CT of the right TMJ area shows a moderately radiopaque homogeneous oval mass *(D),* representing a Delrin condylar prosthesis, anterior to the normal location of the condyle in the closed-mouth position. The metallic radiopaque areas represent the mesh that holds the implant in place. **E,** Parasagittal reformatted view shows the position of the implant *(D)* anterior to the anterior articular eminence *(E)* in the closed-mouth view, confirming the malposition of the implant. **F,** and **G,** Axial view of the right TMJ shows a band of increased radiopacity representing an anteriorly displaced Teflon implant *(T).* There is marked erosion and alteration of the condyle *(C)* and erosion of the anterior border of the glenoid fossa *(F).* The parasagittal reformatted view confirms the anterior displacement of the implant. There is osteophyte formation on the anterior border of the markedly altered head of the condyle.

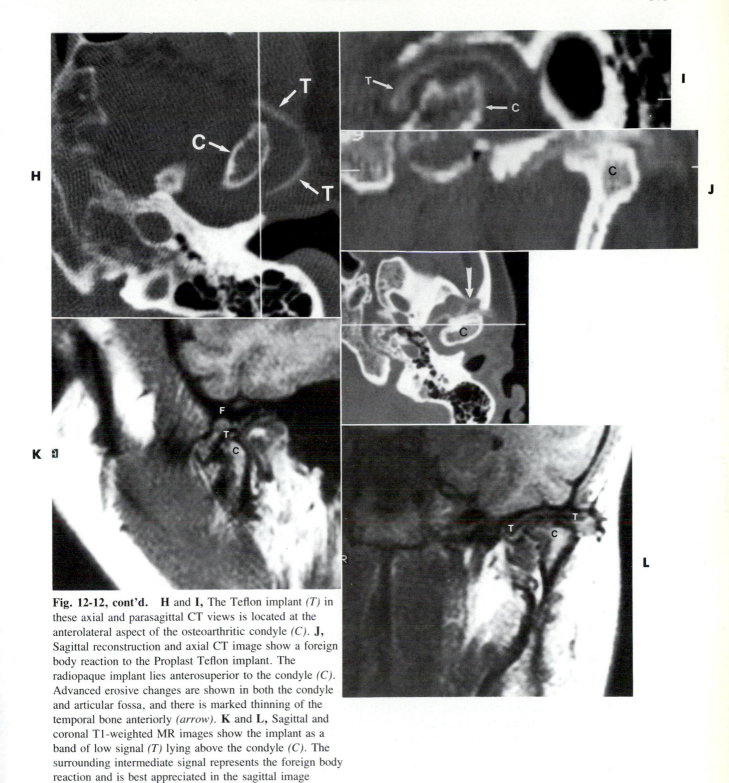

Fig. 12-12, cont'd. **H** and **I,** The Teflon implant *(T)* in these axial and parasagittal CT views is located at the anterolateral aspect of the osteoarthritic condyle *(C).* **J,** Sagittal reconstruction and axial CT image show a foreign body reaction to the Proplast Teflon implant. The radiopaque implant lies anterosuperior to the condyle *(C).* Advanced erosive changes are shown in both the condyle and articular fossa, and there is marked thinning of the temporal bone anteriorly *(arrow).* **K** and **L,** Sagittal and coronal T1-weighted MR images show the implant as a band of low signal *(T)* lying above the condyle *(C).* The surrounding intermediate signal represents the foreign body reaction and is best appreciated in the sagittal image between the implant and the bone of the articular fossa *(F).*

be osteophyte formation. All of these changes may result in slight to massive alterations in joint morphology.

Ancillary Signs

The osseous structures associated with the implant often exhibit the changes of degenerative joint disease (osteoarthrosis), ranging from erosion to osteophyte formation and sclerosis.

Differential Diagnosis

Nonimplant-related degenerative joint disease

MYELOMA TO THE TMJ

Overview

Definition: *Myeloma* refers to single (plasmacytoma) or multiple (multiple myeloma) tumor deposits composed of malignant plasma cells that replace normal bone marrow. These tumors are associated with overproduction of myeloma proteins and polypeptide chains.

Pathogenesis: The cause of plasma cell proliferation is unknown, although both infectious and postinflammatory etiologies have been suggested. Familial multiple myeloma may occur in patterns suggesting a genetic predisposition. The high incidence of myeloma in the mandible has been attributed to its abundance of hematopoietic bone marrow.

Clinical Features

Demographics: The average age of onset is 60 to 70 years; myeloma is rare before 40 years. It is particularly common in blacks and a little more common in men than women.

Signs and symptoms: Local symptoms are pain and tenderness, which can be incapacitating and thus result in limitation of movement. Acute onset of pain may result from pathologic fracture through the condyle. The buccal and gingival mucosa may be affected by plasma cell infiltration or amyloid deposition.

Special tests: Patients with myeloma may show increased total serum protein, usually shown on electrophoresis to result from an increased globulin fraction. Fifty percent of patients are positive for Bence Jones proteinuria.

RADIOLOGIC FEATURES

Cardinal Signs

Conventional radiography and CT.—The most common finding is osteolysis. Cases reported in the mandibular condyle have been mainly of the classic "punched out" type and have been seen in both solitary plasmacytoma and multiple myeloma. However, multiple myeloma can affect both the mandible and temporal bone and may show only a diffuse osteopenic appearance.

Magnetic resonance imaging—Untreated lesions typically show slightly decreased signal on T1-weighted imaging compared to normal fat-containing bone marrow and high signal on T2-weighted imaging, as shown in Fig. 12-13, *A*. Myelomatous lesions enhance with intravenous dimeglumine gadopentetate to show high signal on T1-weighted imaging.

Ancillary Signs

Cases of sclerotic myeloma have been reported but are rare.

The MR appearance of treated myeloma varies because of differing proportions of fatty replacement or fibrosis of marrow.

Bone scintigraphy tends to be unreliable, although a "cold" lesion may be observed. Pathologic fracture may show increased tracer uptake; sclerotic myeloma can show markedly increased tracer uptake.

Differential Diagnosis

Lytic metastatic disease can produce an identical radiologic appearance and effects the same age group. However, unlike myeloma, bony metastases to the mandible are surprisingly uncommon in lytic disease.

Differential diagnosis also includes other lytic processes, including infection and even previous condylectomy.

METASTASIS TO THE TMJ

Overview

Definition: Secondary malignant lesions may be deposited in part of the TMJ from a distant primary malignant neoplasm.

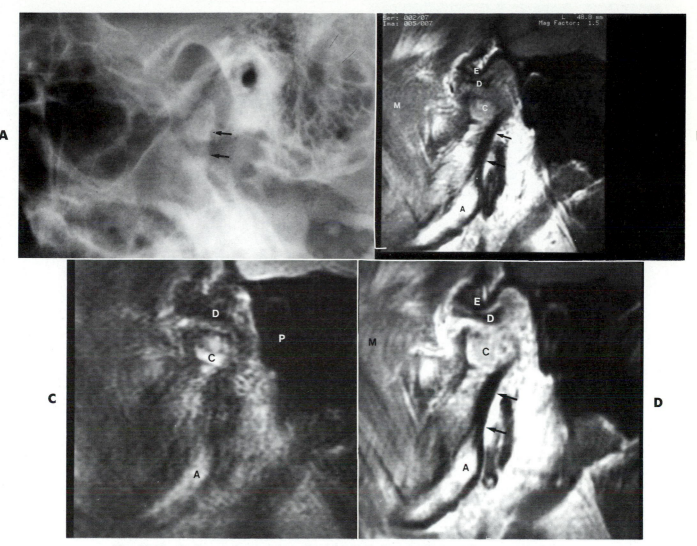

Fig. 12-13 A, Conventional radiograph of the TMJ shows an "empty" fossa as a result of destruction of the condyle by a lesion of multiple myeloma. The posterior aspect of the neck and ramus can be faintly identified *(arrows).* **B,** T1-weighted (TR500, TE25) sagittal MR image of TMJ shows relatively low signal in the condyle *(C)* compared to the normal marrow signal in the angle of the mandible *(A)* and similar signal to that of muscle *(M).* Other anatomic landmarks are the articular disk *(D)* and anterior articular eminence *(E). Arrows* indicate the posterior cortex of the neck and ramus of the mandible. **C,** T2-weighted (TR2000, TE90) sagittal image corresponding to **B** shows relatively high signal in the condyle *(C)* compared to the normal marrow signal in the angle of the mandible *(A).* Other anatomic landmarks are the articular disk *(D)* and the petrous portion of the temporal bone *(P).* **D,** T1-weighted (TR500, TE25) sagittal image following intravenous meglumine gadopentate administration, corresponding to **B** and **C,** shows enhancement of the condyle *(C)* and surrounding tissue. These regions now show higher signal than in the unenhanced T1-weighted image because of the presence of myeloma deposits and adjacent inflammatory tissue. Note that the condyle now shows higher signal than muscle *(M)* and similar signal to normal mandibular marrow. *(A).* Other anatomic landmarks are as in **B.**

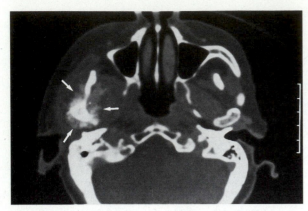

Fig. 12-14 Axial CT scan of the right TMJ shows an osteoblastic metastatic transitional cell carcinoma. There are radiating spicules of bone *(arrows),* mimicking the changes of osteosarcoma. Such changes may be found in other parts of the jaws in association with metastatic carcinomatous lesions.

Pathogenesis: Metastases to the TMJ result from the same metastatic process as at any other site.

Clinical Features

Demographics: Metastases involving the TMJ are relatively rare; less than 20 cases have been reported in the literature. We do know of cases that have not been reported, thus some of the paucity of reports may result from practitioners not knowing that TMJ metastasis is as rare as it seems.

Signs and symptoms: The signs and symptoms are often those of "TMJ dysfunction syndrome": pain, trismus, altered or restricted motion, and swelling.

Special tests: No special tests are required, other than to look for primary lesions. Bone scintigraphy may be done to note activity and uptake.

RADIOLOGIC FEATURES

Cardinal Signs
Changes in condylar morphology, either osteolytic or osteoblastic

Ancillary Signs
Metastatic lesions elsewhere in the body

Differential Diagnosis
Inflammatory destruction resulting from infection or arthritis of various causes

BIBLIOGRAPHY

Hyperplasia of the Mandible and/or Mandibular Condyle

Gray RJ, et al: Histopathological and scintigraphic features of condylar hyperplasia, *Int J Oral Maxillofac Surg* 19:65, 1990.

Henderson MJ, et al: Technetium-99m bone scintigraphy and mandibular condylar hyperplasia, *Clin Radiol* 41:411, 1990.

Iannetti G, et al: Condylar hyperplasia: cephalometric study, treatment planning, and surgical correction (our experience), *Oral Surg Oral Med Oral Pathol* 68:673, 1989.

Lineaweaver W, et al: Posttraumatic condylar hyperplasia, *Ann Plast Surg* 22:163, 1989.

Magnusson T, Ahlborg G, Svartz K: Function of the masticatory system in 20 patients with mandibular hypo- or hyperplasia after correction by a sagittal split osteotomy, *Int J Oral Maxillofac Surg* 19:289, 1990.

Robinson PD, et al: Bone scans and the timing of treatment for condylar hyperplasia, *Int J Oral Maxillofac Surg* 19:243, 1990.

Tommasi AF, Jitomirski F: Congenital crossed hemifacial hyperplasia, *Oral Surg Oral Med Oral Pathol* 67:190, 1989.

Coronoid Process Hyperplasia

Bernstein L, Fernandez B: Bilateral hyperplasia of the coronoid process of the mandible: report of a case, *Arch Otolaryngol* 110:480, 1984.

Giacomuzzi D: Bilateral enlargement of the mandibular coronoid processes: review of the literature and report of a case, *J Oral Maxillofac Surg* 44:728, 1986.

Hall RE, Orbach S, Landberg R: Bilateral hyperplasia of the coronoid processes: a report of two cases, *Oral Surg Oral Med Oral Pathol* 67:141, 1989.

Henriksen LH, Trebo S: Post-traumatic coronoid process impingement on zygomatic arch: CT demonstration, *J Comput Assist Tomogr* 12:712, 1988.

Kreutz RW, Sanders B: Bilateral coronoid hyperplasia resulting in severe limitation of mandibular movement: report of a case, *Oral Surg Oral Med Oral Pathol* 60:482, 1985.

Munk PL, Helms CA: Coronoid process hyperplasia: CT studies, *Radiology* 171:783, 1989.

Tucker MR, Guilford WB, Howard CW: Coronoid process hyperplasia causing restricted opening and facial asymmetry, *Oral Surg Oral Med Oral Pathol* 58:130, 1984.

Hypoplasia of the Mandibular Condyle

Harkness EM, Thorburn DN: Hemifacial microsomia label questioned *Angle Orthod* 60:5, 1990 (letter and comment).

Magnusson T, Ahlborg G, Svartz K: Function of the masticatory system in 20 patients with mandibular hypo- or hyperplasia after correction by a sagittal split osteotomy, *Int J Oral Maxillofac Surg* 19:289, 1990.

Worth HM: Hurler's syndrome: a study of radiologic appearances in the jaws, *Oral Surg Oral Med Oral Pathol* 22:21, 1966.

Mandibular Condyle Dislocation

Ferguson JW, Stewart IA, Whitley BD: Lateral displacement of the intact mandibular condyle: review of literature and report of case with associated facial nerve palsy, *J Craniomaxillofac Surg* 17:125, 1989.

Karabouta I: Increasing the articular eminence by the use of blocks of porous coralline hydroxylapatite for treatment of recurrent TMJ dislocation, *J Craniomaxillofac Surg* 18:107, 1990.

Loh FC, Yeo JF: Subsequent treatment of chronic recurrent dislocation of the mandible after eminectomies, *Int J Oral Maxillofac Surg* 18:352, 1989.

Oatis GW, Huggins R, Yorty JS: *Oral surgery, Dent Clin North Am* 30:583, 1986.

Mandibular Condyle Neck Fractures

Dolan KD, Jacoby CG, Smoker WRK: *Radiology of facial injury,* ed 2, Philadelphia, 1988, Field & Wood, p 57.

Dolan KD, Ruprecht A: Imaging of mandible and tempopomandibular fractures, *Oral Maxillofac Surg Clin North Am* (in press).

Rheumatoid Changes in the TMJ

Goupille P, et al: The temporomandibular joint in rheumatoid arthritis: Correlations between clinical and computed tomography features, *J Rheumatol* 17:1285, 1990.

Koorbusch GF, et al: Psoriatic arthritis of the temporomandibular joints with ankylosis, *Oral Surg Oral Med Oral Pathol* 71:267, 1991.

Krane SM, Simon LS: Rheumatoid arthritis: clinical features and pathogenetic mechanisms, *Med Clin North Am* 70:263, 1986.

Larheim TA, Kolbenstvedt A: Osseous temporomandibular joint abnormalities in rheumatic disease: computed tomography versus hypocycloidal tomography, *Acta Radiol* 31:383, 1990.

Larheim TA, Smith HJ, Aspestrand F: Rheumatic disease of the temporomandibular joint: MR imaging and tomographic manifestations, *Radiology* 175:527, 1990.

Yochum TR, Rowe LJ: *Essentials of skeletal radiology,* Baltimore, 1987, Williams & Wilkins, pp 539-698.

Osteoarthrosis of the TMJ

Katzberg RW, et al: Internal derangements and arthritis of the temporomandibular joint, *Radiology* 146:107, 1983.

Larheim TA, Kolbenstvedt A: Osseous temporomandibular joint abnormalities in rheumatic disease: computed tomography versus hypocycloidal tomography, *Acta Radiol Diagn* 31:383, 1990.

Westesson P, et al: CT and MR of the temporomandibular joint: comparison with autopsy specimens, AJR 148:1165, 1987.

Costochondral Graft in the TMJ

MacIntosh RB: The indications and techniques for autologous temporomandibular joint replacement, *Fortschr Kiefer Gesichtschir* 35:168, 1990.

Mosby EL, Hiatt WR: A technique of fixation of costochondral grafts for reconstruction of the temporomandibular joint, *J Oral Maxillofac Surg* 47:209, 1989.

Matukas VJ, Lachner I: The use of autologous auricular cartilage for temporomandibular joint disc replacement: a preliminary report, *J Oral Maxillofac Surg* 48:348, 1990.

Nelson CL, Buttrum ID: Costochondral grafting for posttraumatic temporomandibular joint reconstruction: a review of six cases, *J Oral Maxillofac Surg* 47:1030, 1989.

Raveh J, Vuillemin T, Sutter F: TMJ dysfunction: surgical management and reconstruction, *J Otolaryngol* 18:334, 1989.

Myeloma to the TMJ

Fruehwald FXJ, et al: Magnetic resonance imaging of the lower vertebral column in patients with multiple myeloma, *Invest Radiol* 23:193, 1988.

Halpern KL, Calhoun NR: Pathological fracture of mandibular condyloid process associated with multiple myeloma: report of a case, *J Oral Surg* 36:560, 1978.

Jagger RG, Helkimo M, Carlsson GE: Multiple myeloma involving the temporomandibular joint: report of a case, *J Oral Surg* 36:557, 1978.

Kaffe I, Ramon Y, Hertz M: Radiographic manifestations of multiple myeloma in the mandible, *Dentomaxillofac Radiol* 5:31, 1986.

Lambertenghi-Deliliers G, et al: Incidence of jaw lesions in 193 patients with multiple myeloma, *Oral Surg Oral Med Oral Pathol* 65:533, 1988.

Temporomandibular Joint Implant and Other Foreign Body Reactions

Acton C, et al: Silicone-induced foreign-body reaction after temporomandibular joint arthroplasty: case report, *Aust Dent J* 34:228, 1989.

AMA Council on Scientific Affairs: Dimethyl sulfoxide: controversy and current status, *JAMA* 248:1369, 1982.

Berarducci JP, Thompson DA, Scheffer RB: Perforation into middle cranial fossa as a sequel to use of a Proplast Teflon implant for temporomandibular joint reconstruction, *J Oral Maxillofac Surg* 48:496, 1990.

Berman DN, Bronstein SL: Osteophytic reaction to a polytetrafluoroethylene temporomandibular joint implant: report of a case, *Oral Surg Oral Med Oral Pathol* 69:20, 1990.

Estabrocks LN, et al: A retrospective evaluation of 301 TMJ Proplast-Teflon implants, *Oral Surg Oral Med Oral Pathol* 70:381, 1990.

Jimenez RAH, Willkens RF: Dimethyl sulfoxide: a perspective of its use in rheumatic diseases, *J Lab Clin Med* 100:489, 1982.

Kligman AM: Topical pharmacology and toxicology of dimethyl sulfoxide–part 1, *JAMA* 193:140, 1965.

Kligman AM: Topical pharmacology and toxicology of dimethyl sulfioxide–part 2, *JAMA* 193:151, 1965.

Kneeland LB, et al: Failed temporomandibular prosthesis: MR imaging, *Radiology* 165:179, 1987.

Sanders B, Buoncristiani RD, Johnson L: Silicone rubber fossa implant removal via partial anthrotomy followed by arthroscopic examination of the internal surface of the fibrous capsule, *Oral Surg Oral Med Oral Pathol* 70:369, 1990.

Schellhas KP, et al: Permanent proplast temporomandibular joint implants: MR imaging of destructive complications, *AJR* 151:731, 1988.

Valentine JD Jr, et al: Light and electron microscopic evaluation of Proplast II TMJ disc implants, *J Oral Maxillofac Surg* 47:689, 1989 (comments).

Wagner JD, Mosby EL: Assessment of Proplast Teflon disc replacements, *J Oral Maxillofac Surg* 48:1140, 1990.

Westermark AH, Sindet-Pedersen, S Boyne-PJ: Bony ankylosis of the temporomandibular joint: Case report of a child treated with Delrin condylar implants, *J Oral Maxillofac Surg* 48:861, 1990.

Willhite CC, Katz PI: Dimethyl sulfoxide, *J Appl Toxicol* 4:155, 1984.

Metastasis to the TMJ

Rubin MM, Jui V, Cozzi GM: Metastatic carcinoma of the mandibular condyle presenting as temporomandibular joint syndrome, *J Oral Maxillofac Surg* 47:507, 1989.

13

DISEASES OF THE PARANASAL SINUSES

CHOANAL ATRESIA

Overview

Definition: In choanal atresia, the nasal cavity on one or both sides does not communicate with the nasopharynx. If the atresia is bilateral, nasal breathing is prevented.

Pathogenesis: Most believe that choanal atresia results from failure of the embryologic nasobuccal membrane to lyse, an event which normally occurs around the seventh week of gestation.

Clinical Features

Demographics: The incidence of choanal atresia has been estimated at 1 in 7,000, with a two-to-one male predominance. From 20% to 50% of those affected have associated anomalies, including cleft palate, Treacher Collins syndrome, and cardiovascular and abdominal malformations.

Signs and symptoms: Choanal atresia is unilateral in two thirds of cases, usually presenting with nasal stuffiness and mucoid discharge. In the other one third, the atresia is bilateral. These patients present at birth with immediate respiratory distress, resulting in asphyxiation unless an oral airway is placed.

RADIOLOGIC FEATURES

Cardinal Signs

A plain lateral radiograph with oily contrast medium instilled into the nose with the patient supine will show obstruction of the choana. This procedure, however, has been rendered obsolete by computed tomography (CT).

A CT scan shows a narrowed choana occluded by a bony plate (80% to 90% of cases) or membranous web (10% to 20%). There is bony thickening of the posterolateral nasal wall and posterior vomer, with both curving toward the obstructed choana.

Differential Diagnosis

Mucosal edema with choanal stenosis may imitate membranous atresia.

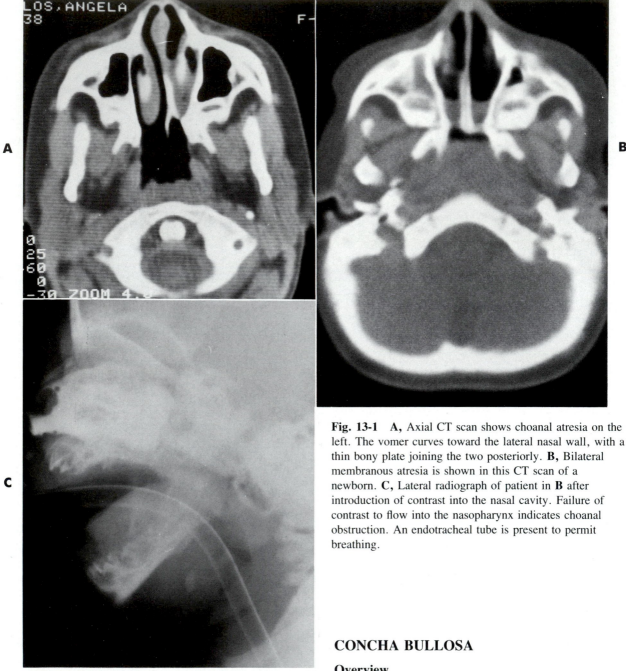

Fig. 13-1 A, Axial CT scan shows choanal atresia on the left. The vomer curves toward the lateral nasal wall, with a thin bony plate joining the two posteriorly. **B,** Bilateral membranous atresia is shown in this CT scan of a newborn. **C,** Lateral radiograph of patient in **B** after introduction of contrast into the nasal cavity. Failure of contrast to flow into the nasopharynx indicates choanal obstruction. An endotracheal tube is present to permit breathing.

CONCHA BULLOSA

Overview

Definition: Concha bullosa is pneumatization of a turbinate by extension of the ethmoid air cells. The middle turbinate is most commonly affected, followed by the lower.

Pathogenesis: By encroaching upon the middle meatus, the enlarged turbinate may obstruct sinus drainage and predispose to sinusitis.

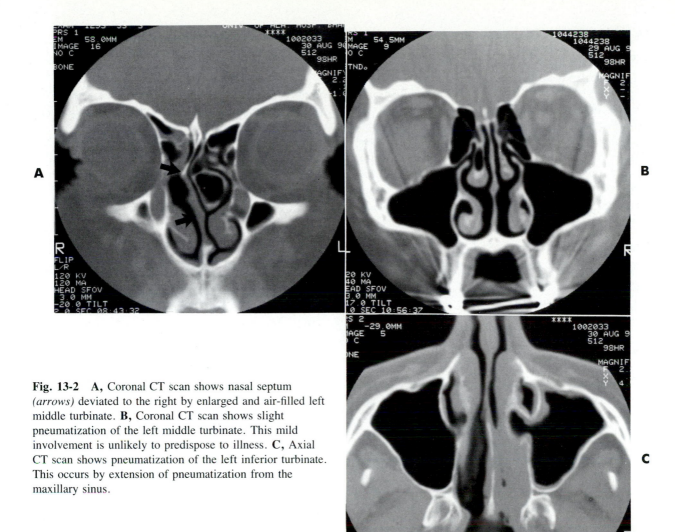

Fig. 13-2   A, Coronal CT scan shows nasal septum *(arrows)* deviated to the right by enlarged and air-filled left middle turbinate. **B,** Coronal CT scan shows slight pneumatization of the left middle turbinate. This mild involvement is unlikely to predispose to illness. **C,** Axial CT scan shows pneumatization of the left inferior turbinate. This occurs by extension of pneumatization from the maxillary sinus.

Clinical Features

Demographics: Concha bullosa is found in 34% of patients with chronic sinusitis, occurring bilaterally in 45% and unilaterally in 55%.

Signs and symptoms Affected patients may present with chronic sinusitis. However, many or most patients with concha bullosa remain asymptomatic throughout life.

RADIOLOGIC FEATURES

Cardinal Signs

Axial and coronal CT show an expanded, air-filled middle turbinate, possibly causing septal deviation or compressing the infundibulum.

Ancillary Signs

In acute infection, the turbinate may appear fluid filled.

Differential Diagnosis

The CT appearance is specific.

ACUTE SINUSITIS

Overview

Definition: Acute sinusitis, one of the most common medical afflictions, is an acute bacterial or viral infection of the paranasal sinuses.

Pathogenesis: The bacteria most often involved are *Haemophilus influenzae* and *Streptococcus pneumoniae*. Viral sinusitis usually occurs in the presence of viral rhinitis. Predisposing factors include upper respiratory infections, nasal masses, trauma, nasal anomalies, dental infections, and allergic mucosal edema.

Clinical Features

Signs and symptoms: Acute sinusitis presents clinically with facial pain, headaches, local tenderness, and purulent nasal drainage.

RADIOLOGIC FEATURES

Cardinal Signs

Plain radiographs (e.g., Waters technique) show air-fluid levels, nodular or smooth mucosal thickening, or complete sinus opacification.

Computed tomography shows air-fluid levels, nodular or smooth mucosal thickening, or complete opacification by fluid (exudate) or soft tissue (mucosal inflammation). There is a concentric ring appearance after intravenous contrast, with thick enhanced mucosa surrounding unenhancing fluid exudate.

Magnetic resonance (MR) imaging shows hyperintensity on T2-weighted images and hypointensity on T1-weighted images. After contrast injection, the inflamed mucosa enhances intensely.

Differential Diagnosis

Air-fluid level
  Hemorrhage
  Antral lavage
  Barotrauma
  Cerebrospinal fluid leak
Mucosal thickening
  Chronic sinusitis
  Polyps
  Early carcinoma (without bone invasion)

CHRONIC SINUSITIS

Overview

Definition: Chronic sinusitis is an infection of the paranasal sinuses that persists beyond the acute stage or fails to respond to therapy. Impaired sinus drainage is a predisposing factor.

Pathogenesis: As opposed to acute sinusitis, anaerobic are organisms more frequently isolated in chronic sinusitis; they are perhaps the most common etiologic agent. Among children, cystic fibrosis is a common predisposing factor.

Clinical Features

Signs and symptoms: Like the acute form, chronic sinusitis is characterized by sinus exudates and mucosal edema and inflammation. With time, reactive sclerosis of the sinus walls and irreversible fibrosis of the sinus lining may develop.

RADIOLOGIC FEATURES

Cardinal Signs

Plain radiographs show a smooth or irregular mucosal thickening. Sclerosis of sinus walls or dystrophic calcification may occur.

Computed tomography shows mucosal thickening, which reflects inflammation or fibrosis sclerosis of the sinus walls (especially the posterior wall of the antrum). Dystrophic calcification with a concentric ring appearance may appear after intravenous contrast injection, with thick, enhanced mucosa surrounding unenhancing fluid exudate.

Magnetic resonance imaging usually shows hyperintensity on T2-weighted images; however, fibrosis is dark on T2-weighted images.

Differential Diagnosis

Acute sinusitis
Polyps
Early carcinoma, without bone erosion
Fibrosis
Wegener granulomatosis

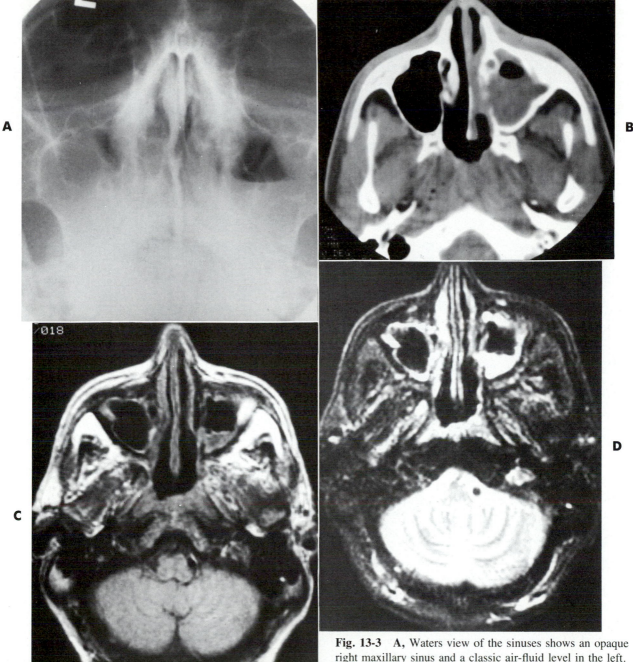

Fig. 13-3 A, Waters view of the sinuses shows an opaque right maxillary sinus and a classic air-fluid level in the left. Both findings are consistent with acute sinusitis, although the appearance on the left is more specific. **B,** Axial CT scan in another patient shows nearly opacified left maxillary antrum with mucosal thickening and an air-fluid level. **C,** Axial T1-weighted MR image in a third case shows thickened mucosa in maxillary antra bilaterally, with an air-fluid level in the left antrum. **D,** Axial T2-weighted MR image shows the markedly hyperintense sinus mucosa (due to edema) and a fluid level in the left antrum.

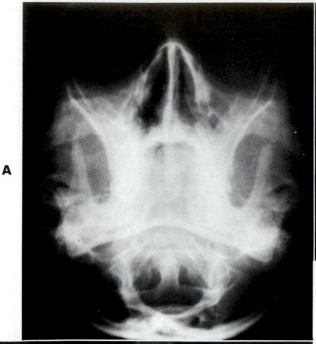

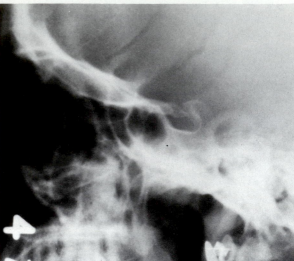

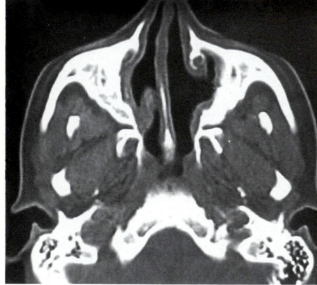

Fig. 13-4   **A,** Waters view of the sinuses shows small, very sclerotic maxillary sinuses bilaterally. **B,** Lateral view of the sinuses also shows bony sclerosis. **C,** Axial CT scan of the same patient as in **A,** shows marked thickening of the maxillary sinus walls with thickened mucosa. The medial wall defects indicate prior nasal antrostomies.

ASPERGILLUS SINUSITIS

Overview

Definition: An opportunistic infection, aspergillus sinusitis presents as chronic sinusitis that does not improve with antibiotics or irrigation.

Pathogenesis: In 90% of cases, *Aspergillus fumigatus* is the offending organism. Aspergillus sinusitis may be noninvasive, invasive, or fulminant. Although it usually occurs in healthy patients, causing little morbidity, a fulminant infection may develop in immunocompromised patients.

Clinical Features

Signs and symptoms: Patients complain of nasal discharge and sinus pain. In immunosuppressed patients the infection may become highly invasive, resulting in bone destruction.

Special tests: The diagnosis is established by histologic examination with fungal stains of the sinus contents.

RADIOLOGIC FEATURES

Cardinal Signs

Plain radiographs show unilateral opacification of the maxillary sinus, with calcifications in approximately 50% of cases. Sometimes the sphenoid or ethmoid sinuses are involved.

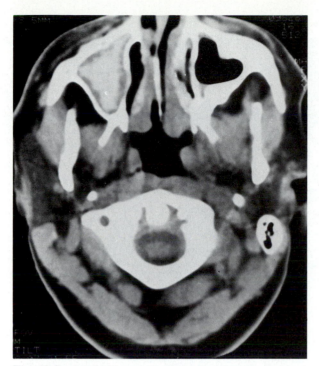

Fig. 13-5 Axial CT scan shows thickened mucosa in the right maxillary antrum. The sinus contents are of high attenuation, reflecting mycetoma. The thickened walls of the left antrum reflect chronic sinusitis.

Computed tomography reveals opacification of the sinuses with hyperdense contents centrally.

Magnetic resonance imaging using T2-weighted images shows hyperintense mucosal edema with central hypointensity as a result of mycetoma.

Differential diagnosis

Hemorrhage
Polyps
Chronic sinusitis
Inspissated mucous
In fulminant form, malignancy

RETENTION CYST

Overview

Definition and pathogenesis The most common mass of the maxillary sinus, retention cysts result from the obstruction of the ducts draining mucous glands.

Clinical Features

Demographics: Retention cysts are considered a complication of sinusitis, with an incidence approaching 10%.

Signs and symptoms: A common incidental finding on CT scans or sinus radiographs, retention cysts are usually asymptomatic. Large retention cysts may have a somewhat flat free surface and mimic an air-fluid level. Unlike air-fluid levels, however, retention cysts will not move freely with a change in position. When very large, they may behave like mucoceles.

RADIOLOGIC FEATURES

Cardinal Signs

Plain radiographs show a smooth, round soft tissue mass, usually in the floor of the maxillary antrum.

Computed tomography reveals a smooth, round mass of the density of water, partly surrounded by air. The sinus is not airless, as it is with mucocele or sinus opacified by exudate.

Retention cysts may be single or multiple.

With MR imaging, retention cysts appear bright on T2-weighted images; they show low, intermediate, or high intensity on T1-weighted images.

Differential Diagnosis

Intrasinus polyp
Periapical cyst

MUCOCELE

Overview

Definition: A mucocele is a an expanded, fluid-filled sinus resulting from obstruction of the sinus ostium with continued mucous secretion. It is lined by sinus mucosa.

Pathogenesis: The ostial obstruction may result from antecedent nasal polyps or inflammatory mucosal thickening.

Clinical Features

Signs and symptoms: Clinically, mucocele causes headaches, unilateral proptosis, and nasal stuffiness. Local pain is unusual.

Demographics: Two thirds occur in the frontal sinus and one third in the ethmoid sinuses. They occur occasionally in the maxillary sinus and rarely in the sphenoid sinus.

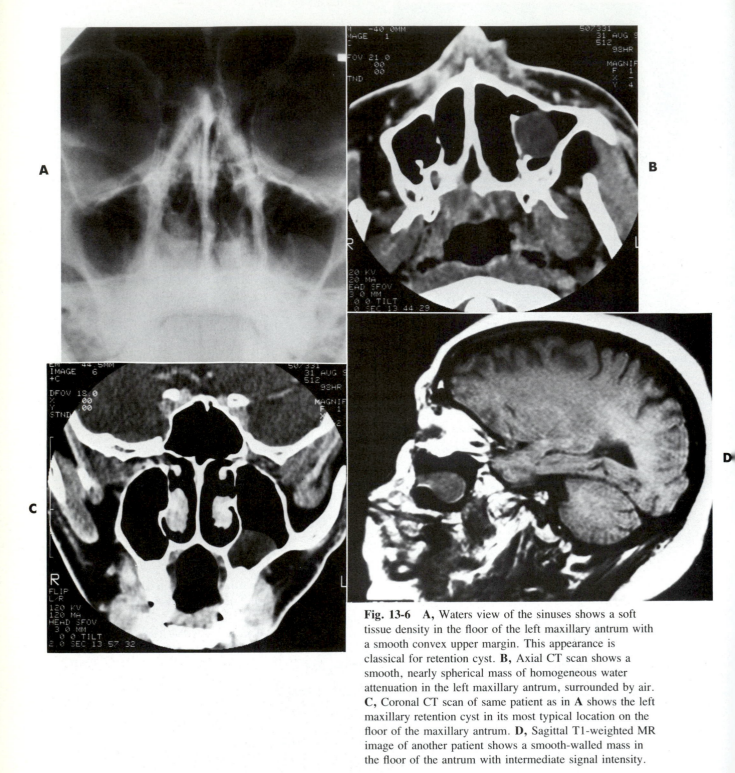

Fig. 13-6 **A,** Waters view of the sinuses shows a soft tissue density in the floor of the left maxillary antrum with a smooth convex upper margin. This appearance is classical for retention cyst. **B,** Axial CT scan shows a smooth, nearly spherical mass of homogeneous water attenuation in the left maxillary antrum, surrounded by air. **C,** Coronal CT scan of same patient as in **A** shows the left maxillary retention cyst in its most typical location on the floor of the maxillary antrum. **D,** Sagittal T1-weighted MR image of another patient shows a smooth-walled mass in the floor of the antrum with intermediate signal intensity.

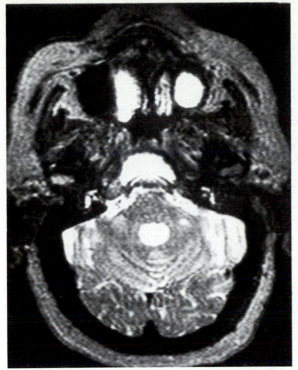

Fig. 13-6, cont'd. **E,** Axial T2-weighted MR image shows a round mass in the left antrum of very high signal intensity, reflecting its high water content.

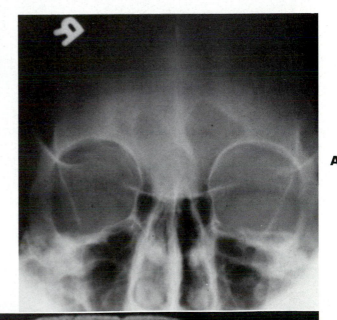

A

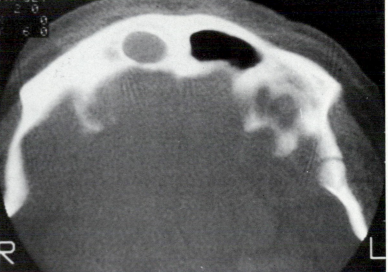

B

Fig. 13-7 A, Anteroposterior view of the frontal sinuses shows opacification of the right frontal sinus with a faintly sclerotic rim. **B,** Axial CT scan of same patient as **A** shows a small, opacified right frontal sinus. The margins are rounded, indicating expansion, with a sclerotic rim.

Continued.

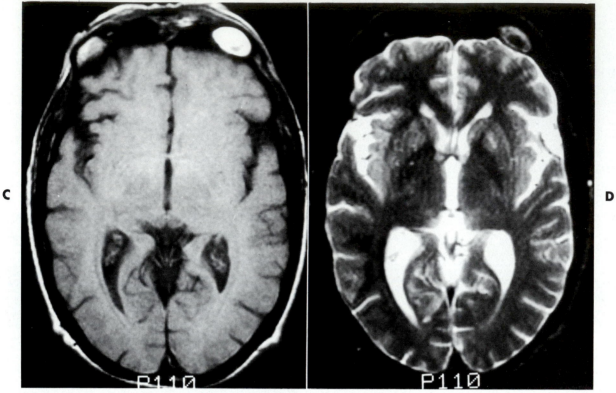

Fig. 13-7, cont'd. C, Axial T1-weighted MR image in another patient shows hyperintensity in a rounded frontal air cell. The brightness results from a high protein content. **D,** Axial T2-weighted MR image shows low signal intensity in the mucocele. This indicates inspissation of the mucocele contents, which occurs with increasing age.

RADIOLOGIC FEATURES

Cardinal Signs

Plain radiographs show an opacified, expanded sinus.

Growth leads at first to bone remodelling and sclerosis of the sinus wall; progressive growth eventually results in erosion of the walls.

Computed tomography shows an airless, fluid-filled sinus.

Continued mucus secretion leads to sinus expansion. Pressure erosion of bony margins may cause rim enhancement, especially if infected.

Magnetic resonance imaging evidences variable signal intensity on T1- and T2-weighted images, depending on age and protein concentration.

Differential Diagnosis

Acute sinusitis
Retention cyst
Adenocarcinoma
Pyomucocele
Giant cell granuloma

NASAL POLYPS

Overview

Definition and pathogenesis: The most common nasal mass, nasal polyps develop from chronic inflammation of upper respiratory mucosa. This results in the formation of polyps composed of edematous mucosa.

Clinical Features

Demographics: The frequency of nasal polyps in the general population is approximately 4%. Sixty per cent of patients are male, and children are rarely affected.

Signs and symptoms: Patients present with nasal stuffiness and sometimes hypertelorism. Predisposing factors include atopy, cystic fibrosis, chronic infection, and asthma. The latter may be present in up to 71% of patients with polyps. When polyps occur in children, consideration should be given to undiagnosed cystic fibrosis.

Special tests: Histologic examination reveals edema, inflammatory cells, and fibrous proliferation.

RADIOLOGIC FEATURES

Cardinal Signs

Plain radiographs show a well-circumscribed, rounded soft tissue mass.

Computed tomography reveals a soft tissue mass of mucoid attenuation, which increases with time, expansion, and opacification of ethmoids with preservation of septae ("ethmoidmucocele"). Cascading, fingerlike soft tissue masses with mucoid background is the most specific appearance.

Magnetic resonance imaging shows a low to intermediate signal on T1-weighted images and a high signal on T2-weighted images.

Chronic polyps have very heterogeneous MR signal characteristics.

Ancillary Signs

Expansion of nasal cavity
Bone remodeling
Ethmoid opacification
Hypertelorism

Differential Diagnosis

Aspergillosis
Chronic sinusitis
Inverted papilloma
Esthesioneuroblastoma
Angiofibroma
Antrochoanal polyp

WEGENER GRANULOMATOSIS

Overview

Definition and pathogenesis: Wegener granulomatosis is an immunologically mediated disease characterized by granulomatous inflammation and a necrotiz-

ing vasculitis. It was originally described by Wegener as a disease with necrotizing granulomas of the upper and lower respiratory tracts, systemic vasculitis, and focal necrotizing glomerulitis.

Clinical Features

Signs and symptoms: Wegener granulomatosis affects the nose and sinuses, lungs, and kidneys. Patients often come to attention with epistaxis or nasal obstruction. Other common symptoms include vague nasal pain, weakness, chills, and cough. In later stages, the presentation may reflect pulmonary or renal involvement.

Demographics: Nasal involvement occurs in 91% of cases, favoring the turbinates. The sinuses are affected in 95%, affecting in decreasing order the maxillary, ethmoid, frontal, and sphenoid sinuses. Secondary staphylococcal infections are common. At one time, the 2-year survival was less than 10%. With the advent of cytotoxic and immunosuppressive therapy, the prognosis is now excellent.

RADIOLOGIC FEATURES

Cardinal Signs

Computed tomography reveals mucosal thickening, air-fluid levels, or soft tissue mass involving the nose and sinuses, usually bilaterally.

There is destruction of the nasal septum, turbinates, and medial antral wall, as well as reactive sclerosis of the antral walls, which may be severe.

Magnetic resonance imaging shows mucosal thickening, hyperintense on T2-weighted images. Bone destruction is seen better on CT.

Fibrosis may be present; it is hypointense on T1- and T2-weighted images.

Ancillary Signs

Concomitant orbital masses in 10% to 15%

Differential Diagnosis

Vasculitis
Granulomatous or fungal infections
Lymphoma
Lymphoepithelioma
Sarcoidosis
Cocaine abuse

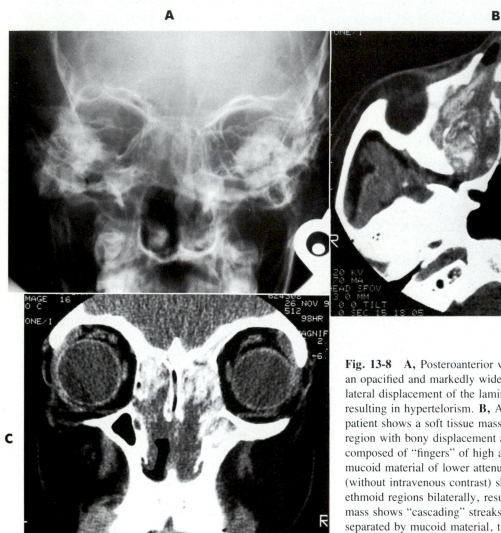

Fig. 13-8 **A,** Posteroanterior view of the sinuses shows an opacified and markedly widened ethmoid complex with lateral displacement of the lamina papyracea bilaterally, resulting in hypertelorism. **B,** Axial CT scan of a different patient shows a soft tissue mass occupying the nasoethmoid region with bony displacement and erosion. The mass is composed of "fingers" of high attenuation separated by mucoid material of lower attenuation. **C,** Coronal CT scan (without intravenous contrast) show expansion of the ethmoid regions bilaterally, resulting in hypertelorism. The mass shows "cascading" streaks of high attenuation separated by mucoid material, the appearance most specific for nasal polyposis.

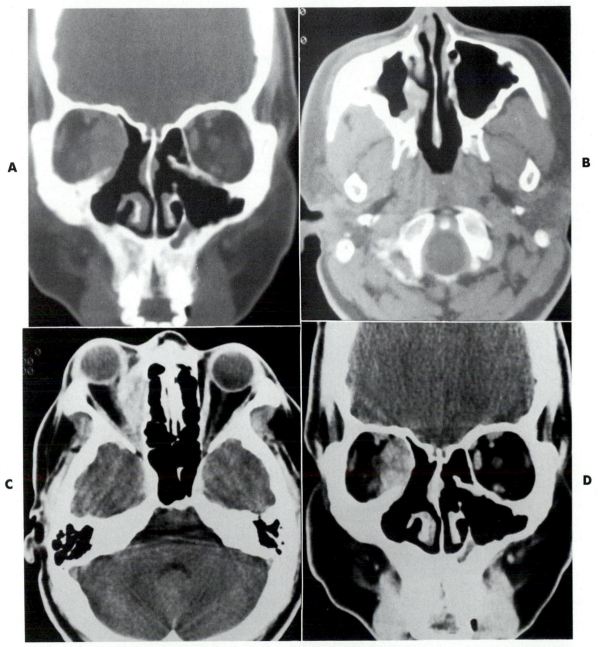

Fig. 13-9 **A,** Coronal CT scan shows mucosal thickening of the nasal septum and destruction of the middle turbinates, ethmoid septae, medial maxillary walls, and right inferior and medial orbital walls. **B,** Axial CT scan shows marked sclerosis of the right anterior and posterior maxillary sinus walls, often seen in Wegener granulomatosis. **C** and **D,** Axial *(C)* and coronal *(D)* CT scans show an orbital mass encasing the medial rectus muscle on the right and causing proptosis.

ANGIOFIBROMA

Overview

Definition: The most common benign nasopharyngeal neoplasm, angiofibroma is a vascular tumor composed of ectatic capillaries and fibrous connective tissue.

Clinical Features

Demographics: Affected patients present at a median age of 15 years old.

Signs and symptoms: Symptoms consist of nasal stuffiness and recurrent, severe epistaxis. Angiofibroma occurs almost exclusively in young males and normally regresses during adulthood. The neoplasm usually arises from the posterolateral wall of the nasal cavity, near the sphenopalatine foramen. From there it may spread into the nasal cavity, retromaxillary space, and maxillary sinus.

RADIOLOGIC FEATURES

Cardinal Signs

Plain radiographs reveal a soft tissue mass in the nasal cavity, erosion of lateral nasal walls or pterygoid plates, and opacification of the sinuses.

Computed tomography shows a soft tissue mass in the nasal cavity, nasopharynx, maxillary sinus, and/or parapharyngeal spaces.

Bone erosion is common.

There is intense enhancement following intravenous contrast with CT and MR.

"Antral sign" may be present—anterior bowing of posterior maxillary sinus wall and posterior bowing of pterygoid plates.

From the pterygoid fossa, the neoplasm may spread into orbit or cranium.

Magnetic resonance imaging shows an homogeneous mass of intermediate intensity on T1-weighted images and moderate hyperintensity on T2-weighted images. "Signal voids" may result from extreme vascularity of these tumors.

Angiography reveals an highly vascular mass with predominantly external carotid supply supplied primarily by the internal maxillary, ascending pharyngeal, and ascending palatine arteries.

Differential Diagnosis

Hemangioma

Inverting papilloma
Esthesioneuroblastoma
Polyposis
Meningioma

OSTEOMA OF THE PARANASAL SINUSES

Overview

Definition: An osteoma is a common lesion of the sinonasal region composed of mature cortical bone. Osteomas are the most frequently occurring osseous tumors of the maxilla and mandible and are very slow growing. Most sinus osteomas occur in the frontal sinus, followed by the ethmoid and maxillary sinuses. Osteomas have been divided into three groups based on their architecture and degree of mineralization: ivory, mature, or fibrous.

Clinical Features

Signs and symptoms: Osteomas are usually asymptomatic throughout life; they are a common incidental finding on radiography or CT. They normally present between the ages of 15 and 40 years. Lesions of the frontal or ethmoid sinuses may cause headaches. Frontal osteomas may invade the posterior wall of the sinus, leading to cerebrospinal fluid rhinorrhea or pneumocephalus. Osteomas also may occlude the sinus ostia, causing sinusitis or mucocele formation.

RADIOLOGIC FEATURES

Cardinal Signs

On CT or plain radiography, osteoma appears as an intrasinus mass of uniformly high attenuation. Ivory osteomas are denser than adjacent bone, and fibrous osteomas are more variable in density

Eighty percent are in the frontal sinus.

Osteoma is usually small, a common incidental finding.

Osteoma may be attached to sinus wall by short pedicle.

On MR imaging the lesions appear inhomogeneous, with low to intermediate signal intensity on all sequences.

Differential Diagnosis

Nonossifying fibroma
Rhinolith
Gardner syndrome (intestinal polyposis type II)

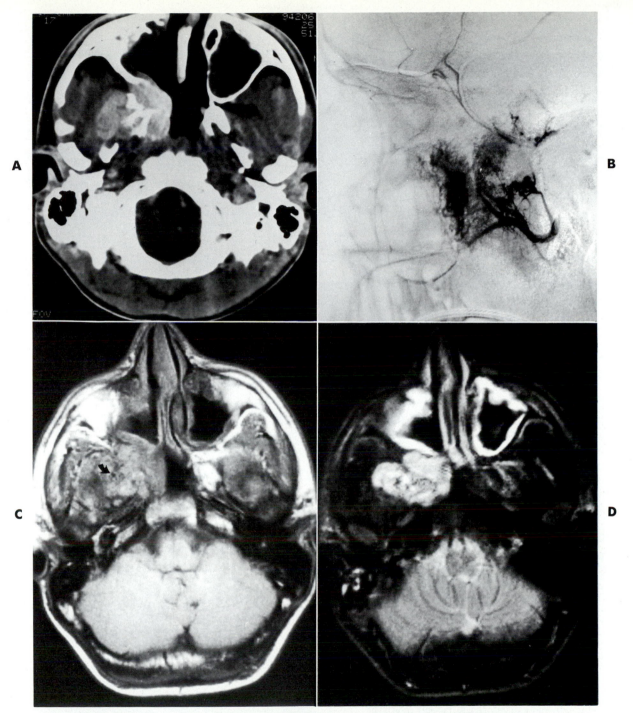

Fig. 13-10 **A,** Axial contrast-enhanced CT scan shows an enhancing mass in the pterygopalatine fossa, lateral nasopharynx, and infratemporal fossa. There is erosion of the posterior maxillary sinus wall and postoperative absence of the medial maxillary sinus wall. **B,** Selective angiogram of the internal maxillary artery shows a hypervascular mass with staining supplied by multiple distal branches. **C,** Axial T1-weighted MR image (same patient in **A**) shows mass of intermediate signal intensity occupying the right pterygopalatine fossa, parapharyngeal space, and infratemporal fossa. Note signal void *(curved arrow)* from enlarged feeding vessel. **D,** Axial T2-weighted MR image (shows hyperintense mass in the paraphyngeal space and pterygopalatine fossa. Mucosal edema is present in both maxillary sinuses, consistent with sinusitis.

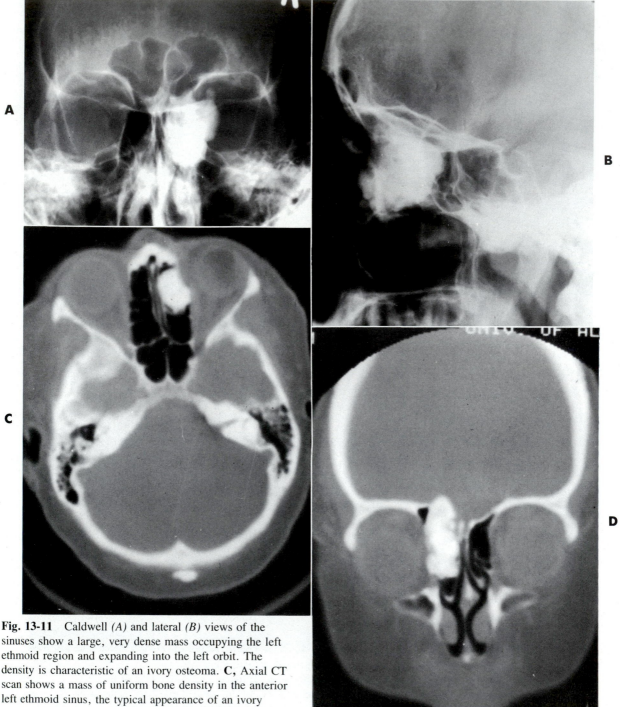

Fig. 13-11 Caldwell *(A)* and lateral *(B)* views of the sinuses show a large, very dense mass occupying the left ethmoid region and expanding into the left orbit. The density is characteristic of an ivory osteoma. **C,** Axial CT scan shows a mass of uniform bone density in the anterior left ethmoid sinus, the typical appearance of an ivory osteoma. **D,** Coronal CT scan shows a mass of bone density occupying the anterior ethmoid and growing up to involve the frontal bone at the floor of the anterior cranial fossa.

INVERTED PAPILLOMA

Overview

Definition: Inverted papilloma is a neoplasm of the nasal cavity composed of a core of vascular connective tissue covered by well-differentiated stratified squamous epithelium. The word *inverted* applies to the tumor's endophytic growth pattern, as it tends to grow under the mucosa and elevate it.

Clinical Features

Demographics: Papillomas are much less common than allergic polyps, with a relative incidence of 2.7%. Inverted papilloma occurs most commonly in 40- to 70-year-old men.

Signs and symptoms: Inverted papilloma usually arises from the lateral nasal wall near the ethmoids and is typically unilateral. With continued growth, it commonly extends into the maxillary and ethmoid sinuses. Patients may have nasal stuffiness or obstruction, epistaxis, or anosmia. Secondary bacterial sinusitis may develop and contribute to the patient's symptoms. The rate of postoperative recurrence is approximately 35% to 40%.

Associations: The average rate of associated malignancy is about 13%, including patients in whom malignant disease coexists at the time of diagnosis and those in whom malignancy, particularly squamous cell carcinoma, ultimately develops.

RADIOLOGIC FEATURES

Cardinal Signs

Lesion is seen on CT as a tissue mass, ranging from a small nasal polypoid mass to an expansile mass with bony remodeling that deviates, but does not cross, the nasal septum. The mass may extend into the ethmoid or maxillary sinuses.

On MR lesion appears as a soft tissue mass of homogeneous, intermediate intensity on T1- and T2-weighted images.

Moderate enhancement is seen on contrast MR imaging.

Differential Diagnosis

Allergic polyps
Esthesioneuroblastoma
Adenocarcinoma
Squamous cell carcinoma

SQUAMOUS CELL CARCINOMA

Overview

Definition: Squamous cell carcinoma is the most common malignant neoplasm of the nose and sinuses. In 80% of cases, the maxillary antrum is involved either primarily or secondarily.

Clinical Features

Demographics: Squamous cell carcinoma constitutes 50% to 80% of all malignant sinus lesions. Men are more commonly affected by a ratio of 2:1, with an average age of 60 years. Over 60% of these tumors originate in the maxillary antra, followed by the nasal cavity and ethmoid sinuses.

Signs and symptoms: Common presenting features of all malignant sinus lesions are facial or dental pain, nasal obstruction, and epistaxis. Other presenting symptoms may include diplopia, epiphora, facial swelling, malocclusion, trismus, neck mass, hearing loss, and facial numbness. Proposed risk factors for squamous cell carcinoma of the sinus include certain occupations (particularly those involving exposure to nickel), chronic sinusitis, and inverted papilloma. The disease is usually advanced by the time of presentation, when 80% of patients have bone destruction. The cumulative survival rate with combined radiation therapy and surgery is approximately 25% to 30%.

RADIOLOGIC FEATURES

Cardinal Signs

Mass in sinus, usually with bone destruction
Computed tomography shows soft tissue mass, usually with bone destruction.
Tumor destroys bone in its path, leaving small fragments behind.
Contrast enhancement on CT is usually minimal to moderate.
Magnetic resonance imaging shows intermediate signal on T1-weighted images and hypointense to intermediate intensity on T2-weighted images.
Tumor shows moderately homogeneous in intensity throughout on MR.

Differential Diagnosis

Lymphoma
Lymphoepithelioma
Adenocarcinoma
Sarcoma
Carcinoma of palate
Fulminant mycotic infection

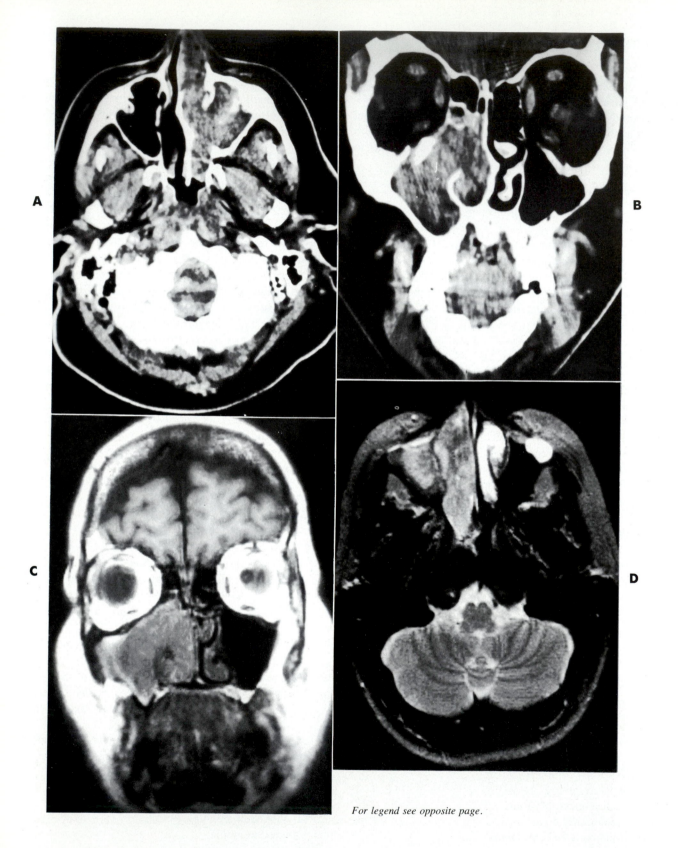

For legend see opposite page.

Fig. 13-12, opposite page, A, Soft tissue mass occupying the left nasal cavity and maxillary antrum. Though the mass has grown through and enlarged the maxillary ostium, the nasal septum and outer sinus walls show no evidence of bone destruction. **B,** Coronal CT scan shows a soft tissue mass occupying the nasal cavity and maxillary antrum. The outer bony margins remain intact. **C,** Coronal T1-weighted MR image in another patient shows mass of intermediate signal intensity occupying the right maxillary antrum and nasal cavity. **D,** Axial T2-weighted MR image shows mass of intermediate signal intensity in the right antrum and nasal cavity. Note the hyperintense mucosa of the turbinate on the left (from nasal cycle) and the hyperintense retention cyst in the left antrum.

Fig. 13-13, right, A, Waters view of the sinuses shows opacification of the left maxillary antrum with destruction of the lateral wall and left orbital floor. **B,** Axial CT scan in another patient shows a large soft tissue mass with a central air-filled cavity occupying the right maxillary antrum. The mass has invaded the retroantral fat pad *(arrowheads),* the nasal cavity, and the malar soft tissues *(arrows).*

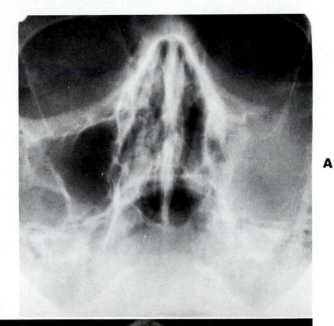

A

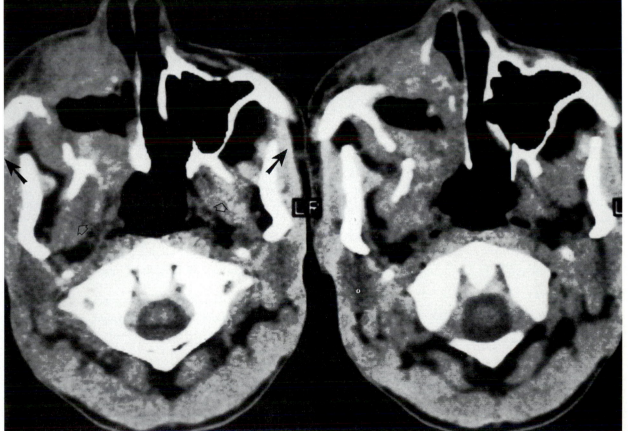

B

Continued.

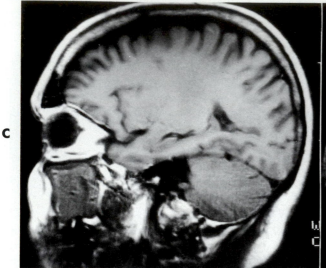

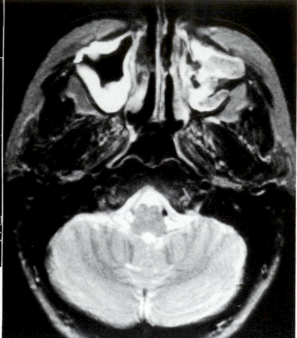

Fig. 13-13, cont'd.   C, Sagittal T1-weighted MR image of a different patient shows a mass of intermediate signal intensity occupying the left maxillary sinus. The sinus walls appear intact. **D,** Axial T2-weighted MR image shows hyperintense thickened mucosa in the antra bilaterally, indicating benign inflammation. A mass of intermediate signal intensity occupies the lateral portion of the left antrum, representing squamous carcinoma. In most cases, MR permits easy differentiation between malignant neoplasm and coexistent inflammation.

ADENOID CYSTIC CARCINOMA

Overview

Of all malignant sinonasal tumors, 10% are glandular in origin. The most common adenocarcinoma of the upper respiratory tract, adenoid cystic carcinoma arises from small submucosal salivary glands. It is slow growing but locally invasive, spreading along nerve sheaths. Up to 20% of cases metastasize, especially to the lungs.

Clinical Features

Demographics: Adenoid cystic carcinoma most commonly starts in the ethmoid sinuses and nasal vault. It is more common in men, age 30 to 60 years.

Signs and symptoms: Adenoid cystic carcinoma usually presents with nasal obstruction and epistaxis. Patients may have cranial nerve deficits or dull pain from perineural invasion. The short-term prognosis is good, with a 5-year survival of 75%; however, late recurrence is common, and the 15-year survival drops to 25%.

RADIOLOGIC FEATURES

Cardinal Signs

Best seen on CT. Tumor initially expands sinus walls, leading to remodelling of bone without breakthrough, thus resembling a mucocele.

Tumor is usually inhomogeneous as a result of cystic degeneration, necrosis, or serous and mucous collections. More cellular tumors are homogeneous.

Magnetic resonance imaging shows intermediate signal intensity on T1-weighted images and intermediate to bright intensity on T2-weighted images.

Differential Diagnosis

Mucocele
Mucoepidermoid carcinoma
Giant cell granuloma

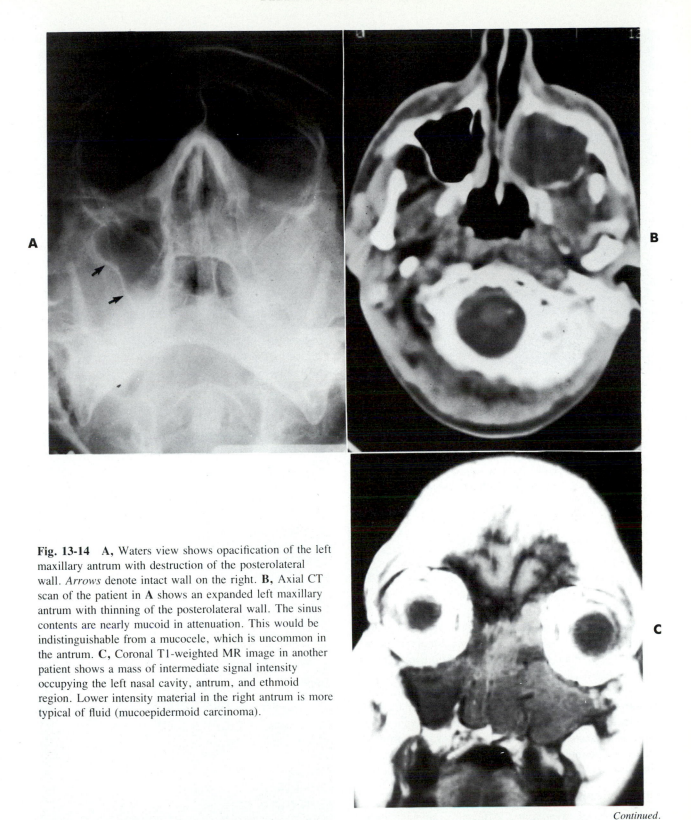

Fig. 13-14 **A,** Waters view shows opacification of the left maxillary antrum with destruction of the posterolateral wall. *Arrows* denote intact wall on the right. **B,** Axial CT scan of the patient in **A** shows an expanded left maxillary antrum with thinning of the posterolateral wall. The sinus contents are nearly mucoid in attenuation. This would be indistinguishable from a mucocele, which is uncommon in the antrum. **C,** Coronal T1-weighted MR image in another patient shows a mass of intermediate signal intensity occupying the left nasal cavity, antrum, and ethmoid region. Lower intensity material in the right antrum is more typical of fluid (mucoepidermoid carcinoma).

Continued.

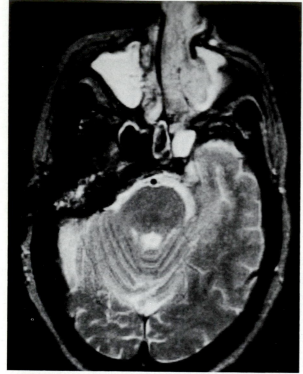

Fig. 13-14, cont'd **D,** Axial T2-weighted MR image in the same patient as in **C** shows a mass of intermediate to high signal intensity in the left nasal cavity and antrum. The T2 images show the tumor extent in the left antrum more clearly, with benign mucosal edema laterally. Benign inflammatory disease is present in the right antrum and left sphenoid sinuses.

RHABDOMYOSARCOMA

Overview

Demographics and definition: The most common malignant neoplasm of the upper respiratory tract in children less than 15 years old, rhabdomyosarcoma occurs only occasionally in adults. Seventy eight percent of those affected are less than 12 years old. Rhabdomyosarcoma is an aggressive neoplasm characterized by rapid progression; it is frequently advanced at time of diagnosis. In the head and neck, the orbit is the most common site of origin, followed by the sinonasal region.

Clinical Features

Signs and symptoms: Affected patients may present with nasal bleeding, rhinorrhea, nasal obstruc-

tion, otalgia, or ear obstruction. The 3-year survival is approximately 70% with combined therapy. Metastases occur by hematogenous, lymphatic, direct, and meningeal spread.

RADIOLOGIC FEATURES

Cardinal Signs

Best seen on CT as a soft tissue mass with both remodeling and destruction of bone.

Mass has a homogeneous appearance, with little or moderate enhancement on CT.

Magnetic resonance imaging shows an homogeneous mass of intermediate signal intensity on all sequences.

Differential Diagnosis

Esthesioneuroblastoma
Metastatic neuroblastoma
Nasal polyposis
Angiofibroma

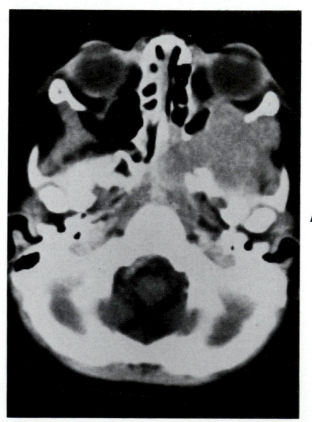

For legend see opposite page.

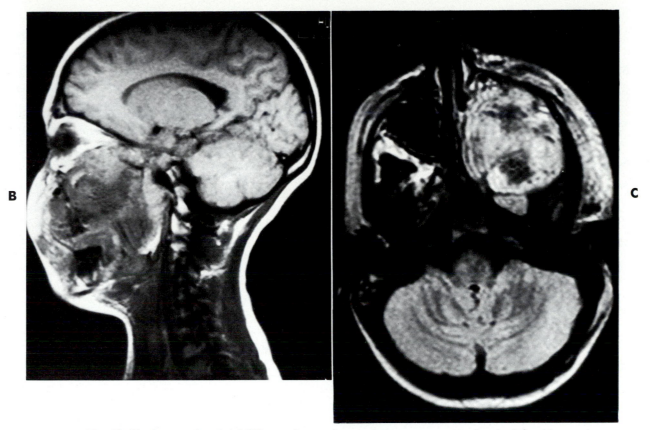

Fig. 13-15 A, opposite, Axial CT scan shows a large soft tissue mass occupying the left orbit, infratemporal fossa, pterygopalatine fossa, and lateral nasal cavity with destruction of the base of the sphenoid (compare to opposite side). **B,** above, Sagittal T1-weighted MR image of a different patient shows a heterogeneous mass of intermediate signal intensity occupying the maxillary antrum, displacing the left orbital floor *(arrows),* and invading the parapharyngeal spaces posteriorly. **C,** Axial MR image shows a large, heterogeneous, hyperintense mass centered on the left maxillary antrum with extension into the infratemporal fossa. The hyperintensity of the malar soft tissues may reflect tumor or lymphedema.

BIBLIOGRAPHY

Choanal Atresia

Harner SG, McDonald TJ, Reese DF: The anatomy of congenital choanal atresia, *Otolaryngol Head Neck Surg* 89:7, 1981.

Tadmor R, et al: Computed tomographic demonstration of choanal atresia, *AJNR* 5:743, 1984.

Concha Bullosa

Zinreich SJ, et al: Concha bullosa: CT evaluation, *J Comput Assist Tomogr* 12:778, 1988.

Acute Sinusitis

Weber AL: Inflammatory diseases of the paranasal sinuses and mucoceles, *Otolaryngol Clin North Am* 21:421, 1988.

Chronic Sinusitis

Weber AL: Inflammatory diseases of the paranasal sinuses and mucoceles, *Otolaryngol Clin North Am* 21:421, 1988.

Aspergillus Sinusitis

Kopp W, et al: Aspergillosis of the paranasal sinuses, *Radiology* 156:715, 1985.

Zinreich SJ, et al: Fungal sinusitis: diagnosis with CT and MR imaging, *Radiology* 169:439, 1988.

Retention Cyst

Gardner DG: Pseudocysts and retention cysts of the maxillary sinus, *Oral Surg Oral Med Oral Pathol* 58:561, 1984.

Ruprecht A, Batniji S, El-Neweihi E: Mucous retention cyst of the maxillary sinus, *Oral Surg Oral Med Oral Pathol* 62:728, 1986.

Mucocele

Hasso AN: CT of tumors and tumor-like conditions of the paranasal sinuses, *Radiol Clin North Am* 22:119, 1984.

Van Tassel P, et al: Mucoceles of the paranasal sinuses: MR imaging with CT correlation, *AJNR* 10:607, 1989.

Nasal Polyps

Som PM, et al: Computed tomography appearance distinguishing benign nasal polyps from malignancies, *J Comput Assist Tomogr* 11:129, 1987.

Wegener Granulomatosis

Lloyd GAS, et al: Magnetic resonance imaging in the evaluation of nose and paranasal sinus disease, *Br J Radiol* 60:957, 1987.

Simmons JT, et al: CT of the paranasal sinuses and orbits in patients with wegener's granulomatosis, *Ear Nose Throat J* 66:134, 1987.

Angiofibroma

Lloyd GAS, Phelps PD: Juvenile angiofibroma: imaging by magnetic resonance, CT, and conventional techniques, *Clin Otolaryngol* 11:247, 1986.

Osteoma of the Paranasal Sinuses

Grove AS: Osteomas of the orbit, *Ophthal Surg* 9:23, 1978.

Weber AL: Tumors of the paranasal sinuses, *Otolaryngol Clin North Am* 21:439, 1988.

Inverted Papilloma

Hasso AN: CT of tumors and tumor-like conditions of the paranasal sinuses, *Radiol Clinics North Am* 22:119, 1984.

Squamous Cell Carcinoma

Som PM, et al: Sinonasal tumors and inflammatory tissues: differentiation with MR imaging, *Radiology* 167:803, 1988.

Weber AL, Stanton AC: Malignant tumors of the paranasal sinuses: radiologic, clinical, and histopathologic evaluation of 200 cases, *Head Neck Surg* 6:761, 1984.

Adenoid Cystic Carcinoma

Hasso AN: CT of tumors and tumor-like conditions of the paranasal sinuses, *Radiol Clin North Am* 22:119, 1984.

Som PM, et al: Sinonasal tumors and inflammatory tissues: differentiation with MR imaging, *Radiology* 167:803, 1988.

Rhabdomyosarcoma

Latack JT, Hutchinson RJ, Heyn RM: Imaging of rhabdomyosarcomas of the head and neck, *AJNR* 8:353, 1987.

C H A P T E R

14

SALIVARY GLAND DISEASES

DEVELOPMENTAL DISTURBANCES

Overview

Developmental disturbances of the salivary glands include agenesis and aplasia. These lesions occur only very rarely.

Definition: Aplasia is the congenital absence of salivary gland formation. It may be unilateral or bilateral. Absence of both the parotid and the submandibular glands bilaterally has also been reported.

Clinical Features

In aplasia the amount of salivary flow decreases in proportion to the degree of the lack of gland formation, possibly leading to xerostomia.

RADIOLOGIC FEATURES

Cardinal Signs

Computed tomographic (CT) image shows a lack of gland development.
Salivary gland scintigrams with ^{99m}Tc-0$_4$ do not show any accumulation in the defective glands.

SIALOLITHIASIS

Overview

Definition: Sialolithiasis is a formation of sialoliths, or "stones," in the secretory portions and ducts of the salivary glands. The presence of such sialoliths causes inflammation in the secretory portions and ducts. Sialoliths occur most often in the major salivary glands, with the greatest frequency in the submandibular glands.

Clinical Features

Signs and symptoms: Sialolithiasis produces various symptoms according to the site of the sialolith and stage of the disease. Common symptoms are salivary gland pain and local swelling. The long-term presence of a ductal sialolith may induce infection. When suppurative sialoadenitis occurs, erythema and purulence may be found at the ductal orifices.

RADIOLOGIC FEATURES

Cardinal Signs

Sialoliths in the ducts of submandibular gland image as opaque round or elliptic structures

Differential Diagnosis

In panoramic x-ray films the shadows of sialoliths sometimes overlap the mandible or maxilla. In such cases it is necessary to differentiate this disease from enostosis, exostosis, osteosclerosis, sclerosing osteitis, and other similar diseases. An occlusal film will aid in the diagnosis of the location of the lesion, whether it is inside or outside of the jaw bones. Sialoliths may occasionally need to be distinguished from phleboliths, or calcified submandibular lymph nodes.

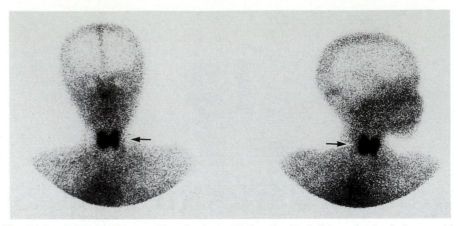

Fig. 14-1 Aplasia of the parotid and submandibular glands. Salivary gland scintigram with technetium 99m pertechnetate. Note normal positive uptake in the thyroid glands *(arrows),* whereas both the parotid and submandibular glands show negative uptake.

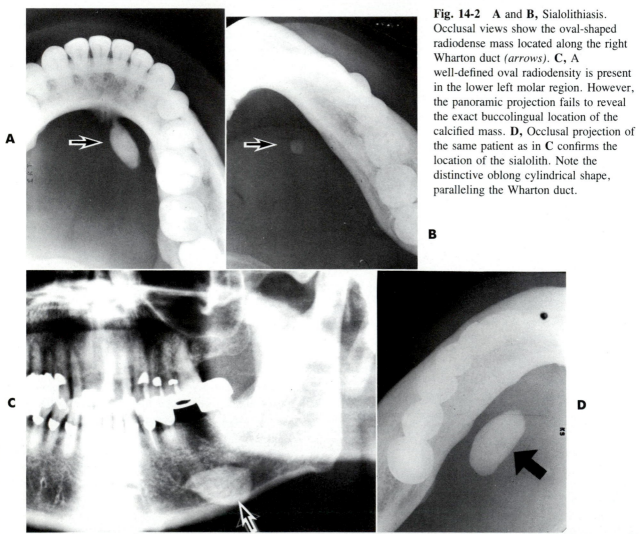

Fig. 14-2 A and **B,** Sialolithiasis. Occlusal views show the oval-shaped radiodense mass located along the right Wharton duct *(arrows).* **C,** A well-defined oval radiodensity is present in the lower left molar region. However, the panoramic projection fails to reveal the exact buccolingual location of the calcified mass. **D,** Occlusal projection of the same patient as in **C** confirms the location of the sialolith. Note the distinctive oblong cylindrical shape, paralleling the Wharton duct.

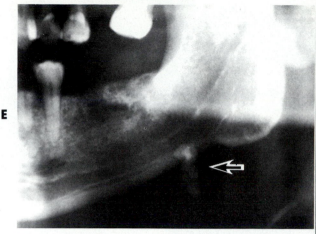
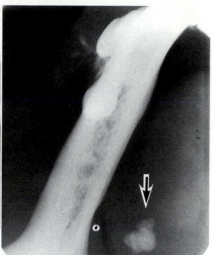
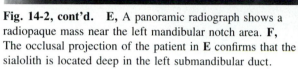

Fig. 14-2, cont'd. **E,** A panoramic radiograph shows a radiopaque mass near the left mandibular notch area. **F,** The occlusal projection of the patient in **E** confirms that the sialolith is located deep in the left submandibular duct.

SIALOADENITIS

Overview

Definition: Sialoadenitis is inflammation of the salivary glands, generally caused by infection.

Clinical Features

Sialoadenitis tends to occur in elderly persons and children. This disorder occurs most commonly in the parotid glands, secondly in the submandibular glands, and only infrequently in the sublingual gland.

ACUTE SIALOADENITIS

Acute sialoadenitis (also known as acute suppurative sialoadenitis, epidemic parotiditis, acute allergic sialoadenitis) predominantly occurs in the parotid glands, generally bilaterally. This disease is often caused by retrograde infection, especially when the systemic resistance is low. Painful, firm swelling of the parotid glands usually is present, with erythema and swelling of the opening of the ducts, hyposalivation, and discharge of purulent secretions. Many of the patients diagnosed as having acute suppurative sialoadenitis are in the acute exacerbation stage of chronic sialoadenitis.

Radiologic assessment: Radiology is not indicated. Sialography should not be done in the acute in-flammation phase, because it is likely to exacerbate these symptoms.

Generally, in cases of true acute sialoadenitis, such as mumps and acute allergic sialoadenitis, a sialogram after the resolution of symptoms shows no specific findings.

CHRONIC SIALOADENITIS

Chronic sialoadenitis (also known as chronic recurrent parotitis, Kuttner tumor) may occur in the parotid glands and submandibular glands. Its causes include sialolithiasis, inflammation of the adjacent tissues, and abnormalities of the duct. Retrograde infection from the glandular orifice with nonspecific normal flora of the oral cavity is also considered a direct cause.

Clinical Features

The disease mostly runs a chronic course and is usually symptomless. The acute transformation is repeated many times, attributable to reduced physical health. During the acute stage, symptoms of acute suppurative sialoadenitis are found. These symptoms disappear with the recovery of physical health.

Chronic recurrent parotitis, which is also a nonspecific bacterial sialoadenitis, is frequently found in childhood.

Text continued on page 408.

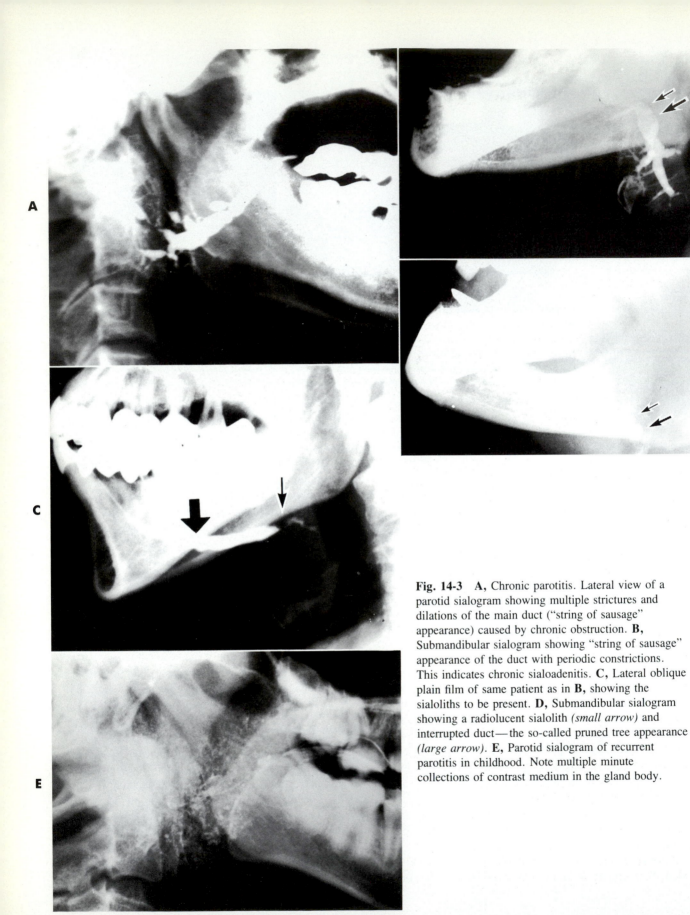

Fig. 14-3 **A,** Chronic parotitis. Lateral view of a parotid sialogram showing multiple strictures and dilations of the main duct ("string of sausage" appearance) caused by chronic obstruction. **B,** Submandibular sialogram showing "string of sausage" appearance of the duct with periodic constrictions. This indicates chronic sialoadenitis. **C,** Lateral oblique plain film of same patient as in **B,** showing the sialoliths to be present. **D,** Submandibular sialogram showing a radiolucent sialolith *(small arrow)* and interrupted duct—the so-called pruned tree appearance *(large arrow)*. **E,** Parotid sialogram of recurrent parotitis in childhood. Note multiple minute collections of contrast medium in the gland body.

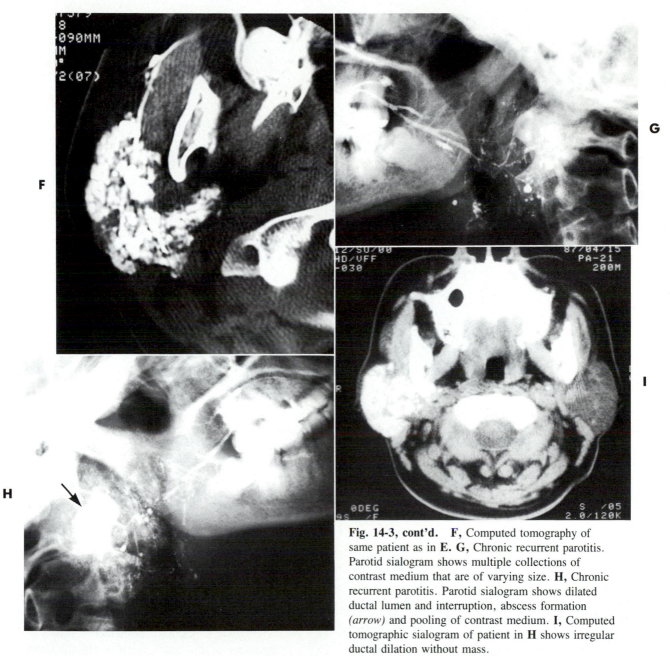

Fig. 14-3, cont'd. F, Computed tomography of same patient as in **E. G,** Chronic recurrent parotitis. Parotid sialogram shows multiple collections of contrast medium that are of varying size. **H,** Chronic recurrent parotitis. Parotid sialogram shows dilated ductal lumen and interruption, abscess formation *(arrow)* and pooling of contrast medium. **I,** Computed tomographic sialogram of patient in **H** shows irregular ductal dilation without mass.

Continued.

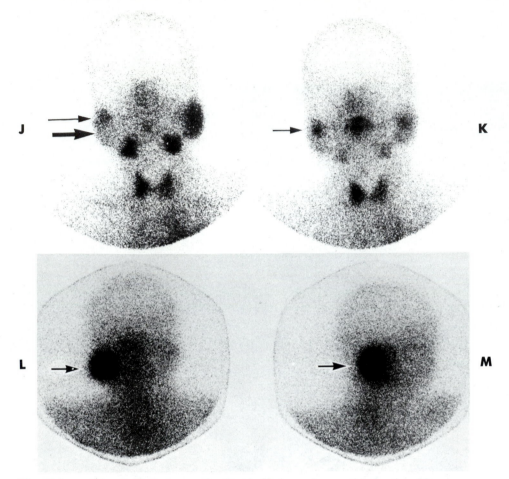

Fig. 14-3, cont'd.   J, Static image of patient in **H** shows decreased technetium 99m pertechnetate activity *(large arrow)* compared with left parotid gland. **K,** Washout image of patient in **H** demonstrates greatly retained activity *(small arrow)* in region of the abscess formation in the abnormal right parotid gland. **L,** Gallium-67 scintigram of patient in **H** shows strong positive uptake *(arrow).*

Chronic sclerosing sialoadenitis, or Kuttner tumor, is a sialoadenitis of the submandibular glands unilaterally. The gland enlarges painlessly and becomes sclerosed over a period of several months to several years.

Radiologic assessment: Generally sialography should not be performed during the acute exacerbation stage of chronic sialoadenitis. If sialography is done immediately after acute symptoms resolve, the clinician should gently flush the inside of the glands with sterile saline to remove pus and mucus before taking the sialogram.

RADIOLOGIC FEATURES

Cardinal Signs

The sialogram of chronic sialoadenitis shows enlargement of the ducts, particularly thickening of the main duct, first branch, and second branch.

The remarkably dilated ducts exhibit "sausage" or "string of sausages" appearance.

In radionuclide salivary imaging of chronic sialoadenitis, a $^{99m}Tc\text{-}0_4$ image manifests decreased activity, and its washout image shows retained activity.

Gallium #67 (^{67}Ga) image manifests positive uptake in proportion to the degree of inflammation.

Ancillary Signs

Sialolith obstruction of the duct may be present. In cases of relatively large sialoliths the duct breaks in the parotid transitional region or the submandibular transitional region, and the plain radiograph reveals a "pruned tree" appearance.

In chronic recurrent parotitis in childhood sialograms display many small round shadows in the secretory portion, similar to those seen in Sjögren syndrome.

Chronic sclerosing sialoadenitis, or Kuttner tumor, shows a slight enlargement of the main or secondary duct, irregularities of the duct wall, and the disappearance of the terminal duct.

Differential Diagnosis

Trauma
Malignant tumors
Sialolithiasis
Mucous plugging
Sjögren syndrome

BENIGN LYMPHOEPITHELIAL LESION (MIKULICZ DISEASE AND MIKULICZ SYNDROME)

Overview

History and definition: In 1892, Mikulicz reported a lesion that presents as a bilateral swelling of the lacrimal glands and salivary glands. It appeared to be caused by chronic infection. Subsequently lesions with clinical findings similar to this have been reported, including those caused by specific inflammations, such as tuberculosis, syphilis, leukemia, and malignant lymphoma. Thus lesions resulting from any obvious cause and characterized by secondary bilateral enlargement of the major salivary and lacrimal glands are known as *Mikulicz syndrome*. Lesions with similar findings but of unknown origin are known as *Mikulicz disease*. Later, on the basis of a report by Godwin in 1962, Mikulicz disease became commonly known by the term *benign lymphoepithelial lesion*.

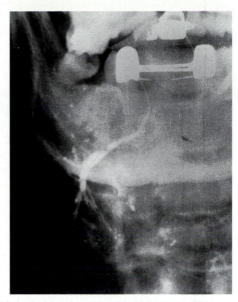

Fig. 14-4 Benign lymphoepithelial lesion. Frontal submandibular sialogram showing the distended Wharton duct. Smaller terminal ducts are not visualized.

Clinical Features and Comparison with Sjögren Syndrome

Some authors think that benign lymphoepithelial lesions and Sjögren syndrome lesions may be essentially the same kind because of pathologic similarities. However, patients with Sjögren syndrome complain of severe dryness of the eyes and oral cavities, whereas those with benign lymphoepithelial lesions complain mainly of swelling, induration, and xerosis. In Sjögren syndrome atrophic induration is found; in benign lymphoepithelial lesion, there is painless swelling. In addition, some cases of benign lymphoepithelial lesion may result in malignant lymphoma or cancerous changes in the epithelial islands. As a result, this disease is considered to have a tendency toward malignancy.

RADIOLOGIC FEATURES

Cardinal Signs

The early sialographic features of this disease include irregular dilation or partial disappearance of peripheral ducts and maculation. In this stage the sialogram shows dilation of the main ducts and extensive disappearance or diffuse defects of peripheral ducts.

Ancillary Signs

Punctuate shadows

SJÖGREN SYNDROME

Overview

History and definition: In 1933, Sjögren reported a case characterized by keratoconjunctivitis sicca (conjunctivitis sicca), dry mouth, chronic rheumatoid arthritis, and swelling of the salivary glands. Thereafter similar cases have been reported as Sjögren's syndrome. The etiology of this syndrome has remained a mystery.

Clinical Features

The syndrome occurs most commonly in middle-aged women. It is a systemic disease, with the above symptoms complicated by rheumatoid arthritis, collagen diseases, and autoimmune diseases, which lead to various clinical manifestations. Xerostomia is caused by hyposalivation, which may bring about atrophy, erosion, or ulcers of the oral mucosa.

RADIOLOGIC FEATURES

Cardinal Signs

Sialographic findings include the presence of numerous small round shadows, called the "branchless fruit-laden tree" appearance. The degree of distention in the peripheral parts of the ducts is divided into four stages. Stage I is classified as the punctuate pattern; stage II, the globular pattern; stage III, the cavitary pattern; and stage IV, the destructive pattern.

Salivary gland scintigram with ^{99m}Tc-0_4 shows a decrease in the uptake into the parotid and submandibular glands bilaterally. The washout image displays the retained radioactivity in the salivary gland.

Differential Diagnosis

Progressive systemic sclerosis
Rheumatoid arthritis
Systemic lupus erythematous
Polymyositis
Chronic recurrent parotitis

Special Tests

Other techniques used to diagnose Sjögren syndrome include biopsy of minor salivary glands and sialochemistry.

SALIVARY GLAND TUMORS

Overview

Salivary gland tumors occur in the parotid glands in 75% to 85% of all cases, with the remainder occurring in the minor salivary glands and submandibular glands. Sublingual gland tumors are very rare. Most minor salivary gland tumors originate in the palate. Histologically epithelial tumors are most common, 60% to 70% being pleomorphic adenomas. The box below shows the World Health Organization (WHO) histologic classification.

The preoperative diagnostic evaluation to determine whether a lesion is benign or malignant is very significant. Table 14-1 shows the diagnostic point of distinction between benign and malignant tumors of the salivary glands.

WORLD HEALTH ORGANIZATION CLASSIFICATION OF SALIVARY GLAND TUMORS (1972)

Epithelial tumors
  Adenomas
    Pleomorphic adenomas (mixed tumors)
    Monomorphic adenomas
      Adenolymphoma
      Oxyphilic adenoma
      Other types
Mucoepidermoid tumor
Acinic cell tumor
Carcinomas
  Adenoid cystic carcinoma
  Adenocarcinoma
  Epidermoid carcinoma
  Undifferentiated carcinoma
  Carcinoma in pleomorphic adenoma (malignant mixed tumor)
Nonepithelial tumors
Unclassified tumors
Allied conditions

From Thackray AC, Sobin LH: Geneva, 1972, World Health Organization.

TABLE 14-1   Features of Benign and Malignant Salivary Gland Tumors

	Benign tumor	Malignant tumor
Clinical features		
	Benign tumor	Malignant tumor
	Rate of tumor growth slow	Rate of tumor growth rapid
	No symptoms	Feeling of pressure and pain
		Other facial neuropathy
Features of diagnostic images		
Contrast sialogram	Pressure, shift of duct system	In addition to findings of benign tumor:
	Filling defect of gland parenchyma	Cutoff of duct
	Stretching of duct in marginal region of pressure	Leakage of contrast medium
	("ball in hand" appearance)	
CT or CT sialogram	Clearly defined border from surrounding tissue	Unclear border from surrounding tissue
	Smooth tumor margin and oval shape	Irregular tumor margin
Scintigram	^{67}Ga scintigram shows normal uptake.	^{67}Ga scintigram shows positive uptake.
	With ^{99m}Tc-0_4 relatively large tumor represents a defect.	Care is needed after sialography with oily contrast media.
	With ^{99m}Tc-0_4 adenolymphoma shows positive uptake.	With ^{99m}Tc-0_4 tumor region shows negative uptake.
	(Washout image also has positive uptake.)	
Ultrasonogram	Clear border and smooth margin	Unclear border and irregular margin
	No echoes from boundaries or regular linear echoes on all sides	Echoes from boundaries irregular and strong
	Internal echoes absent or even and weak	Internal echoes absent or uneven, rough, and strong
	Posterior echoes enhanced	Posterior echoes reduced or absent
MR imaging	Clearly defined border from surrounding tissue	Unclear border from surrounding tissue
	Smooth tumor margin and oval shape	Irregular tumor margin
	On T2-weighted image, intensity of malignant tumor frequently lower than that of benign tumor	

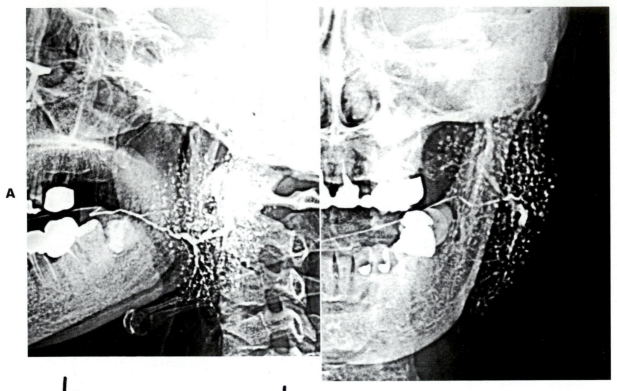

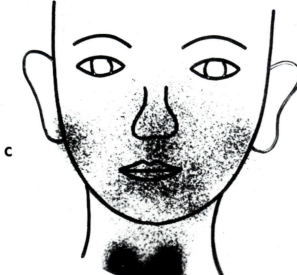

Fig. 14-5 Sjögren syndrome. Parotid sialograms using storage phosphors and computed radiography clearly demonstrate the "branchless fruit-laden tree" appearance. Lateral view. **B,** Sjögren syndrome, posteroanterior view. **C,** Sjögren syndrome, Technetium-99m pertechnetate salivary scintigram. In contrast to strong uptake in the thyroid glands, both submandibular and parotid glands show minimal uptake, indicating hypofunction.

BENIGN SALIVARY GLAND TUMORS

Pleomorphic Adenoma (Mixed Tumor)

Pleomorphic adenoma, also known as a mixed tumor, is the most common benign tumor in salivary glands. It accounts for 60% to 70% of all salivary gland diseases.

Clinical Features

The growth of a pleomorphic adenoma is slow and painless. The onset of disease is usually in the second to fifth decades of life.

RADIOLOGIC FEATURES

Cardinal Signs

When a tumor exists in the center of the secretory portion and is relatively large, it produces the typical sialographic appearance of the so-called ball in hand. This finding is caused by a dislocation of and pressure on the duct resulting from a benign tumor with a capsule or pseudocapsule. The ducts appear to surround the tumor. This is accompanied by a filling defect in the gland parenchyma. Because of pressure by the tumor, the duct is extended, and the distance between furcations becomes longer. Interruption of the extended duct may also be present.

On CT and MR imaging, this tumor appears as a round lesion with a distinct boundary line between it and the surrounding tissue. The margin is smooth, and the inside is more homogeneously of high density than the surrounding tissues. Sometimes its central part has a slightly lower density. CT sialography clearly shows the relation among the tumor, the secretory portion, and the surrounding tissue. Therefore CT sialography is very effective for the diagnosis of tumor localization (topographic diagnosis).

On ultrasonography, internal echoes are absent or homogeneous and weak. The posterior echoes are enhanced.

^{99m}Tc-0$_4$ scintigrams show areas of decreased radioactivity that correspond to the neoplasm.

Differential Diagnosis
Adenolymphoma (Warthin tumor)
Lipoma

Adenolymphoma (Warthin Tumor)

Adenolymphoma is also known as papillary adenocystoma lymphomatosum, or Warthin tumor.

Clinical features: The growth of an adenolymphoma is slow and painless. The tumor most frequently involves the parotid gland. Its peak incidence for detection occurs between the ages of 40 and 60 years.

RADIOLOGIC FEATURES

Cardinal Signs

CT, sialographic, and ultrasonographic findings are similar to those of pleomorphic adenoma.

For the qualitative diagnosis of adenolymphoma, ^{99m}Tc-0$_4$ scintigraphy is effective, especially the washout image, which provides the characteristic finding of residual radioactivity in the tumor.

MALIGNANT SALIVARY GLAND TUMORS

Mucoepidermoid Tumor (Mucoepidermoid Carcinoma)

This tumor was termed *mucoepidermoid tumor* by Stewart et al. in 1945, who considered it to be divided into benign and malignant types. However, some authors have concluded that all of these tumors are malignant and that they should be classified as low-grade or high-grade mucoepidermoid carcinoma. The WHO regards this tumor as a lesion with malignant potential but believes it is irrelevant to call any of these tumors carcinomas in a variety of clinical instances. Thus the WHO, which has also adopted the term *mucoepidermoid tumor,* feels this tumor is intermediate between adenoma and carcinoma.

Clinical features: Mucoepidermoid tumors account for almost 30% of the malignancies that occur in the salivary glands and appear most commonly in the third to fourth decades of life. The growth of the tumor is relatively slow. The mass frequently forms in the parotid glands.

Text continued on page 423.

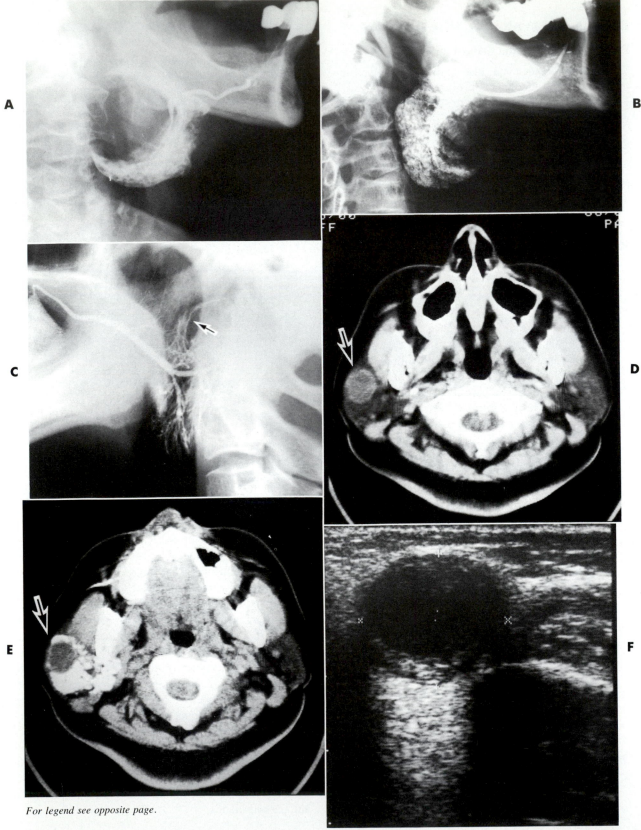

For legend see opposite page.

Continued.

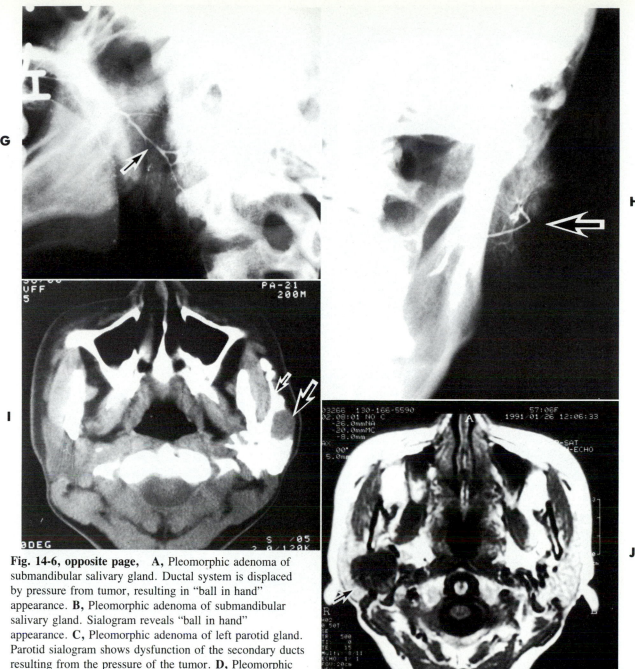

Fig. 14-6, opposite page, **A,** Pleomorphic adenoma of submandibular salivary gland. Ductal system is displaced by pressure from tumor, resulting in "ball in hand" appearance. **B,** Pleomorphic adenoma of submandibular salivary gland. Sialogram reveals "ball in hand" appearance. **C,** Pleomorphic adenoma of left parotid gland. Parotid sialogram shows dysfunction of the secondary ducts resulting from the pressure of the tumor. **D,** Pleomorphic adenoma of the left parotid gland. Computed tomographic image shows round, encapsulated, well-circumscribed lesion. **E,** Computed tomographic sialogram of patient in **D** confirms the position of the tumor *(arrow).* **F,** Ultrasonographic examination of patient in **D** demonstrates findings characteristic of a benign tumor—a well-circumscribed circular tumor mass with no internal echoes and slightly intensified posterior echoes. **G,** above, Pleomorphic adenoma of left parotid gland. Lateral view of parotid sialogram shows the low density of the contrast medium *(arrow).* **H,** Frontal view of parotid sialogram of patient in **G** shows the ductal system affected by the tumor pressure *(arrow).* **I,** Computed tomographic sialogram of patient in **G** indicates that the tumor *(large arrow)* is located lateral to the Stenson duct *(small arrow),* indicating that this tumor is in the superficial portion of the parotid gland. **J,** Pleomorphic adenoma. Transverse T1-weighted MR scan shows sharply defined, low-intensity mass in right parotid gland *(arrow).*

Continued.

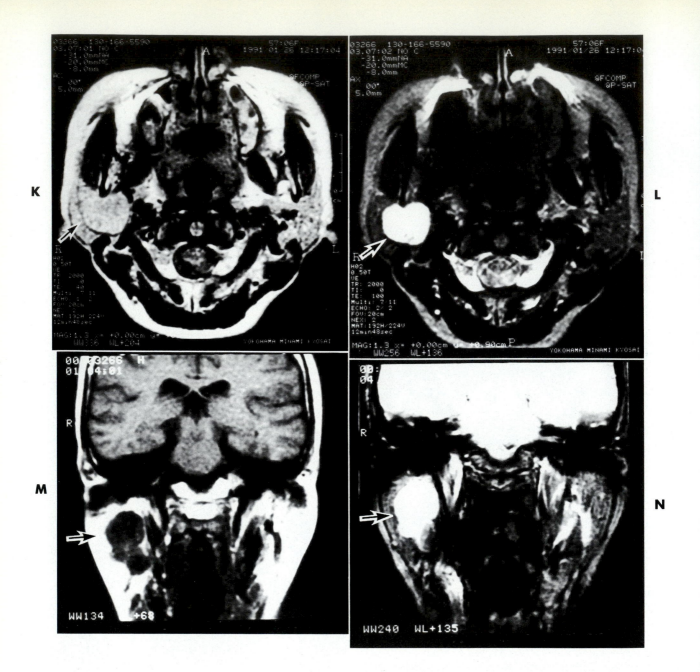

Fig. 14-6, cont'd. **K,** Transverse proton-weighted MR scan of patient in **J** shows moderate-intensity signal for the tumor *(arrow)*. **L,** Transverse T2-weighted MR scan of patient in **J** shows high-intensity signal for tumor *(arrow)*. **M,** Coronal T1-weighted MR image of patient in **J** shows low-intensity signal for tumor *(arrow)*. **N,** Coronal T2-weighted MR image of patient in **J** shows high-intensity signal for tumor *(arrow)*.

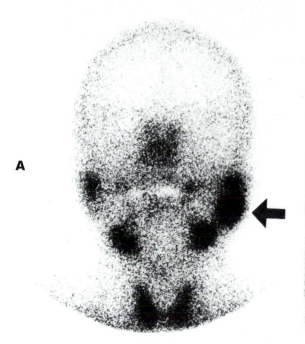

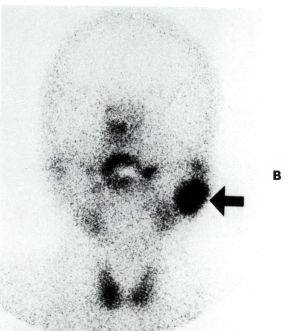

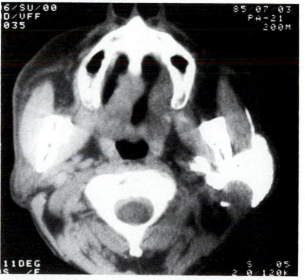

Fig. 14-7 **A,** Adenolymphoma (Warthin tumor) of the left parotid gland. Static Technetium-99m pertechnetate image shows marked uptake in the inferior portion of the left parotid gland corresponding to the tumor *(large arrow),* as compared with the normal parotid gland. **B,** Washout image of patient in **A** shows marked retained radiopharmaceutical activity in the inferior portion of the left parotid gland corresponding to the tumor after stimulation *(arrow).* **C,** Adenolymphoma (Warthin tumor) of the left parotid gland. Computed tomographic sialography shows a filling defect corresponding to the tumor in the inferior portion of the left parotid gland.

Continued.

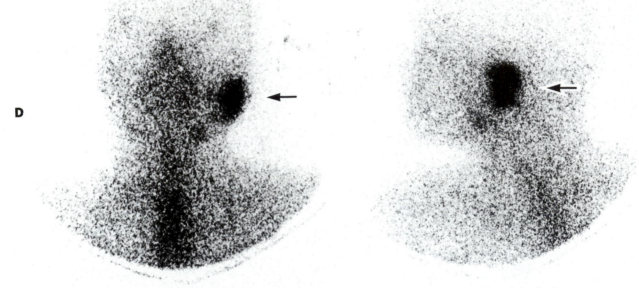

Fig 14-7, cont'd. D, Gallium 67 scintigram of patient in **C** shows strong radioactivity in the normal portion of the left parotid gland *(arrows)*.

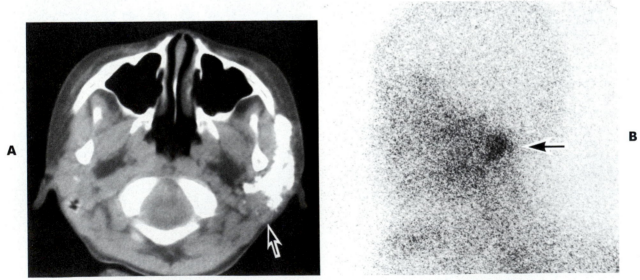

Fig. 14-8   A, High-grade mucoepidermoid tumor. Computed tomographic sialogram shows filling defect with ill-defined margins *(arrow)*. **B,** Gallium 67 scintigram of patient in **A** shows increased radioactivity *(arrow)*.

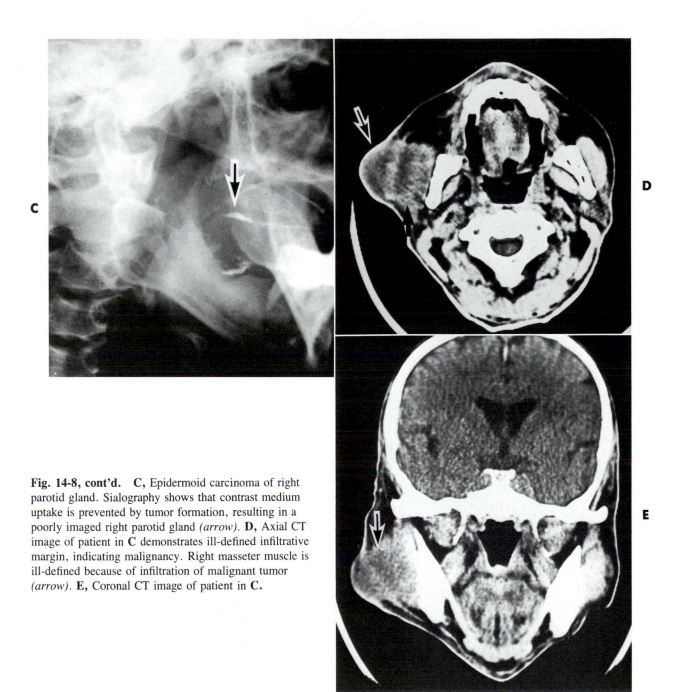

Fig. 14-8, cont'd. **C,** Epidermoid carcinoma of right parotid gland. Sialography shows that contrast medium uptake is prevented by tumor formation, resulting in a poorly imaged right parotid gland *(arrow)*. **D,** Axial CT image of patient in C demonstrates ill-defined infiltrative margin, indicating malignancy. Right masseter muscle is ill-defined because of infiltration of malignant tumor *(arrow)*. **E,** Coronal CT image of patient in C.

Continued.

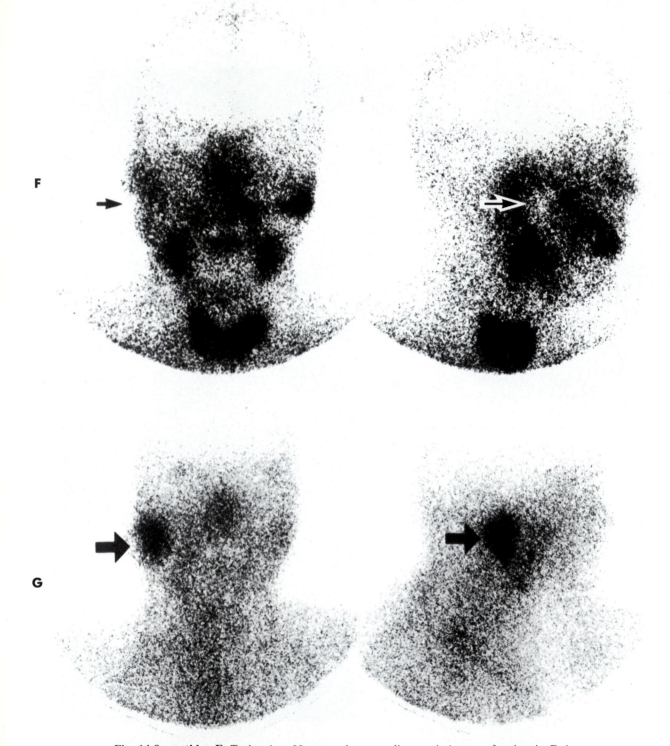

Fig. 14-8, cont'd.   F, Technetium-99m pertechnetate salivary scintigrams of patient in **C** show area of decreased activity *(arrows)*. **G,** Gallium-67 scintigrams of patient in **C** show strong positive uptake at the site of the tumor *(arrows)*.   *Continued.*

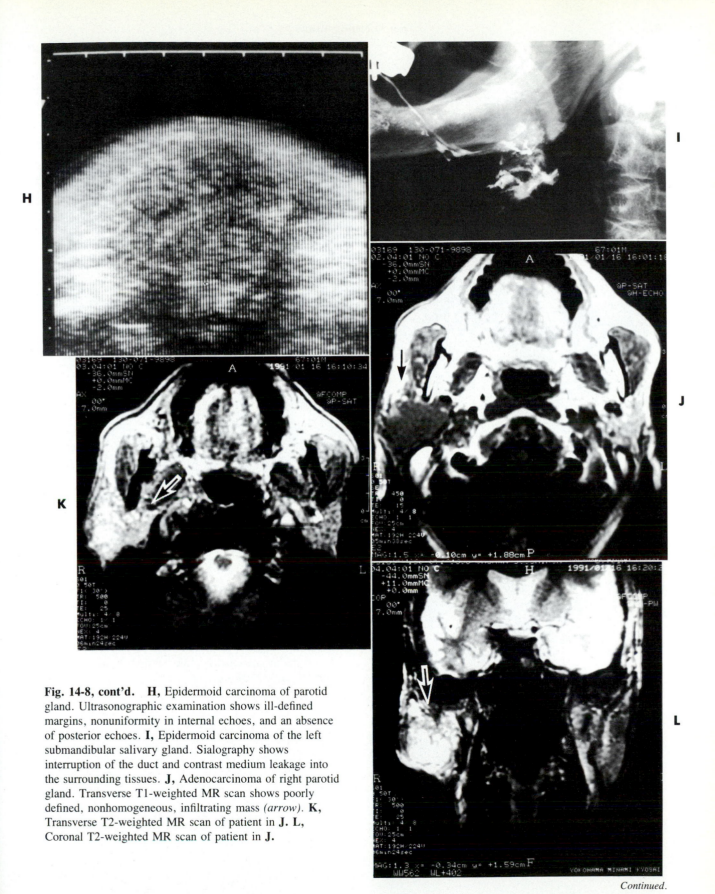

Fig. 14-8, cont'd. **H,** Epidermoid carcinoma of parotid gland. Ultrasonographic examination shows ill-defined margins, nonuniformity in internal echoes, and an absence of posterior echoes. **I,** Epidermoid carcinoma of the left submandibular salivary gland. Sialography shows interruption of the duct and contrast medium leakage into the surrounding tissues. **J,** Adenocarcinoma of right parotid gland. Transverse T1-weighted MR scan shows poorly defined, nonhomogeneous, infiltrating mass *(arrow)*. **K,** Transverse T2-weighted MR scan of patient in **J. L,** Coronal T2-weighted MR scan of patient in **J.**

Continued.

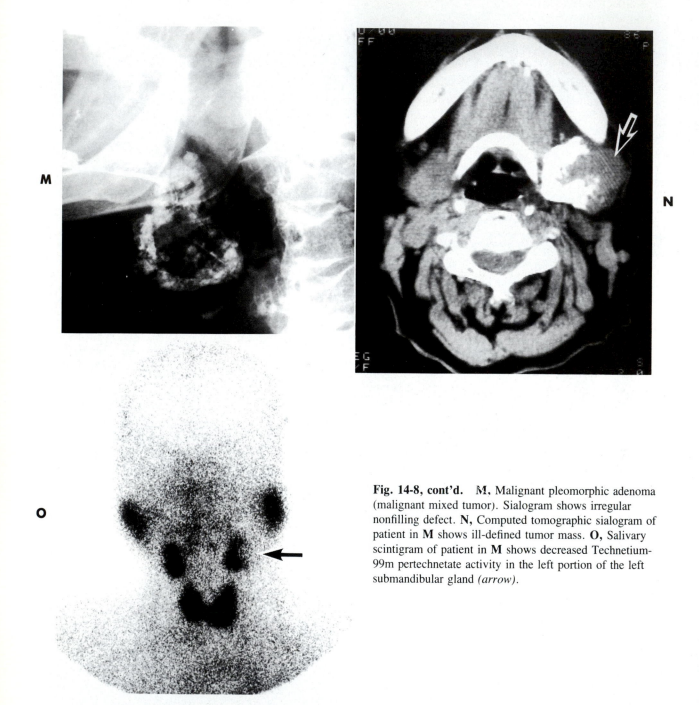

Fig. 14-8, cont'd.   M, Malignant pleomorphic adenoma (malignant mixed tumor). Sialogram shows irregular nonfilling defect. **N,** Computed tomographic sialogram of patient in **M** shows ill-defined tumor mass. **O,** Salivary scintigram of patient in **M** shows decreased Technetium-99m pertechnetate activity in the left portion of the left submandibular gland *(arrow).*

Epidermoid Carcinoma (Squamous Cell Carcinoma)

Epidermoid carcinoma is a relatively rare salivary gland tumor occurring mainly in the parotid and submandibular glands. It is found predominantly in men older than 50 years. Its growth is very fast. In some cases it adheres to the cutaneomucosal region and leads to ulceration. The histologic features are usually similar to squamous cell carcinoma, except for a decreased tendency for keratinization.

Adenocarcinoma

Adenocarcinoma most commonly involves the minor salivary glands and submandibular glands, accounting for 5% to 10% of salivary gland tumors. It occurs most frequently between the fourth and seventh decades of life and is slightly more common in females. The growth is relatively slow and often painful.

This tumor accounts for about 5% of salivary gland tumors. It primarily involves the parotid glands but is sometimes found in the submandibular and minor salivary glands. The growth is fast and painful. It may occur after the prime of life and is slightly predominant in males. Its histologic features are similar to those of other glandular tissues. This carcinoma includes tubular adenocarcinomas, myxadenocarcinomas and papillary adenocarcinomas.

Acinic Cell Tumor (Acinic Cell Carcinoma)

Previously considered benign, acinic cell tumors have proved to be malignant. Thus they are usually called acinic cell carcinoma.

Clinical features: Acinic cell tumors are very rare and frequently involve the parotid glands. They occur most commonly between the ages of 40 and 50 years, predominantly in women.

Malignant pleomorphic adenoma

Pathologically, malignant pleomorphic adenoma results from the transformation of the epithelial tissue in a pleomorphic adenoma. Malignant pleomorphic adenoma occurs predominantly in patients older than 50 years.

RADIOLOGIC FEATURES

At present, it is impossible to differentiate these tumors on imaging studies.

Cardinal Signs

Break in the duct and leakage indicates malignant changes.

Computed tomographic sialogram shows the irregular filling defect of the peripheral gland body.

Ultrasonographic findings include unfixed contour, unclear boundary, and irregular margin. The internal echoes are uneven, rough, and strong, but the posterior echoes are frequently attenuated or absent.

^{99m}Tc-0$_4$ scintigram shows a tumor region with negative uptake.

Positive uptake of ^{67}Ga citrate occurs.

MR imaging shows unclear boundaries and irregular margins. T2-weighted images are frequently very high-intensity signal.

As in benign tumors, sialography also reveals pressure on and shifting of the duct caused by the tumor and filling defects of the gland parenchyma.

Ducts in contact with the tumor are extended, and the distance between furcations becomes long.

Cutoff of ducts is seen.

Differential Diagnosis

A break in the duct and leakage of contrast media, which are sialographic signs of malignancy, are usually found in epidermoid carcinoma (squamous cell carcinoma), adenocarcinoma, and high-grade mucoepidermoid carcinoma. However, most of the malignant tumors in salivary glands (low-grade mucoepidermoid carcinoma, malignant pleomorphic adenoma, and adenoid cystic carcinoma) have a low rate of malignancy. Since the malignant signs of these neoplasms often include a break in thin ducts, such as the third or fourth branch, and a small amount of punctate leakage occurs, careful observation is required. A ^{67}Ga-citrate scintigram, after a sialogram with oily contrast media, shows a positive uptake in the salivary gland. Therefore the clinician should be careful not to mistake this uptake for a malignant lesion.

BIBLIOGRAPHY

Developmental Disturbances

Vogel C, Reichart P: Aplasie der Glandulae parotides und submandibularis mit Atresie der Canaliculi lacrimales, Ein kasuistischer Beitrag *Dtsch Zahnaeztl Z* 33:415, 1978.

Sialolithiasis

Rauch S, Golin RJ: *Disease of salivary glands.* In Golin RJ, Goldman HM, editors: *Thoma's oral pathology,* ed 6, St Louis, 1970, CV Mosby, pp 997-1001.

Benign Lymphoepithelial Lesion

Batsakis JG: The pathology of head and neck tumors: the lymphoepithelial lesion and Sjögren's syndrome, part 16, *Head Neck Surg* 5:150, 1982.

Lapes M, et al: Conversion of a benign lymphoepithelial salivary gland lesion to lymphocytic lymphoma during dilantin therapy, *Cancer* 38:1318, 1976.

Sjögren Syndrome

Ben-Aryeh H, et al: Sialochemistry for diagnosis of Sjögren's syndrome in xerostomic patients, *Oral Surg Oral Med Oral Pathol* 52:487, 1981.

Daniels TE, et al: An evaluation of salivary scintigraphy in Sjögren's syndrome, *Arthritis Rheum* 22:809, 1979.

Greenspan JS, et al: The histopathology of Sjögren's syndrome in labial saliva in severe xerostomia, *Int J Oral Surg* 37:217, 1974.

Rubin P, Holt JF: Secretory sialography in disease of major salivary glands, *AJR* 77:575, 1957.

Tarpley TM, Anderson LG, White CL: Minor salivary gland involvement in Sjögren's syndrome, *Oral Surg Oral Med Oral Pathol* 37:64, 1974.

Salivary Gland Tumors

Ballerini G, Mantero M, Sbrocca M: Ultrasonic patterns of parotid masses, *JCU* 12:273, 1984.

Higashi H, et al: Identification of Warthin's tumor with technetium-99m pertechnetate, *Clin Nucl Med* 12:796, 1987.

Higashi hi T, et al: Salivary gland uptake of gallium-67 citrate after sialography, *Clin Nucl Med* 13:110, 1988.

Kashima I, Ikuta H: Diagnostic value of salivary gland scintigraphy with technetium-99m pertechnetate, *Bull Kanagawa Dent Coll* 17:191, 1989.

Kassel EE: CT sialography. II. Parotid masses, *J Otolaryngol* 11:11, 1982.

Mandelblatt SM, et al: Parotid masses: MR imaging, *Radiology* 163:411, 1987.

Mirich DR, McArdle CB, Kulkarni MV: Benign pleomorphic adenomas of salivary glands: surface coil MR imaging versus CT, *J Comput Assist Tomogr* 11:620, 1987.

Sone S, et al: CT of parotid tumor, *AJNR* 3:143, 1982.

Thackray AC, Sobin LH: Histological typing of salivary gland tumors, Geneva, 1972, World Health Organization.

GLOSSARY

Abrasion (Tooth): Nonphysiologic wearing away of the teeth, usually as a result of habits, such as improper toothbrushing, or occupational hazards.

Acrocephaly: Malformation of the head, consisting of a high or pointed cranial vault, resulting from premature closure of the sagittal, coronal, and lambdoid sutures.

Acute Apical Abscess: Circumscribed collection of pus at the apical periodontal ligament of a tooth, resulting from inflammatory disease of the dental pulp.

Acute Apical Periodontitis: Acute inflammation in the apical periodontal ligament as a result of reaction to inflammatory degradation products from an infected dental pulp.

Acute Dentoalveolar Abscess: Acute inflammation leading to necrosis and pus formation in the tissues around the apex of the tooth.

Acute Subperiosteal Osteomyelitis: Pus-producing inflammation of the bone marrow occurring when inflammatory exudate, usually from an infected tooth, elevates the periosteum of the bone, leading to local necrosis and resorption of the cortical plate.

Acute Suppurative Osteomyelitis: Acute inflammation of the bone marrow that produces clinically apparent pus and secondarily affects the calcified component of the bone.

Adenoamelobastoma: See *adenomatoid odontogenic tumor*. Not related to ameloblastoma.

Adenomatoid Odontogenic Tumor: Probably a developmental overgrowth of odontogenic tissue rather than a true neoplasm. The lesion is frequently associated with an unerupted tooth.

Albers-Schönberg Disease: See *osteopetrosis*.

Albright Syndrome: Condition featuring Fibrous dysplasia of multiple bones, pigmented skin lesions (café au lait spots), and various endocrine disturbances, most commonly precocious puberty, goiter, hyperthyroidism, hyperparathyroidism, Cushing syndrome, and acromegaly.

Ameloblastic Fibroma: Benign mixed odontogenic tumor arising from both epithelial and mesenchymal elements of the tooth germ.

Ameloblastic Fibroodontoma: Lesion consisting of elements of ameloblastic odontoma and compound odontoma. See *ameloblastic odontoma* and *odontoma, compound*.

Ameloblastic Odontoma: Rare type of hamartoma of odontogenic tissues in which some of the odontogenic epithelial component fails to differentiate histologically, producing a lesion in which undifferentiated ameloblastoma-like epithelium mixes with the other dental tissues (enamel, dentin, cementum) of the lesion.

Ameloblastoma: Aggressive benign tumor, apparently arising from the remnants of the dental lamina and dental origin, with an appearance similar to the early cap-stage ameloblastic elements of developing teeth.

Amelogenesis Imperfecta: Developmental disturbance of tooth formation, usually hereditary, that results in marked defects in the enamel of all or nearly all teeth in both dentitions. Major types include generalized hypoplasia, localized hypoplasia, and hypomineralization.

Amputation Neuroma: See *neuroma*

Aneurysmal Bone Cyst: Tumorlike reactive lesion of bone that probably represents an exaggerated, localized, proliferative response of vascular tissue. Its name is a misnomer, because it contains no vascular aneurysms and is not a true bony cyst.

Ankylosis: Stiffening or fixation of a joint. May result from osseous union (true ankylosis) or from fibrous bands between the bones forming the joint (fibrous or false ankylosis).

Anodontia: Failure of all teeth to develop.

Antrolith: Calcified mass found in the maxillary sinus as a result of calcification of stagnant mucus, root fragments, or foreign objects.

Aplasia: Lack of development of a part.

Arteriovenous Fistula: Direct communication between an artery and a vein that bypasses the intervening capillary bed. Also called arteriovenous (AV) shunt, aneurysm, or malformation.

Attrition (Tooth): Physiologic wearing away of the dentition, resulting from occlusal contact between the teeth during mastication.

Avulsion (Tooth): Complete displacement of a tooth from its alveolus.

Basilar Invagination: Condition seen in Paget disease in which the bones of the base of the skull become softened, leading to possible herniation of vertebral structures into the skull and compression of nerves.

"Bays Within Bays": Pattern of bone destruction in which smaller areas of erosion are present within larger areas of destruction at the margin of a lesion.

Beak: Projection of bone, resembling the beak of a bird.

"Beaten Copper" Marks: Term sometimes used to describe the radiographic appearance of the skull in children with hypophosphatasia. The skull radiograph may demonstrate multiple small radiolucent areas with relatively round radiopaque markings around them, in a pattern similar to that produced by beating on a sheet of copper with a small mallet.

Bifid: Cleft into two parts or branches.

Blastic: Term describing the production or formation of tissue.

Blow-Out: A type of orbital fracture, caused by conversion of the kinetic energy carried by an object striking the globe into hydraulic energy by the fluid-filled globe. This energy is then transmitted to the orbital walls, leading to a bursting of the bone. This is most common in the posterior area of the floor, medial to the infraorbital suture and anteromedial to the inferior orbital fissure.

Bossing: Uneven, variable bulging or undulation of the cortical contour of bone.

Botryoid Cyst: Multilocular variant of lateral periodontal cyst.

Brachycephaly: Reduced anteroposterior dimension of the skull with increased skull width.

Branchial: Related to the embryonic branchial clefts, arches, or pouches in the lateral portion of the neck.

Bright: Term describing an area of high signal strength on a magnetic resonance image; white in appearance.

Bright Light: Radiographic sign of facial fracture describing a bone fragment within the maxillary sinus.

Brown Tumor: A giant cell tumor of the skeleton associated with hyperparathyroidism.

Burkitt Lymphoma: Malignancy of the lymphoreticular cells that is the most common childhood malignancy in east central Africa, although it can occur elsewhere. The African form usually involves the jaw, whereas the American form involves the abdomen more frequently.

Caffey Syndrome: See *infantile cortical hyperostosis*.

Calcifying Epithelial Odontogenic Cyst: Benign odontogenic lesion of the jaws with some features of a neoplasm, such as continued growth, and some features of a cyst. Also called *Gorlin cyst*. This lesion is distinct from calcifying epithelial odontogenic tumor.

Calcifying Epithelial Odontogenic Tumor: Benign tumor of distinctive microscopic appearance that appears to arise from either the reduced enamel epithelium or dental epithelium. Also called *Pindborg tumor*.

Cementifying Fibroma: Encapsulated benign fibroosseous neoplasm of the jaws. There is no clear-cut distinction between cementifying and ossifying fibroma. The lesion may appear radiolucent, radiopaque, or mixed, depending on the amount of calcification present.

Cementoblastoma: Benign neoplasm, derived from the periodontal ligament, that produces a large bulbous mass of cementum on the roots of an affected tooth.

Central: Arising within the jaws, rather than invading the jaws from the periphery.

Central Giant Cell Granuloma: Lesion of the jaws that occurs mainly in children and young adults. Theories as to its nature of include a reparative response to intrabone hemorrhage and inflammation, a neoplasm related to the giant cell tumor of long bones, and a developmental anomaly closely related to aneurysmal bone cyst.

Central Giant Cell Lesion of Hyperparathyroidism: Late manifestation of hyperparathyroidism. Occurring in about 10% of the cases, the lesion is associated with raised serum calcium and alkaline phosphatase and decreased serum phosphate. It is identical microscopically to the central giant cell granuloma. Also called Brown tumor.

Charcot Joint: Enlargement of a joint with osteoarthritis resulting from trophic disturbances in patients with tabes dorsalis.

Cherubism: Inherited fibroosseous disease of the jaws in children characterized by bilateral multilocular cystlike radiolucencies of the mandible, and sometimes the maxilla, that enlarge and coalesce. Clinical signs include firm enlargement of the jaws with intact and nonpainful mucosa. Teeth may be displaced.

Chondroma: Benign tumor of cartilage, relatively common in parts of the skeleton but not found often in the jaws.

Chondrosarcoma: Malignant tumor of cartilaginous origin.

Chronic Apical Periodontitis: Low-grade reaction to an infection or to inflammatory products of relatively long duration and low virulence, confined to the periodontal ligament at the apex of a tooth root.

Chronic Suppurative Osteomyelitis: Localized and persistent purulent infection of the bone marrow, milder than in the acute form.

Clastic: Term describing destruction of tissue.

Cleidocranial Dysplasia (Dysostosis): Developmental anomaly of the skeleton and teeth characterized by brachycephaly; delayed or failed closure of the fontanelles; open skull sutures; multiple wormian bones; undeveloped maxilla; varying degrees of underdevelopment of the clavicles, up to complete absence; prolonged retention of the primary dentition; and delayed eruption of the permanent dentition.

Codman Triangle: An appearance highly suggestive of osteosarcoma. The tumor strips the periosteum from the bone and new bone is laid down between the tumor and the periosteum, forming triangular projections from the surface of the bone.

Comminuted: Fracture with two or more fragments at the fracture site.

Compound: Fracture that is exposed to the external environment through a wound in the skin or mucous membrane.

Concresence: Union of roots of two or more teeth by cementum below the cementoenamel junction.

Condensing Osteitis: Circumscribed proliferation of bone at the apex of a tooth as a result of low-grade periapical inflammation. New bone is deposited along existing trabeculae, leading to a more radiopaque appearance of the apical bone. Also called *focal sclerosing osteomyelitis*.

Corticated: Term describing the radiographic appearance of a lesion with a circumscribed, well-defined radiopaque border.

Cotton Wool Appearance: Term describing the fluffy, roundish radiopaque masses of abnormal bone within the jaw lesions of Paget disease.

Craniofacial Dysostosis: Developmental anomaly of unknown cause, characterized by early closure of all cranial sutures leading to a bulging of the frontal bone in the midline over the nose and a downward sloping of the back of the head. Eyes may be set wide apart or protrude. Blindness as a result of increased intracranial pressure is not uncommon. Also called *Crouzon disease*.

Crouzon Disease: See *craniofacial dysostosis*.

Cystlike: Lesion with the radiographic features of a cyst: a smooth, rounded radiolucent lesion with a well-defined border.

Degenerative Joint Disease: See *osteoarthritis*.

Dens Evaginatus: Enamel-covered tubercle on the occlusal surface of a molar or premolar as a result of evagination of the enamel organ during tooth development.

Dens in Dente: Disturbance in tooth formation in which the outer surface of the tooth is folded into the interior, giving the radiographic appearance of a "tooth within a tooth."

Dens Invaginatus: See *Dens in Dente*.

Dental Cyst: See *periapical cyst*.

Dentigerous: Having or containing teeth.

Dentigerous Cyst: Cyst arising from the reduced enamel epithelium around the crown of an unerupted or impacted tooth. Also called *follicular* or *pericoronal cyst*.

Dentin Dysplasia: Autosomal dominant developmental anomaly of teeth, characterized by short, poorly developed roots; obliterated pulp chambers and root canals; and periapical radiolucencies associated with noncarious teeth.

Dentinogenesis Imperfecta: Autosomal dominant disturbance of tooth development characterized by an amberlike translucency of teeth, which are a variety of colors from yellow to blue-gray; easy fracture of enamel from the dentin; constricted cervical portion of the tooth; short and slender roots; and partial or complete obliteration of pulp chambers. Some forms are associated with osteogenesis imperfecta. Also called *hereditary opalescent dentin*.

Dentinoma: Rare benign odontogenic tumor of immature connective tissue, odontogenic epithelium that has failed to histodifferentiate, and irregular or dysplastic dentin.

Developmental Salivary Gland Defect: A deep, well-defined depression, usually in the posterior body of the mandible, containing an aberrant lobe of the submandibular gland. Similar depressions occasionally found in the molar-premolar and canine areas contain portions of the sublingual gland. Also called *latent bone cyst, stafne bone cyst,* or *static bone cavity*.

Diastasis: Separation of an epiphysis from the shaft of a long bone occurring in the young without fracture of the bone. Any simple separation of normally joined parts.

Diastrophic: Distortion occurring in an object as a result of bending.

Diffuse Sclerosing Osteomyelitis: Low-grade infection of bone characterized primarily by reactive proliferation of bone rather than necrosis and pus formation.

Dilaceration: Disturbance in tooth formation that results in a sharp bend or curve in the tooth.

Dislocation of Condyle: Translation of a condylar head to a position anterior and superior to the articular eminence. Usually requires professional treatment to reduce.

Distodens: Supernumerary tooth occurring distal to the third molar. Also called *distomolar*.

Distomolar: See *distodens*.

Dolichocephaly: Condition of having a disproportionately long head.

Driven Snow Appearance: Term sometimes used to describe the radiographic appearance of a calcifying epithelial odontogenic tumor: that of scattered radiopaque foci of varying size and density within a unilocular or multilocular radiolucent lesion.

Dyscephaly: Syndrome of bony anomalies of the calvaria, face and jaw, with birdlike face; narrow curved nose; multiple eye defects including microphthalmia, microcornea, and cataract; and often alopecia overlying skull sutures or alopecia areata and hypoplasia or absence of eyebrows.

Eagle Syndrome: Elongation and/or mineralization of the styloid process associated with symptoms such as pain on swallowing, referred pain to the ear on the affected side, tinnitus, neck pain in the anterior cervical triangle, and transient light-headedness on turning the neck.

Ectodermal Dysplasia: Developmental abnormalities of tissues of ectodermal origin, including congenital absence of sweat glands; malformed and missing teeth; sparse fragile hair, sometimes with deformed nails; absent breast tissue; mental retardation; or syndactyly. The condition is sex-linked recessive in inheritance.

Ely Cysts: Minute areas of degeneration and fibrous replacement of bone tissue occurring just below the surface of the bone in a joint affected by osteoarthrosis.

Enamel Pearl: Small globule of enamel occurring on the roots of molars.

Endosteal: Pertaining to the membrane lining the surface of bone in the medullary cavity.

Enostosis: Localized growth of compact bone extending from the inner surface of cortical bone into the cancellous bone.

Eosinophilic Granuloma: Localized form of histiocytosis X, a disease considered to be an inflammatory reticuloendothelial condition that might be related to some type of infection.

Epidermoid Carcinoma: Malignant neoplasm derived from stratified squamous epithelium.

Erosion (Bone): Irregular, generally shallow, loss of bony tissue, as if eaten away.

Erosion (Tooth): Loss of tooth structure from a chemical action not involving bacteria.

Ewing Sarcoma: Malignancy of bone derived from mesenchymal connective tissue of the bone marrow.

Exostosis: Localized growth of compact bone extending outward the surface of a bone.

Facet: Small, smooth area on a bone or other firm structure.

Favorable Fracture Line: Fracture direction in which the actions of the various muscles tend to keep the fracture fragments in satisfactory alignment for healing to occur.

Fibroosseous Lesion: One of a family of lesions in which normal bone is replaced by benign fibrous tissue containing various amounts of mineralization.

Fibrous Dysplasia: Localized benign developmental anomaly of the skeletal system of unknown cause. It arises from bone-forming mesenchyme in the spongiosa and develops by proliferation of fibrous tissue. Irregular trabeculae form and increase in number and size as the lesion matures.

Fibrous Dysplasia, Monostotic: Fibrous dysplasia affecting a single bone and presenting no extraskeletal effects other than occasional pigmented skin lesions.

Fibrous Dysplasia, Polyostotic: Fibrous dysplasia involving multiple bones and other extraskeletal signs. Divided into two forms: *Jaffe type* and *Albright syndrome*.

Fibrous Healing Defect: Abnormal healing of bone wound in which there is a fibrous rather than bony union. This may occur when there is a loss of cortical plate and periosteum or movement of bony fragments after fracture or surgery.

Floating Tooth: Loss of normal alveolar bone structure so that tooth roots are completely surrounded by a radiolucency. This may be seen in advanced periodontitis as well as in malignant neoplasms of the jaws and surrounding structures.

Flocculent: Resembling tufts of cotton or wool.

Florid Osseous Dysplasia: Widespread form of periapical cemental dysplasia. The lesions are usually seen as a radiolucent cavity filled with dense masses of lobular or lumpy shape and fluffy radiopaque character. There are usually multiple lesions in one or both jaws that may coalesce as they enlarge.

Focal Osteoporotic Bone Marrow Defect: Localized area of hematopoietic or fatty marrow, usually found in the jaws during routine radiographic examination. Appearance is variable. No treatment is necessary once the diagnosis is established.

Focal Sclerosing Osteomyelitis: See *condensing osteitis*.

Follicular Cyst: See *dentigerous cyst*.

Follicular Sac: Pericoronal radiolucency seen around the crowns of normally erupting teeth.

Fusion (Tooth): Mingling of cells of adjacent tooth germs, resulting in union of developing teeth. Appearance is variable, depending on the stage of odontogenesis at time of fusion.

Gardner Syndrome: Hereditary condition characterized by multiple osteomas, cutaneous sebaceous cysts, subcutaneous fibromas, and multiple polyposis of the small and large intestine. Multiple unerupted supernumerary and permanent teeth may also be occur.

Garré Osteomyelitis: A nonsuppurative sclerosing osteomyelitis of the jaws characterized by the formation of a hard, bony swelling at the periphery of the jaw. See *proliferative periostitis*.

Gemination: Developmental anomaly occurring when the bud of a single tooth attempts to divide. Appearance varies with the degree of twinning.

Ghost Image: Image formed when the object is located between the x-ray source and the center of rotation in a panoramic x-ray machine.

Ghost Teeth: See *odontodysplasia*.

Giant Cell Granuloma: See *central giant cell granuloma*.

Globulomaxillary Cyst: Cyst of disputed origin. Classically thought to arise from embryonal epithelium in the globulomaxillary region, now thought to be either a primordial cyst of a supernumerary tooth or apical periodontal cyst of an adjacent nonvital tooth.

Globulomaxillary Region: Area of fusion between the embryonic globular portion of the median nasal process and the maxillary process.

Gorlin Cyst: See *calcifying epithelial odontogenic cyst*.

Gorlin-Goltz Syndrome: See *odontogenic keratocyst–basal cell nevus syndrome*.

Granular Appearance (of Bone): Radiographic pattern produced by many closely arranged, small trabeculae. Also called *"ground glass," "orange peel,"* or *"salt-and-pepper" appearance* Used to describe the radiographic appearance of fibrous dysplasia, hyperparathyroidism, and other diseases affecting the bone.

Greenstick: Fracture in which only one cortex of the bone is broken while the opposite side is bent.

Ground Glass Appearance: See *granular appearance.*

Hair-on-End Appearance: Radiographic appearance of the skull in which the diploic space is widened, the outer table is lost, and the bone in the space is arranged vertically in parallel rows resembling hair standing out from the head. It may be seen in sickle cell or other hemolytic anemias.

Hallermann-Streiff Syndrome: Syndrome including dyscephaly, parrot nose, mandibular hypoplasia, hypostichosis, blue sclera, and multiple supernumerary teeth.

Hallux (Halluces): The great toe, the first digit of the foot.

Hand-Schüller-Christian Disease: A chronic disseminated form of histiocytosis X, characterized by two or more of the following abnormalities: osteolytic skull lesions, diabetes insipidus, and exophthalmos.

Hemangioma, Central: Benign tumor of blood vessels occurring most often in the vertebrae and skull. It may be developmental or traumatic in origin.

Hemifacial Hypoplasia: Reduced growth of half of the face. It commonly affects the whole of one side of the face but may affect the mandible alone.

Hereditary Opalescent Dentin: See *dentinogenesis imperfecta.*

Histiocytosis X: Inflammatory reticuloendothelial condition that may be a reaction to some type of infection. It has multiple clinical presentations.

Honeycomb Appearance: Term describing the radiographic appearance of a multilocular lesion when the compartments are small and tend to be uniform in size.

Hutchinson Teeth: Hypoplasia of permanent incisors resulting from congenital syphilis. The mesial and distal surfaces of the crown taper from the middle of the crown to the incisal edge, giving the appearance of a screwdriver.

Hypercementosis: Regressive change in teeth manifested by excessive deposition of cementum on the roots.

Hyperdontia: Increased number of teeth, beyond that described by the normal dental formula of two incisors, one canine, two premolars, and three molars.

Hyperostotic Border: Thin radiopaque border of a radiolucent lesion.

Hyperplasia: Abnormal increase in the number of cells.

Hypertrophy: Increase in size of a part resulting in an increase in size of its constituent cells.

Hypondontia: Failure of development of one or a few teeth.

Hypoplasia: Defective or incomplete development of a part.

Impacted: Pressed closely together so as to be immovable, such as in a fracture in which the jagged ends of the broken bone are wedged together. The term denotes a tooth so placed in the alveolus as to be incapable of erupting into normal position. It also describes teeth driven upward into the alveolar process or surrounding tissues as a result of trauma.

Incisive Canal Cyst: Developmental cyst arising from epithelial remnants of the nasopalatine duct. More correctly called *nasopalatine duct cyst.*

Infantile Cortical Hyperostosis: A disease of infants in which the cortex of affected bones—typically mandible, clavicle, and ulna—thickens. The bone changes usually follow a period of fever and soft tissue swelling in the region of future bone proliferation. The cause is unknown, although an infectious origin has been proposed. Also called *Caffey syndrome.*

Jaffe Type: Fibrous dysplasia involving multiple bones and areas of increased skin pigmentation called cafe au lait spots.

Jug Handle: Term sometimes used to describe an underexposed submentovertical radiographic projection that demonstrates the zygomatic arches ("jug handles") well.

Keratinizing and Calcifying Odontogenic Cyst: See *calcifying epithelial odontogenic cyst.*

Lamina Dura: Thin white lining of the tooth socket seen on radiographs of the jaws.

Latent Bone Cyst: See *developmental salivary gland defect.*

Lateral Periodontal Cyst: Cyst arising from embryonic epithelial tissue remnants of Serres in the periodontal ligament.

LeFort: Classification system for fractures of the facial skeleton.

LeFort I: Horizontal fracture in the body of the maxilla resulting in detachment of a maxillary tooth-bearing fragment from the middle face. The fracture line passes above the teeth, below the zygomatic process, through the maxillary sinuses, and through the tuberosities to the inferior portion of the pterygoid processes.

LeFort II: Pyramidal fracture separating the maxilla from the base of the skull. The fracture line usually starts in the region of the nasion, extends obliquely through the medial aspect of the orbit and inferior orbital rim, and continues posteriorly in a horizontal fashion above the hard palate to involve the pterygoid plates. The zygoma remains attached to the cranium.

Lefort III: Fracture involving complete separation of the middle third of the facial skeleton from the cranium. The fracture line usually extends through the nasal bones and the frontal processes of the maxillary or nasofrontal and maxillofrontal sutures, across the floors of the orbits, and through the ethmoid and sphenoid sinuses and the zygomaticofrontal suture. It passes across both pterygomaxillary fissures and separates the pterygoid plates where they arise from the sphenoid bone.

Letterer-Siwe Disease: Acute disseminated form of histiocytosis X occurring in infancy, characterized by soft tissue and bony granulomatous lesions throughout the infant's body.

Lipping: Formation of shelflike extensions of the anterior border of the mandibular condyle as a result of osteoarthrosis.

Lordosis: Anteroposterior curvature of the spine, generally the lumbar spine, with the convexity facing anteriorly.

Luxation (Tooth): Dislocation of the articulation between tooth and bone (periodontal ligament). A luxated tooth is both abnormally mobile and displaced.

Macrodontia: Presence of teeth that are larger than the upper limits of the normal range.

Malignant Lymphoma: One of a group of malignant immunologic neoplasms that generally arise in lymphoid tissue.

Mandibulofacial Dysostosis: Developmental anomaly that is often inherited as an autosomal dominant trait but may arise spontaneously. The anomalies are variable but most commonly include underdevelopment of the zygomatic bones, downward inclination of the palpebral fissures, underdevelopment of the mandible with a steep mandibular angle, macrostomia, malformation of the external ears, absence of the external auditory canal, and occasional facial clefts. Also called *Treacher Collins syndrome.*

Marble Bones: See *osteopetrosis.*

MD: Term describing a type of internal derangement of the temporomandibular joint in which the disk (meniscus) is displaced anteriorly to the condyle in the closed-mouth position and does not reduce in the open-mouth position.

MDR: Term describing a type of internal derangement of the temporomandibular joint in which the disk (meniscus) is displaced anteriorly to the condyle in the closed-mouth position but reduces to a normal superior location in the open-mouth position.

Medial Sigmoid Depression: Osseous depression in the medial portion of the ramus just below the sigmoid notch area as an anatomic variant.

Mesiodens: Supernumerary tooth occurring between or just posterior to the central incisors.

Metatrophic: Deriving sustenance from dead organic matter; same as saprophytic when applied to bacteria.

Metopic: Relating to the forehead or anterior portion of the cranium.

Metopism: Persistence of the frontal suture in adults.

Microdontia: Presence of teeth that are smaller than the lower limits of the normal range.

Micrognathia: Smallness of the jaws, especially the mandible.

Mixed Lesion: Radiographically, a lesion containing both radiolucent and radiopaque parts.

Moth Eaten Appearance: Term describing the radiographic appearance of a destructive lesion of calcified tissue, characterized by a lack of smoothly contoured borders. Also called *ragged appearance.*

Mottled: Term describing the radiographic appearance of poorly defined aggregates of small spicules of bone distributed throughout a radiolucent area.

Mucocele: Expanding, destructive lesion that begins with the development of a mucous retention cyst in a sinus with a blocked ostium. It may destroy sinus walls and occurs most often in the ethmoid and frontal sinuses.

Mucoepidermoid Carcinoma: Low-grade malignant neoplasm of the salivary glands, composed of both epidermoid and mucus-secreting cells from the salivary duct system.

Mucositis: Inflammatory reaction in a mucosal surface; sometimes used to describe the thickened mucosa in the maxillary sinus resulting from sinusitis or the penetration of organisms into the sinus from an infected tooth.

Mucous Retention Cyst (Phenomenon): Cystic lesion formed in the paranasal sinuses as a result of obstruction of the ducts of the seromucinous glands in the lamina propria of the sinus lining. The cystic fluid is gland secretion.

Mulberry Molars: Hypoplasia of permanent first molars as a result of congenital syphilis. The crowns are small, with a constricted occlusal third of the crown, reduced cusps, and irregular globules of enamel on the occlusal surface, resembling the surface of a mulberry.

Multilocular: Term describing a lesion that appears to be formed of multiple adjacent compartments within bone.

Multiple Cementoma: See *periapical cemental dysplasia*.

Multiple Myeloma: Malignant neoplasm with proliferation of a single clone of abnormal plasma cells in the bone marrow.

Myofascial Pain Dysfunction Syndrome: Disease complex of the temporomandibular joint region characterized by pain of myofascial origin arising from trigger points located within the muscle or its tendinous attachments.

Nasopalatine Duct Cyst: See *incisive canal cyst*.

Neurilemmoma: Benign tumor of neuroectodermal origin, arising from the Schwann cells that make up the inner layer covering the peripheral nerves.

Neurofibroma: Benign mixed ectodermal arising from the connective tissue of the sheath of Schwann as well as other components of nerves, including the axons.

Neurofibromatosis: Autosomal-dominant inherited syndrome that includes multiple neurofibromas, cutaneous cafe au lait macules, bone abnormalities, central nervous system changes, and other stigmata. Also called *von Recklinghausen's disease*.

Neuroma: Overgrowth of a severed nerve attempting to regenerate when it has been blocked from reaching its distal end. Also called *amputation* or *traumatic neuroma*.

Nevoid Basal Cell Carcinoma Syndrome: See *odontogenic keratocyst–basal cell nevus syndrome*.

Nevoid Basalioma: See *odontogenic keratocyst–basal cell nevus syndrome*.

Odontodysplasia: Disturbance of tooth formation resulting in localized arrest of tooth development with hypoplasia and hypocalcification of all tooth elements. Also called *ghost teeth*.

Odontogenic: Related to development of the teeth.

Odontogenic Keratocyst: One of a group of cysts that have a highly characteristic microscopic appearance, produce abundant keratin, and have the highest recurrence rate of any odontogenic cyst. It probably arises from dental lamina remnants in the jaws.

Odontogenic Keratocyst–Basal Cell Nevus Syndrome: Collection of abnormalities most consistently including multiple basal cell carcinomas of the skin; multiple odontogenic keratocysts; and skeletal anomalies, the most common being bifid rib. Other skeletal changes can include agenesis, deformity, and synostosis of the ribs; kyphoscoliosis, vertebral fusion; polydactyly; shortening of the metacarpals; temporoparietal bossing; minor hypertelorism; mild prognathism; and calcification of the flax cerebri and other parts of the dura. Also called *Gorlin-Goltz syndrome,* and *nevoid basal cell carcinoma syndrome*.

Odontogenic Myxoma: Benign odontogenic tumor, probably arising from the dental papilla, follicular mesenchyme, or periodontal ligament. Also called odontogenic myrofibroma.

Odontoma, Complex: Mixed ectodermal-mesodermal hamartoma of odontogenic tissues, containing nondescript masses of dental tissue.

Odontoma, Compound: Mixed ectodermal-mesodermal hamartoma of odontogenic tissues, containing multiple teeth or toothlike masses.

Oligodontia: Agenesis of numerous teeth.

Onion skin Appearance: Formation of periosteal new bone in layers.

Opacification: Pathologic or physiologic change in a structure or lesion to a whiter or more radiopaque appearance on radiographs.

Orange Peel Appearance: See *granular appearance.*

Orofaciodigital Syndrome (Dysostosis): Inherited syndrome with varying combinations of defects of the oral cavity, face, and hands, including lobulated or bifid tongue, cleft or pseudocleft palate, tongue tumors, missing or malpositioned teeth, pug nose, depressed nasal bridge, brachydactyly, clinodactyly, incomplete syndactyly, and frequently mental retardation.

Ossifying Fibroma: Encapsulated benign fibroosseous neoplasm of the jaws arising from the periodontal ligament. There is no clear-cut distinction between ossifying and cementifying fibroma. The lesion may appear radiolucent, radiopaque, or mixed, depending on the amount of calcification present.

Ossifying Subperiosteal Hematoma: Rapid ossification of a subperiosteal hematoma induced by trauma or fracture. It usually occurs in people under age 15, in whom the bones are still growing.

Osteitis Deformans: See *Paget disease.*

Osteitis Fibrosa Cystica: Increased osteoclastic resorption of calcified bone with replacement by fibrous tissue, the result of primary hyperthyroidism or other causes of rapid mobilization of mineral salts. Also called *osteitis fibrosa generalisata.*

Osteitis Fibrosa Generalisata: See *osteitis fibrosa cystica.*

Osteoarthritis: Inflammation of the articular extremity of a bone involving the contiguous joint structures, resulting in erosion and fibrillation of the cartilages and eburnation of the bones with osteophytic growths. Also called *degenerative joint disease.*

Osteoblastic: Relating to the bone-forming cell.

Osteoblastoma: Benign tumor of bone-forming tissues that is composed of osteoid and newly formed trabeculae. It is closely related to osteoid osteoma, but considered more progressive.

Osteochondroma: Benign tumor consisting of a pedicle of normal bone protruding from the cortex and covered with a rim of proliferating cartilage cells.

Osteogenic: Relating to the formation of bone.

Osteoid Osteoma: Benign tumor that may be a variant of osteoblastoma. The tumor core is composed of osteoid and newly formed trabeculae within a highly vascularized osteogenic connective tissue.

Osteolytic: Relating to the softening, absorption, and destruction of bony tissue.

Osteoma: Benign tumor or hamartoma producing compact or cancellous bone or both. It may arise from cartilage or embryonal periosteum and occurs almost exclusively on the skull and facial skeleton on membrane bone.

Osteomyelitis: Inflammatory reaction of the bone marrow that clinically produces pus.

Osteopenia: Decrease in bone mass resulting from other diseases or drug use, rather than the classic, age-related loss of bone. Results from a deficit of bone matrix rather than a deficit of mineral.

Osteopetrosis: Rare bone disease with abnormal persistence of calcified cartilage. Following development of the skeletal system, the spongy portion of an affected bone ultimately becomes a solid block of calcified cartilage, leaving inadequate space for hematopoiesis. Also called *Albers-Schönberg disease* and *marble bones.*

Osteophyte: Bony outgrowth.

Osteoporosis: Reduction in the quantity of bone. The remaining bone is normally mineralized.

Osteoporosis Circumscripta: Discrete radiolucent areas seen on skull radiographs in the early lytic stage of Paget disease.

Osteoradionecrosis: Tissue necrosis and pus formation resulting from injury or infection in bone that has been exposed to intense irradiation in the past (40 to 80 Gy).

Osteosarcoma: Malignant tumor of bone derived from osteoblasts. Also called *Osteogenic sarcoma.*

Osteosclerosis: Asymptomatic area of exceptionally dense bone in the jaws. The cause is unknown but does not seem to be related to the sequelae of infection.

Oxycephaly (Hypsicephaly): Occurrence of a skull with a high vertical index. Also called *turricephaly.*

Paget Disease: General skeletal disease of older people of unknown cause, in which bone resorption and formation are both increased, leading to thickening and softening of bones such as those in the skull and bending of weight-bearing bones. Also called *osteitis deformans*.

Pagetoid Osteitis: Resorption of calcified bone with replacement by fibrous tissue resulting from primary hyperparathyroidism (osteitis fibrosa cystica), with marked deformity of the bones.

Panoramic Anterior Median Radiolucent Pseudolesion: Round radiolucent area seen in the anterior mandible on panoramic radiographs. It occurs in when an especially prominent depression in the labial mental area is located in the panoramic focal zone.

Panoramic Innominate Line: Thin, vertical, radiopaque line in the posterior portion of the maxillary sinus seen on panoramic radiographs. The lower portion is formed by the thin cortical outline of the posterior surface of the zygomatic process of the maxilla and the upper half by the thin cortical outline of the posterior surface of the frontal process of the zygoma. It is different from the innominate line seen in the Caldwell view.

Paramolar: Supernumerary tooth occurring in the molar area.

Parosteal: Relating to the tissues immediately adjacent to the periosteum of the bone.

Penetrance: The frequency, usually expressed as a percentage, with which a mutant gene produces its characteristic effect in those possessing it.

Periapical Cemental Dysplasia: Reactive fibroosseous lesion derived from odontogenic cells in the periodontal ligament, with a predilection for the periapical region of mandibular anterior teeth. The lesions are frequently multiple. Previously called *multiple cementoma*.

Periapical Cyst: Late stage in the sequence of inflammatory conditions occurring at the apex of an infected tooth. The cystic lining is derived from the proliferation of rests within a periapical granuloma. Also called *dental* or *radicular* cyst.

Periapical Granuloma: Chronic inflammatory lesion at the apex of an infected tooth in which bone and necrotic soft tissue are replaced with granulation tissue.

Periapical Rarefying Osteitis: Term sometimes used to describe the radiographic appearance of loss of lamina dura and bone at the apex of an infected tooth in a periapical granuloma.

Periapical Scar: Dense scar formation at the apex of a pulpless tooth that has been successfully treated endodontically.

Pericoronal Cyst: See *dentigerous cyst*.

Peridens: Supernumerary tooth that erupts buccally or lingually to the normal arch.

Periodontal Ligament Space: Radiolucent line seen between a tooth and the lamina dura of the tooth socket on radiographs of the jaws.

Periosteal: Relating to the periosteum, the thick fibrous membrane covering the entire surface of a bone except for its articular cartilage.

Periostitis Ossificans: See *proliferative periostitis*.

Peripheral: Related to, situated at, or originating from the outside of a body rather than from the center or within.

Phantom Bone Disease: Progressive resorption of bone of unknown cause. Also known as massive osteolysis.

Phlebolith: Concretion in a vein resulting from the calcification of an old thrombus.

Pindborg Tumor: See *calcifying epithelial odontogenic tumor*.

Polyp: Accentuated thickening of the mucosa that is already thickened by chronic inflammation. When it occurs in the paranasal sinuses, bone displacement or destruction may result.

Poorly Circumscribed: Term describing the radiographic appearance of a lesion whose borders are fuzzy, indistinct, or difficult to delineate. Also called *poorly delineated*.

Poorly Defined: See *poorly circumscribed*.

"President's Tumor": Panoramic anterior median radiolucent pseudolesion that occurred in a former president of the United States.

Primordial Cyst: Cyst arising from a developing tooth that undergoes cystic degeneration before calcification.

Prognathia: Abnormal forward projection of one or both jaws.

Progressive Systemic Sclerosis: Generalized connective tissue disease of unknown origin that causes sclerosis of the skin and other tissues. Formerly called scleroderma when it was thought to involve primarily the skin.

Proliferative Periostitis: Type of osteomyelitis characterized by the formation of new bone on the periphery of the cortex over an area of infected bone. Also called *periostitis ossificans*. Previously known as *Garré osteomyelitis*.

Proptosis: Forward displacement of any organ; specifically, exophthalmos, or protrusion of the eyeball.

Pseudocyst: Small radiolucent area just below the bony surface of a joint, representing replacement of bone tissue with fibrous tissue in osteoarthritis.

Pseudocyst of Condyle (Panoramic): Radiolucency on the mandibular condyle seen on panoramic radiographs. It is a normal anatomic variant that represents a cupped-out depression on the surface of the condyle.

Pseudohyperostosis: An apparent buildup of alveolar bone distal to the last tooth in the mandible.

Pulp Stone: Localized area of calcification in the pulp chamber of a tooth.

Pulpal Sclerosis: Diffuse calcification in the pulp chamber and pulp canals of teeth.

Punched out: Term describing the radiographic appearance of a well-defined radiolucent lesion without a radiopaque border.

Pyknodysostosis: Rare disease having many similarities with osteopetrosis.

Radicular Cyst: Cyst forming at the apex of a tooth as a result of pulpal death from infection. The epithelial lining develops from the rests of Malassez in the periodontal ligament. Also called *periapical cyst*.

Radiolucent: Term describing an object that absorbs little radiation and thus casts a dark shadow on a radiograph.

Radiopaque: Term describing a dense object that absorbs large amounts of radiation, causing its radiographic image to be light.

Railroad Track Appearance: Radiographic sign describing an additional oblique line on the lateral aspect of the orbit following a tripod fracture. It occurs as a result of rotation of the zygoma so that the x-ray beam is tangential to the fractured edge of the frontal process of the zygoma. A linear radiopaque line is formed parallel to the innominate line.

Rarefaction: The process of becoming less dense; increasing radiolucency (blackness) on a radiograph.

Real Image (Panoramic): Image formed when the object is between the film and the rotation center of the beam in a panoramic x-ray machine.

Remodeling: Physiologic alteration of bone in response to environmental demands occurring without loss of articular surface of the bone.

Renal Osteodystrophy: Bone changes occurring as a result of chronic renal failure and secondary hyperparathyroidism.

Residual: Relating to or of the nature of a residue; left behind.

Residual Cyst: Periapical (radicular) cyst that either remained in the jaw when its associated tooth was removed or formed in residual epithelial rests from the periodontal ligament of the involved tooth.

Resorption of bone: Loss of bone by lysis.

Retrognathia: Abnormal retrusion of one or both jaws.

Rheumatoid Arthritis: Autoimmune inflammatory condition of joints in which the inflamed and hypertrophic synovial membrane grows onto the articulating surfaces. Also called *Still disease*.

Rhinolith: Calcareous concretion in the nasal cavity.

Salt and Pepper Appearance: See *granular appearance*.

Scalloped: Term describing the border of a lesion that appears as multiple, regular, rounded indentations or protrusions.

Scaphocephaly: Having a long narrow skull with a more or less prominent ridge along the prematurely ossified sagittal suture.

Scoliosis: Lateral curvature of the spine.

Septum: Thin wall dividing two cavities or masses of softer tissue.

Sequestrum: Piece of necrosed bone that has become separated from the surrounding healthy osseous tissue.

Serous Retention Cyst: Cyst arising in the paranasal sinuses from cystic degeneration within an inflamed, thickened mucosal lining or polyp. The fluid in the lesion is a transudate from the capillaries damaged by the inflammation.

Sialolith: Stone within the major or minor salivary glands or in the ducts of these glands.

Sickle Cell Anemia: Hereditary form of chronic hemolytic anemia affecting mainly North American blacks.

Simple Bone Cyst: See *traumatic bone cyst*.

Soap Bubble Appearance: Term describing the radiographic appearance of a multilocular lesion when the compartments are circular and vary in size, and usually appearing to overlap somewhat.

Socket Sclerosis: Repair of a tooth socket after extraction with exceptionally dense bone that appears whiter than usual on radiographs.

Solitary Bone Cyst: See *traumatic bone cyst*.

Spur: Small projection from a fracture.

Stafne Bone Cyst: See *developmental salivary gland defect*.

Static Bone Cavity: See *developmental salivary gland defect*.

Step Defect: Cortical discontinuity occurring when the fragments of a fractured bone are displaced.

Stepladder Pattern: Bone pattern occurring when the trabeculae in the interdental areas of the jaw bones are coarse and arranged parallel to each other, appearing like the rungs on a ladder. Seen occasionally in sickle cell or other hemolytic anemias.

Still Disease: See *rheumatoid arthritis*.

Stria: Stripe, band, streak, or line, distinguished from the tissue in which it is found, by color, texture, depression, or elevation.

Subchondral Cyst: Radiolucent cystlike area seen in bones affected with osteoarthritis in which a portion of the bone beneath the cartilaginous surface is replaced with fibrous tissue.

Subchondral Sclerosis: Increasing radiographic density of bone under the cartilaginous surface of the mandibular condyle or articular fossa as a result of a degenerative process in the joint.

Subluxation of Condyle: Translation of the head of a condyle to a position anterior and superior to the articular eminence. Distinguished from dislocation in that with subluxation the patient can reduce the mandible without professional treatment.

Sunburst: Term describing a bone pattern in which the bone is formed in perpendicular columns from the cortex outward. Also called sunray.

Supernumerary: Exceeding the normal number.

Synodontia: Fusion of adjacent tooth germs resulting in union of developing teeth. Variable in appearance, depending on stage of odontogenesis at the time of fusion.

Synostosis: Fusion of bone (bony ankylosis) or synarthrosis (union of bone by fibrous tissue).

Taurodontism: Anomalous tooth form that includes a clinical and anatomic crown of normal size and shape, an elongated body, short roots, and a longitudinally enlarged pulp chamber.

Temporomandibular Disease: One or more of a series of disorders affecting the craniomandibular articulation and its musculature.

Tennis Racket Appearance: Term describing the radiographic appearance of a multilocular lesion with angular rather than rounded compartments.

Thanatrophic: Form of dwarfism.

Thistle-Tube Pulp: A feature of some forms of dentin dysplasia, in which the pulp chamber in anterior and premolar teeth extends into the root.

Torus Mandibularis: Slow-growing bony hyperplasia occurring on the lingual surface of the mandible, above the mylohyoid line, in the incisor-canine-premolar region.

Torus Palatinus: Slow-growing bony hyperplasia occurring in the central portion of the hard palate.

Transposition: Teeth occupying an unusual position in relation to other teeth in the dental arch, such that it appears that two teeth have exchanged position.

"Trap Door" Sign: Radiographic sign of a blow-out fracture of the floor of the orbit in which a bone fragment is partially avulsed from the floor of the orbit (roof of the maxillary sinus) and hangs into the sinus.

Traumatic Bone Cyst: Empty cavity in the bone of unknown origin but hypothesized to occur when a trauma-induced intramedullary hematoma results in bone resorption and cavitation during hematoma resolution. Not a true cyst. Also called *simple* or *hemorrhagic bone cyst*.

Traumatic Neuroma: See *neuroma*.

Treacher-Collins Syndrome: See *mandibulofacial dysostosis*.

Tripod Fracture: Fractures or diastases in the region of the zygomaticotemporal, zygomaticomaxillary, and zygomaticofrontal articulations.

Turner Hypoplasia: Term describing a succedaneous tooth with a local hypoplastic defect in its crown. Also called *Turner tooth*.

Turner Tooth: See *Turner hypoplasia*.

Turricephaly: See *oxycephaly*.

Unerupted: Tooth that is located totally within bone and has not yet emerged into the oral cavity.

Unfavorable Fracture Line: Fracture direction in which the action of the various muscles inserting on the different fracture fragments will result in distraction at the fracture site.

Unicameral: See *unilocular*.

Unilocular: Lesion composed of a single compartment in the bone. Also called *unicameral*.

von Recklinghausen's Disease: See *neurofibromatosis*.

Well Circumscribed: Term describing the radiographic appearance of a lesion whose borders are distinct and easy to delineate. Also called *well defined*.

Well Defined: See *well circumscribed*.

Wolff's Law: Changes in the form or function of a bone are followed by definite changes in its internal architecture and secondary alterations in its external form.

Wormian Bones: Small irregular bones in the sutures of the skull that are formed by secondary centers of ossification in the suture lines.

Xerostomia: Dryness of the mouth.

INDEX

Italic page numbers indicate illustration.